Obesity in Childhood and Adolescence

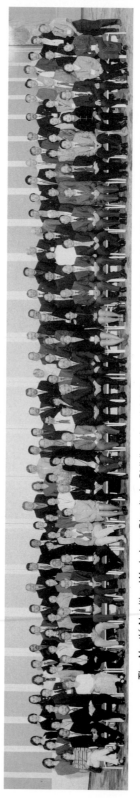

The Nestlé Nutrition Workshop, Obesity in Childhood and Adolescence, was held in Shanghai, China, 22–26 April 2001.

Nestlé Nutrition Workshop Series
Pediatric Program Volume 49

Obesity in Childhood and Adolescence

Editors

Chunming Chen   *Chinese Center for Disease Control and Prevention, Beijing, China*

William H. Dietz   *Division of Nutrition and Physical Activity, Centers for Disease Control and Prevention, Atlanta, Georgia, USA*

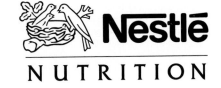

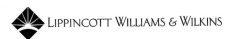

Acquisitions Editor: Beth Barry
Developmental Editor: Maria McAvey
Production Editor: Melanie Bennitt
Manufacturing Manager: Colin Warnock
Compositor: Maryland Composition
Printer: Maple Press

Nestec Ltd., 55 Avenue Nestlé
CH-1800 Vevey, Switzerland
Lippincott Williams & Wilkins,
530 Walnut Street
Philadelphia, PA 19106 USA
LWW.com

Printed in the USA

Library of Congress Cataloging-in-Publication Data

Nestlé Nutrition Workshop (49th : 2001 : Shanghai, China)
    Obesity in childhood and adolescence / editors, Chunming Chen, William H. Dietz.
      p. ; cm. — (Nestlé Nutrition workshop series. Pediatric Program ; v. 49)
    Includes bibliographical references and index.
    ISBN 0-7817-4132-7
      1. Obesity in children—Congresses. 2. Obesity in adolescence—Congresses. 3. Children—Nutrition—Congresses. 4. Teenagers—Nutrition—Congresses. I. Chen, Chunming. II. Dietz, William H. III. Title. IV. Nestlé Nutrition workshop series, Pediatric Program ; v. 49.
    [DNLM: 1. Obesity—Adolescence—Congresses. 2. Obesity—Child—Congresses. WD 210 N468o 2002]
    RJ399.C6 N48 2001
    618.92′398—dc21

                    2002023584

10 9 8 7 6 5 4 3 2 1

Preface

Thirty years ago, severe childhood obesity was an unusual problem that confronted few pediatricians. Today, childhood obesity is epidemic. For example, in the United States between the completion of the second National Health and Examination Survey (NHANES) in 1980 and NHANES 3 in 1994, the prevalence of overweight children and adolescents doubled. Over the same time period, the prevalence of obesity in adults increased by 50%, indicating that the problem of excess weight in children and adolescents was deteriorating much more rapidly than in adults. Such increases are not limited to the USA. As this nutrition workshop and other publications have illustrated, every country that has collected longitudinal data has found an increased prevalence of childhood overweight. Countries undergoing a nutritional transition appear equally vulnerable, because children whose growth has been stunted are now becoming overweight. Although morbidity and mortality from obesity in childhood and adolescence are rare, the increase in type 2 diabetes among overweight adolescents in the USA, the high frequency of biochemical precursors of adult disease among overweight children, and the impact of childhood onset overweight on the severity of obesity in adults suggest that childhood obesity has already begun to affect health care costs directly.

The rapidity with which the prevalence of childhood and adolescent overweight has increased excludes genetic causes as a source of the obesity epidemic, and rightfully focuses attention on broad potential cultural and environmental causes. In both developed and developing countries, television has become widely available, and several countries have now reported data that link television viewing to childhood or adolescent overweight. The food supply has changed dramatically. Fast food has become global, and advertising promoting the consumption of fast food is pervasive. In the USA, soda and sugared beverage consumption now accounts for 6% of the average child's daily energy intake. The variety of foods available has increased dramatically, and experimental data suggest that increased variety increases consumption. Safe opportunities for physical activity have declined. In 1999, only 29% of American teens participated in daily physical education programs, a decrease of almost 30% since 1991. The frequency with which American children and teenagers include physical activity as part of their daily lives has also declined. Less than one third of children who live within one mile of their school walk to school, and although 25% of all the trips we make are less than one mile, 75% of those trips are by car. Urbanization may have begun to reduce physical activity levels among children and adolescents in the developing world. Improved water supplies, larger numbers of immunized children, reduced infectious diseases, and increased availability of low-cost cooking oils may be contributory factors in the developing world. Nonetheless, despite these trends, few longitudinal studies enable us to argue that any of these environmental trends are causal.

Identification of the causes and the development of effective prevention and treatment strategies will be essential to reduce the prevalence of obesity and its associated health care costs. Although good surveillance data are available to track the progression of the epidemic, we lack the longitudinal studies to link most of the food and activity behaviors outlined above to the development or persistence of obesity. Likewise, although the natural history of childhood obesity has become clearer, the environmental, behavioral, and physiologic factors that predispose children and adolescents to the development of obesity at critical periods remain uncertain. A reasonably sound scientific basis underlies the preventive strategies of breast feeding, reduced television time, and physical activity. However, how these strategies can be successfully implemented and what impact their implementation will have on the prevalence of childhood obesity requires further research. Elements of therapy that appear effective include a family-based approach, meetings with children and parents in separate groups, as well as meetings with the parent and child, a focus on reduced television viewing, reduction or elimination of high-energy-density foods, and behavior modification to reinforce these strategies. However, the effectiveness of these strategies in primary care settings has not yet been examined.

In the absence of a public health program that focuses on policy and environmental strategies to improve diet and activity levels and reduce television viewing, clinical approaches will not likely reduce the prevalence of obesity. How to mobilize the resources necessary to change the food and activity environment will provide the biggest challenge to the successful elimination of obesity.

Professor William H. Dietz, USA

Foreword

Obesity is increasing not only in the developed countries but recently also in some developing countries. It was therefore important to organize the 49th Nestlé Nutrition Workshop in China, where important clinical work in this field has been done by Professor Chunming Chen, one of the chairmen of this workshop.

As obesity has long been an issue in the industrialized countries, the scientific study of this problem has a longer tradition in those countries than in the developing countries. Thus many speakers at this workshop came from the USA and Europe.

We thank the two chairmen, Professor Chunming Chen and Professor William Dietz, who are outstanding experts in the field of obesity research and who undertook the task to select appropriate topics and find speakers for this workshop. Invited scientists from 26 countries contributed substantially to the discussions, which are printed at the end of each chapter. Mrs. KeLan Liu and her team from Nestlé China provided the logistical support and introduced the participants to Chinese hospitality. Dr. Anne-Lise Carrié-Fässler, from the Nutrition Strategic Business Division in Vevey, Switzerland, was responsible for the scientific coordination. Her cooperation with the chairmen was essential for the success of the workshop.

PROFESSOR WOLF ENDRES, M.D.
Nestec Ltd.
Vevey, Switzerland

Contents

Contributing Authors

Speakers

Linda G. Bandini
Massachusetts Institute of Technology
Cambridge, Massachusetts
USA

Mary C. Bellizzi
Health Promotions
Aberdeen, Scotland
United Kingdom

Leann L. Birch
Department of Human Development
*   and Family Studies*
The Pennsylvania State University
University Park, Pennsylvania
USA

Chunming Chen
Chinese Center for Disease Control and
*   Prevention*
Beijing, China

Timothy J. Cole
Center for Pediatric Epidemiology and
*   Biostatistics*
Institute of Child Health
London, England
United Kingdom

William H. Dietz
Division of Nutrition and Physical Activity
Centers for Disease Control and
*   Prevention*
Atlanta, Georgia
USA

Abdul G. Dulloo
Department of Medicine
Institute of Physiology
University of Fribourg
Fribourg, Switzerland

David S. Freedman
Division of Nutrition and Physical Activity
Centers for Disease Control and
*   Prevention*
Atlanta, Georgia
USA

Steven L. Gortmaker
Department of Health and Social Behavior
Harvard School of Public Health
Boston, Massachusetts
USA

Anna Jacob
Food and Nutrition Specialists Pte Ltd.
Singapore, China

Juliana Kain
Institute of Nutrition and Food Technology
*   (INTA)*
University of Chile
Santiago, Chile

Guansheng Ma
Institute of Nutrition and Food Hygiene
Chinese Academy of Preventive Medicine
Beijing, China

Claudio Maffeis
Department of Pediatrics
University of Verona-Polyclinic
Verona, Italy

Thomas N. Robinson
Division of General Pediatrics
Department of Pediatrics and Center for
*   Research in Disease Prevention*
Stanford University School of Medicine
Palo Alto, California
USA

Marie F. Rolland-Cachera
National Institute of Health and Medical
*   Research*

INSERM Group
Paris, France

Atul Singhal
MRC Childhood Nutrition Research
   Centre
Institute of Child Health
London, England
United Kingdom

Kate S. Steinbeck
Departments of Endocrinology and
   Adolescent Medicine
Royal Prince Alfred Hospital and
University of Sydney
Sydney, Australia

Jack A. Yanovski
Unit on Growth and Obesity
Developmental Endocrinology Branch
National Institute of Child Health and
   Human Development
National Institutes of Health
Bethesda, Maryland
USA

Session Chairmen

W. Cai / *China*
S.B. Ning / *China*
W.P. Wang / *China*
X. G. Yang / *China*

Invited Attendees

David Moore / *Australia*
Manzoor Hussain / *Bangladesh*
Sergio Augusto Cabral / *Brazil*
Jose Augusto Taddei / *Brazil*
Oded Bar-Or / *Canada*
Eduardo Atalah / *Chile*
Juan Chen / *China*
Yanhui Chen / *China*
Sitang Gong / *China*
Hongwei Guo / *China*
Yizhen Guo / *China*
Jianguo Hong / *China*

Zhaoyi Hong / *China*
Yu Jin / *China*
Changgang Li / *China*
Xiaomao Li / *China*
Yimin Li / *China*
Li Liang / *China*
Zhugen Liao / *China*
Cuiqing Liu / *China*
Guangming Nong / *China*
Shuixian Shen / *China*
Yuan Shi / *China*
Yanping Wan / *China*
Hongwei Wang / *China*
Wenjing Wang / *China*
Xiaolei Wang / *China*
Yuwei Wang / *China*
Chaoying Yan / *China*
Jianyi Zhang / *China*
Peibin Zhang / *China*
Jasenka Ille / *Croatia*
Mahmoud Bozo / *Dubai (Middle East)*
Mohammed Jan / *Dubai (Middle East)*
Olivier Goulet / *France*
Carl-Peter Bauer / *Germany*
Berthold Koletzko / *Germany*
Konstantinos Samaras / *Greece*
Elaine Kwan / *Hong Kong*
Yn-Tz Rita Sung / *Hong Kong*
Rajendra Nath Srivastava / *India*
Dr. Satriono / *Indonesia*
Damayanti Rusli Sjarif / *Indonesia*
Johannes Capistranus Susanto /
   Indonesia
Guslihan Dasa Tjipta / *Indonesia*
Pier Luigi Duvina / *Italy*
Dong Hwan Lee / *Korea*
Eun Kyung Lee / *Korea*
Olga Zimanaite / *Lithuania*
Zulkifli Ismail / *Malaysia*
Selva Kumar A/L Selvapunniam /
   Malaysia
Norzila Mohamed Zainudin / *Malaysia*
Leticia Buenaluz / *Philippines*
Maria Susana Campos / *Philippines*

Sylvia Estrada / *Philippines*
Ruby Go / *Philippines*
Constança Maria Lima Bentes
  Olkkola / *Portugal*
Adrian Ion Georgescu / *Romania*
Mei Lin Fong / *Singapore*
Kah Yin Loke / *Singapore*
Jacobus C. Van Dyk / *South Africa*
Kurt Baerlocher / *Switzerland*

Marie-Thérèse (Mai) Nguyen Howles
  / *Switzerland*
Michel Roulet / *Switzerland*
Christoph Rutishauser / *Switzerland*
Ladda Mo-Suwan / *Thailand*
Manit Teeratantikanont / *Thailand*
Vallop Thaineua / *Thailand*
Benjamin Caballero / *United States*
Strauss Richard / *United States*

Nestlé Representatives

Louis-Dominique Van Egroo
Norean Sayers
Kevin Acheson

Luis Cantarell
Wolf Endres
Bianca-Maria Exl

Anne-Lise Carrié-Fässler
Evangelos Kaloussis
Ulrich Preysch

Marie-Christine Secretin
Linda Hsieh

Nestlé France, Paris, France
Nestlé Malaysia, Selangor, Malaysia
Nestlé Research Centre, Lausanne,
  Switzerland
Nestec Ltd., Vevey, Switzerland
Nestec Ltd., Vevey, Switzerland
Nestlé Suisse S.A., Vevey,
  Switzerland
Nestec Ltd., Vevey, Switzerland
Nestec Ltd., Vevey, Switzerland
Nestlé Suisse S.A., Vevey,
  Switzerland
Nestec Ltd., Vevey, Switzerland
Nestlé USA, Inc., Glendale, CA, USA

Nestlé Nutrition Workshop Series Pediatric Program

Obesity in Childhood and Adolescence

Obesity in Childhood and Adolescence, edited by
Chunming Chen and William H. Dietz. Nestlé
Nutrition Workshop Series, Pediatric Program,
Vol. 49. Nestec Ltd., Vevey/Lippincott
Williams & Wilkins, Philadelphia © 2002.

Assessment: National and International Reference Standards

Timothy J. Cole

*Center for Pediatric Epidemiology and Biostatistics, Institute of Child Health,
London, England, UK*

Child obesity is a serious and increasing problem worldwide. It has important psychosocial and physical effects during childhood and later, in adult life. There is an important need to quantify the scale of the problem, for three reasons: to establish its prevalence in different parts of the world, to monitor the trends in prevalence over time, and to test the effectiveness of interventions introduced to address the problem.

DEFINITION OF CHILDHOOD OBESITY

Obesity is very simple to define qualitatively. It is an excess of body fat. But a quantitative definition requires wide agreement about how to measure body fat, and what cutoff points to use to separate the obese from the nonobese. An extra requirement in childhood is to link the cutoffs to the child's age and sex, because child growth ensures that body size, and hence the amount of body fat, changes with age in a way that is quite unrelated to obesity. So the definition of obesity throws up two requirements: (a) a way to measure body fat and (b) a set of age- and sex-specific cutoff points. A third requirement is that these two requirements are widely recognized, so that there is a degree of standardization in the definition.

MEASUREMENT OF BODY FAT

Another name for *body fat* is *adipose tissue,* and adiposity is the state of having body fat. Compared with *obesity,* this is a neutral term to describe the spectrum of fatness from obese through very thin. Adipose tissue is spread round the body, some of it subcutaneous and some internal. Subcutaneous fat can be accessed through the skin and so can be measured to reasonable accuracy using skinfold calipers. But internal fat cannot be reached in this way and it requires more expensive whole-body research instruments to measure it. The amount of central body fat—that is, at waist level, both internal and subcutaneous—can be estimated by measuring the waist circumference, though this also involves other internal organs, such as the liver.

There are more complex methods—for example, dual-energy x-ray absorptiometry (DEXA) or isotope dilution—that provide whole-body measures of adipose tissue, either directly or indirectly, but for population use they are impractical, in terms of both cost and availability. This constrains useful population measures of body fat to anthropometry—skinfold thickness measurements, circumferences, weight, and height.

Body Mass and Body Fat

Unlike skinfolds and circumferences, weight and height are whole-body measures. Weight, though related to fat, does not measure it directly, whereas height has little relation to fat. Weight and height are fairly highly correlated, with a correlation coefficient of around 0.7 during childhood; weight adjusted for height has long been considered to be a simple and convenient index of body shape, independent of body size (1).

This view first developed in the field of malnutrition, where weight adjusted for height (or weight-for-height) was used as a measure of wasting—that is, it indicated the amount of body tissue that had been lost because of malnutrition. There was no suggestion that the lost tissue was purely fat; indeed, it was recognized that much of it was fat-free tissue. For this reason malnutrition should not be viewed simply as the opposite of obesity; it is not simply a deficit of body fat. For the same reason, weight-for-height used to assess malnutrition should not be viewed simply as the mirror image of weight-for-height used to assess obesity. The relation between weight-for-height and body fat is important for obesity, but less so for malnutrition.

Weight–Stature Indices

The term *weight-for-height* has been in use for 40 years or more, yet it can be a confusing concept. Many ways exist for statistically adjusting weight-for-height, some better than others, and they all involve slightly different assumptions. A brief description of some of the issues is given here, but for a more complete discussion see Cole (1). It is easier to consider adults and children separately, as age is an important extra confounding variable in children that is less relevant for adults.

Adults

The simplest way to adjust weight-for-height is to identify a reference population, split it into a series of height classes by sex, and average the weights in each height class. An individual's weight can then be compared with this reference weight for his or her height and sex. But although this approach is simple to do, it is inefficient. The mean weights in the different height cells tend to increase smoothly with height, so the means can be smoothed across cells. This allows the mean weights to be represented as a smooth curve drawn on a chart as a function of height. This is traditionally known as the weight-for-height chart. Median rather than mean weight may alternatively be used.

If the weight–height trend is linear, then the linear regression of weight on height provides a compact formula relating expected weight to height, where expected weight is of the form [$a + b \times$ height] and a and b are estimated regression coefficients. This leads to a *difference* index of the form

$$\text{weight} - \text{expected weight-for-height}$$

which is a direct measure of over- or underweight, given height. However, this form of index is less intuitively appealing than the *ratio* index:

$$\text{weight/expected weight-for-height}$$

which is more commonly used.

Linear regression presents two problems in this context: heteroscedasticity and skewness. The first of these is the phenomenon of nonconstant variability of weight; its standard deviation tends to increase as mean weight increases. The second problem, skewness, is the upper tail of the weight distribution tending to be longer and more extended than the lower tail. This is most apparent on a chart where the upper centiles are further apart than the lower centiles. The presence of skewness or heteroscedasticity reduces the validity of the regression equation, and the correct procedure is to find a transformation of weight that will remove them. A popular and effective transformation is to take logarithms, so the regression equation involves log weight and (by symmetry) log height rather than weight and height. This leads to the regression equation log weight = $a + p \times$ log height, and a difference index of the form

$$\text{log weight} - p \times \text{log height}$$

When antilogged this gives the ratio index: weight/height^p.

Two important corollaries arise from this analysis. The first is that the log transform, by converting a difference index to a ratio index, provides a statistical justification for the ratio index. The second relates to the power of height p. Using regression analysis means that the value of p tends to be less than the number 3 implied using dimensional arguments (i.e., the argument that weight is proportional to volume, which is proportional to length^3).

In adults p is close to 2 in men, and somewhat smaller in women. Despite this sexual dimorphism, the value 2 has been preferred, and the index weight/height^2 is now in universal use for assessing overweight and obesity in adults, both men and women (2). It is often called Quetelet's index, after the Belgian mathematician Adolphe Quetelet, who first observed that weight goes as the square of height, but more recently it has become known as the body mass index (BMI) (3).

Children

Moving from adults to children, age becomes a third dimension, in addition to weight and height, that needs to be accounted for. Weight adjusted for height may or may not be adjusted for age as well. The weight-for-height chart described earlier, which ignores the child's age, is useful to monitor malnutrition in areas of the world where age is not recorded. Cutoff points for malnutrition have in the past used the ratio index:

$$\text{weight/expected weight-for-height} \times 100,$$

where less than 80% of expected weight is the definition of wasting (4).

However, in many parts of the world the child's age is known, and ignoring it is inefficient and leads to bias. Weight averaged in narrow height classes can be extended to include tabulation by age as well—that is, the height classes are defined within age classes, though this requires a very substantial sample size. Baldwin (5) used this approach as long ago as 1925 to provide height-, age-, and sex-specific values for weight in American children.

Within each age class the relation between weight and height can be summarized using log-log regression, as described earlier, which leads to the index weight/height^p, where p depends on age. The question then is, "Does p change much with age or is it fairly constant?" Rolland-Cachera *et al.* (6) showed almost 20 years ago that height^2 was appropriate in early childhood but that during puberty the relation was steeper and height^3 was better. Three years earlier, Cole (7) had come to the same conclusion using a different statistical approach, expressing weight and height as weight-for-age and height-for-age, respectively—that is, dividing each measurement by a reference value for the child's age and sex. The regression of log weight-for-age on log height-for-age adjusts for age and estimates the optimal height power p simultaneously.

This age dependence in the value of the height power has led to some soul searching. On the one hand, people have argued on pragmatic grounds that weight/height^2 should be used throughout childhood. This would mean that during puberty the index does not adjust wholly for the effects of height, and taller children will tend to have a larger index—that is, taller children will appear fatter. The same does not hold earlier in childhood, where the index is broadly uncorrelated with height.

On the other hand, there is a feeling that the index should be uncorrelated with height at all ages, even though this involves at least two distinct indices, weight/height^2 and weight/height^3. A more purist approach still is to allow the height power to change smoothly with age (8), which complicates the issue further.

It is useful at this point to ask what the index is for. Is it to measure weight-for-height or is it to identify obesity? If the former, then we are obliged to use the age-related height power, as otherwise the index will not adjust properly for height at all ages. But if our aim is to measure obesity (which it is), then we require the index to measure body fat as best it can.

Before puberty both approaches identify the BMI as the optimal index; it is uncorrelated with height and maximally correlated with body fat. During puberty an association develops between body fat and height; fatter children tend also to be taller, so the optimal index of weight-for-height, weight/height^3 needs to be adjusted further for height. This again leads to the BMI. So for assessing obesity BMI is the optimal index throughout childhood and adolescence, as it is during adulthood.

Weight and Height Centiles and Z Scores

Anthropometry is often expressed in the form of a standard deviation score, SD score, or z score. This is the number of standard deviations that the individual child's measurement is above or below the median of the distribution for age and sex. So a height z score of 0 indicates median height for age, whereas $+2$ z scores is two standard deviations above the mean and corresponds to the 98th centile. Based on the reference population, the z score has a mean of 0 and a standard deviation of 1 and is normally distributed.

Until recently, the z score calculation has required the measurement to be normally distributed, so that weight, BMI, or skinfold thickness—which each have markedly skewed distributions—could not be expressed in z score form. However, this has now become possible using a power transformation of the measurement, so that z scores for weight, height, and BMI are now available. The British and American references are both constructed on this basis, a method known as the LMS method (see later).

The availability of weight z score and height z score provides a new way of defining weight-for-height, using the regression of weight z score on height z score. It is a logical extension of the two regression approaches described earlier: log weight on log height, and log weight-for-age on log height-for-age. But the z score does not need a log transformation, as it is already normally distributed. This regression leads to a difference index of the following form:

$$\text{weight } z \text{ score} - b \times \text{height } z \text{ score}$$

where the coefficient b lies in the range 0.5 to 0.7, depending on age and sex (unpublished data).

This apparently complex formula links directly to the informal process that pediatricians employ to assess a child's fatness from weight and height. They look at the child's weight and height charts, read off the corresponding centiles, and compare the child's deviations from the median. If the two deviations are similar they conclude that the child's weight is appropriate for his or her height. This assessment is a form of difference index that treats the weight and height centiles as equally important.

Statistically speaking, it is more appropriate to compare z scores than centiles, for two reasons: centiles are on a nonlinear scale that is elongated in the tails of the distribution, and in any case z scores provide a direct measure of the deviation from the median. So the informal procedure is equivalent to treating the difference in z score between weight and height as a measure of weight-for-height. But the preceding formula shows that the two z scores should not be given equal importance—height is only half to two-thirds as important as weight.

So the informal process that compares weight and height centiles needs modifying. For children of average fatness, the weight z score is roughly 50% greater than the height z score. If it is appreciably more than 50%, this is a sign of fatness; if it is appreciably less, this indicates thinness. In the simplest case, the child's weight and height are both on the median for age, and this represents average fatness by definition.

The same approach can be extended to BMI expressed as a z score, which it turns out can also be expressed to high accuracy as a difference index of the form [weight z score $- b \times$ height z score] (31).

Body Mass Index: Pros and Cons

The body mass index has now been embraced wholeheartedly for use in children. Since the early 1990s BMI growth charts have been published for several countries, providing population centile curves for BMI by age and sex. These charts allow the individual child's BMI to be expressed as a centile, and where the centile is too high or there is appreciable upward centile crossing over time, the child is at increased risk of obesity.

There are several advantages to the BMI for assessing obesity: It is based on measurements that are simple and cheap to make; it provides an assessment based on the whole body; it is highly correlated with body fat and broadly uncorrelated with height; and it is the index used in adults. Against these advantages there is one major disadvantage—it cannot distinguish between fat mass and fat-free mass. Consider two children matched for age, weight, and height, but one fat and the other lean. Because their weights and heights are the same, they have the same BMI yet they differ considerably in body composition. The excess fat in the one child weighs the same as the extra muscle in the other child, and the BMI is unable to distinguish between them.

This is potentially a serious problem for monitoring trends in obesity. If the trend to increasing fatness over time is matched by a corresponding decrease in muscle mass, the trend will be invisible to the BMI. This switch from fat-free to fat mass is tending to happen, as one of the main risk factors for obesity is sedentary behavior leading to a lack of fitness and reduced muscle mass. The problem does not arise with obesity indices based directly on body fat (e.g., skinfold thickness). Thus Flegal (9) has shown that trends in obesity over time in American adolescents are much more obvious when based on changes in triceps skinfold than when based on changes in BMI. This means that apparent trends in BMI are likely to underestimate the scale of the underlying problem.

REFERENCES AND STANDARDS

Growth charts based on reference standards have been mentioned several times in this chapter, but here they are discussed in more detail. The first issue is what to call them—references or standards. References are normative; that is, they are based on a reference population representative of some geographic or cultural group, whereas standards are prescriptive—they are based on a population selected on the basis of health. The implication is that standards represent optimal growth in some sense, whereas references indicate typical growth.

A practical problem with standards lies in the inclusion and exclusion criteria needed to define the reference population. The criteria are inevitably arbitrary (e.g., should severely asthmatic children be excluded, and if so how is severe asthma defined?), and this weakens the objectivity of the process. In practice, most growth charts are references rather than standards, constructed to be representative of one country. The term *growth standards* is, strictly speaking, incorrect in this context.

Purpose

Growth charts based on growth references are designed to assess measurements at a single moment in time, but in practice they are used to monitor growth over extended periods. This distinction is important to understand the strengths and weaknesses of the growth chart. The reference data underlying the chart usually consist of single measurements from a large sample of children covering the required age range, obtained from a cross-sectional anthropometric survey. Such a dataset contains no information about growth over time, as each child contributes just one measurement. So the term *growth chart* is, strictly speaking, inappropriate—the chart measures body *size* at different ages, not growth.

But doesn't everyone use growth charts to assess growth? Yes, but only in a limited sense. The assumption is that once they are past infancy, children grow along their own chosen centile on the chart. Normal growth is represented by a constant centile, and abnormal growth is seen as centile crossing, either up or down. This is fine so far as it goes, but in practice no child stays on exactly the same centile. Inevitably, some centile crossing occurs from age to age. The key question is, "How much centile crossing is reasonable, and at what point does it become excessive?" This is a question that the conventional growth or "distance" chart fails to answer. What is needed here is a "velocity" chart, which quantifies the change in the measurement (or its z score) over time (10). It is also possible to represent velocity information on the distance chart by adding extra curves with slopes that indicate a given rate of centile crossing (11).

The degree of centile crossing that occurs depends on the correlation among measurements at different ages. Height, for example, tracks very strongly, with children tending to stay close to their chosen centile in late infancy until they reach puberty. The year-on-year correlation for height is about 0.98 in mid-childhood (12). For weight the correlation is slightly lower, and the amount of tracking is less. For BMI, which is weight adjusted for height, the tracking is even less, as the stabilizing effect of height has been adjusted out. So a child's BMI centile is likely to change over time considerably more than for height.

The correlation of 0.98 seems very high, as indeed it is, but the amount of centile crossing over time depends not on the correlation r itself, but on the function $\sqrt{1 - r^2}$ of r, which is the standard deviation of the change in z score over the period (11). So if $r = 0.98$ then $\sqrt{1 - r^2} = 0.20$, and 95% of subjects followed over a year will cross centiles by less than $2 \times 0.20 = 0.40$ z scores up or down, about two-thirds of the width between two centile curves. (This channel width is typically 0.67 z scores 13.) For BMI the correlation r is about 0.94 (Rudolf M, personal communication), so $\sqrt{1 - r^2} = 0.34$ and the 95% confidence interval is $2 \times 0.34 = 0.68$ z scores or one channel width, 50% more than for height. A modest reduction in the correlation leads to a dramatic increase in the amount of centile crossing over 1 year.

Over a 2-year period the correlation for BMI is roughly $0.94 \times 0.94 = 0.89$, which is one-third more centile crossing than for 1 year. And for each successive year that

BMI is monitored, the correlation shrinks by the factor 0.94 and the degree of centile crossing increases accordingly.

This is a weakness of the BMI chart, as centile crossing is a more sensitive risk factor for later obesity than a high centile at any one moment in time. There is as yet no information about the limits of centile crossing to guide the use of the BMI chart. This is an area requiring further research.

Construction

So far we have discussed growth centile charts without considering where they come from. After the reference sample has been identified and the measurements collected, the statistical construction of the centile curves is the logical next stage. The methodology of centile curve construction has developed considerably in the last 15 years and has focused on two distinct approaches. The first, usually termed *quantile regression* (14), estimates the shapes of a series of prespecified centile curves (e.g., the third, 50th, and 97th centiles), using only the rankings of the measurements at each age in the region of the particular centile. Take the third centile, for example: For each of a series of narrow age groups the data are sorted into order and the cutoff point is identified, which separates the smallest 3% from the remainder. These cutoff points are smoothed across ages to provide the third centile curve. The same process leads to the median and 97th centile curves.

An important property of quantile regression is that the shapes of individual curves do not affect the shapes of neighboring curves. There is no guarantee that they will be similar in shape, and in principle the curves can touch or even cross. Quantile regression is most useful when one single centile is of interest (e.g., the 99th centile for wind speed over a period of time). But when the requirement is for a set of several centile curves rather than just one, as here, quantile regression is inefficient. The curves need to be similar in shape and spaced a suitable distance apart. It ought to be possible for curves to "borrow strength" from their neighbors during the estimation process.

This summarizes the other major approach to centile curve construction, which assumes some form of underlying frequency distribution at each age. The distribution ensures that the centiles are appropriately spaced, and equally that the centile curves plotted against age are of similar shape. The frequency distribution may—indeed will—change with age, but as long as the change is smooth and gradual, the centile curves will themselves be smooth.

The simplest distribution is the normal (Gaussian) distribution, and certain measurements (e.g., height) are close to normally distributed. This means that the distribution of height by age can be summarized in terms of the age-specific mean and SD, and these in turn define the required centiles of the distribution. Assume that z_α is the normal equivalent deviate corresponding to a tail area of α, so that $100\alpha\%$ of the distribution is to the left of z_α. The corresponding centile is given by the following:

$$\text{Centile } 100\alpha = \text{Mean} + \text{SD} \times z_\alpha$$

Any required centile can be obtained by setting z_α appropriately. For example, $z_\alpha = -1.88$ corresponds to the 3rd centile and 0.67 to the 75th centile.

Commonly, the standard deviation of the distribution increases in step with the mean, as can be seen on many growth charts—the centiles expand as the mean increases. Another way of describing the standard deviation is to express it as a fraction of the mean. This is known as the coefficient of variation, or CV, where CV = SD/mean. The advantage of the CV is that with child anthropometry it is less dependent on age than the SD, and so is simpler to estimate. The corresponding formula for centile 100α is

$$\text{Centile } 100\alpha = \text{Mean} (1 + \text{CV} \times z_\alpha) \qquad [1]$$

The elegance of this approach lies in its simplicity and parsimony. It depends only on two variables, the mean and CV, each of which can be represented as smooth curves plotted against age; it produces *any* required centiles, depending only on the choice of z_α, and it is much more efficient than quantile regression (15). Its main problem in the past has been that many anthropometric variables are not normally distributed, which has ruled it out.

Statisticians often have to deal with data that are not normally distributed, where one tail of the distribution (usually the right) is longer than the other—known as skewness. They commonly use a transformation (e.g., taking logarithms) to make them more normally distributed. The transformation alters the shape of the distribution by stretching the lower half and shrinking the upper half. In this way it removes the skewness and "pulls" the distribution closer to normality. The log transformation is only one of a whole family of power transformations (16) that allow the stretching-shrinking process to be tailor made to the individual distribution, to ensure that after transformation the two tails are of equal length. The transformation involves creating a new variable Y from the original variable X such that $Y = X^L$. The log transformation is a special case where $L = 0$, while other popular transformations are the square root ($L = 0.5$) and the reciprocal ($L = -1$).

To ensure that the transformation removes the skewness in the distribution it needs to take nonintegral values, and it needs to change smoothly with age. This is because the degree of skewness itself changes with age. So the power L can be thought of as a third age-varying variable, after the mean and the CV, which is represented as a smooth curve plotted against age.

The three curves allow centiles to be constructed for any anthropometric data with a normal or a skew normal distribution. (*Skew normal* means that a power transformation makes the distribution normal.) In practice this covers virtually all anthropometry. It has been named the *LMS method*, the letters of the name indicating the three underlying curves: L the power, M the mean (actually the median), and S the CV (17,18). M is the median rather than the mean because it is calculated as the mean on the normal transformed scale and back-transformed. The mean of a normal distribution is also the median, and on back-transformation it retains its position in the middle of the distribution. The formula for centile 100α is

$$\text{Centile } 100\alpha = M(1 + L \times S \times z_\alpha)^{1/L} \qquad [2]$$

where the values for L, M, and S are read off the corresponding curves for a child of given age and sex. The centile curve is obtained by calculating centiles over a range

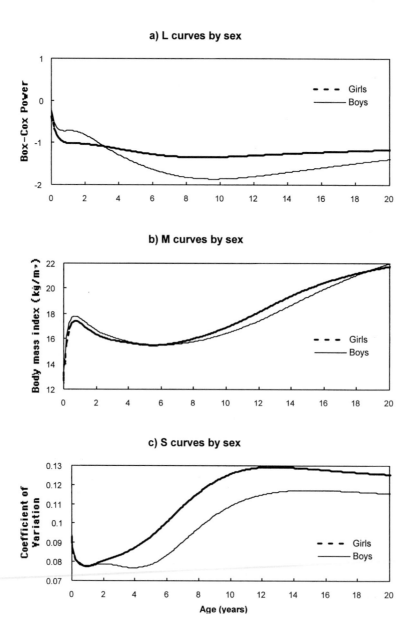

FIG. 1. Body mass index *LMS* curves by sex for British children, 1990 (23).

of ages. Substituting $L = 1$ into this formula gives the simpler case $M(1 + S \times z_\alpha)$ for normally distributed data, as shown in formula (1).

Other approaches to centile construction have used the same principle of a third curve to represent skewness, though with different parameterizations (19–21). Apart from the parameterization another issue is the form of the smooth curves that are to be fitted—polynomial, cubic spline, or kernel smoother. The LMS method in its most recent form (22) uses cubic splines, which allow for quite complicated curve shapes but at the cost of requiring a table of values by age rather than providing a simple formula.

An important advantage of all these distribution-based approaches is that anthropometric measurements can be converted with full accuracy to z scores. With the LMS method, for example, a measurement *Anth* is converted to a z score Z with the following formula:

$$Z = \frac{(Anth/M)^L - 1}{L \times S}$$ [3]

where L, M, and S are read from the curves and are appropriate for the child's age and sex.

As an example of the LMS method, Fig. 1 shows the fitted L, M, and S curves for the British BMI reference by sex (23). The M curves show median BMI for boys and girls, with the familiar rise then fall during the first year, the adiposity rebound at 6 years, and the subsequent rise to adulthood. The S curve is the coefficient of variation of BMI, which is near 0.08, or 8%, before puberty and then jumps to 12% during and after puberty. The L curve shows the changing degree of skewness. Already at birth the distribution is sufficiently skewed to require a log transformation ($L = 0$), but soon afterward the skewness increases and a reciprocal transformation ($L = -1$) becomes necessary. The reciprocal of BMI is height^2/weight, and so surprisingly this upside-down index is close to normally distributed. There are two obvious sex differences in the curves: During puberty, median BMI increases faster and flattens earlier in girls than in boys; and the variability of BMI is consistently greater in girls than in boys from as early as 2 years of age.

The centile curves that result from the LMS curves of Fig. 1 are shown in Fig. 2. The current British growth charts use centiles that are equally spaced, two-thirds of a unit apart on the z score scale. This leads to the following (approximate) centiles as seen in Fig. 2: 2, 9, 25, 50, 75, 91, and 98. Each centile curve is the same shape as the M curve, but the centiles splay out with increasing age, and the spacings between them are much greater above the median than below, indicating the presence of appreciable skewness. The age of the second rise in adiposity, known as the adiposity rebound (24), occurs 3 to 4 years earlier on the 98th than on the 2nd centile, suggesting that an earlier adiposity rebound is associated with greater fatness.

CHOICE OF CUTOFF POINTS

Risk-Based Cutoff Point

The definition of *obesity* requires a cutoff for BMI, with obesity deemed to be present above the cutoff and absent below it. A second, less extreme cutoff defining

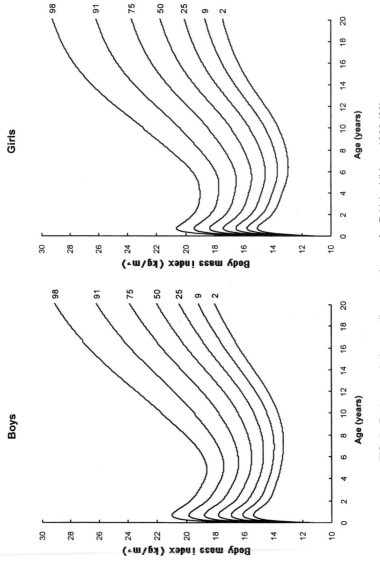

FIG. 2. Body mass index centile curves by sex for British children, 1990 (23).

overweight or the risk of overweight may also be required. But how is this cutoff to be identified?

The most obvious approach is to place it at the point on the BMI distribution that identifies the small number of individuals who, because of their obesity, are at risk of future ill health. But the problem is that this point cannot be identified with any confidence—the link between current fatness in childhood or adolescence and a later adverse outcome (e.g., adult hypertension, diabetes, or cardiovascular disease) is simply too weak to be useful. The risk increases steadily with increasing fatness, but there is no obvious "shoulder" on the plot of risk versus BMI that would indicate a demarcation between low risk and high risk. And even if there were a clear link between child/adolescent fatness and later morbidity/mortality, it would be mediated through adult fatness, which is known to be linked to both. Is a fat child who stays fat at greater risk than a thin child who becomes fat? Or, to put it another way, is the increase in fatness from child to adult a risk factor in its own right?

There are two further practical difficulties with identifying a cutoff based on risk. Cutoff points are required for children of all ages, so a separate cutoff needs to be developed for each age. This requires far more detailed information about the link between current fatness and later outcome than is now available. And the final problem is that the etiology of obesity may have changed in recent years—its steeply increasing prevalence may indicate a different form of the condition from that in the past. If true, this means that the available retrospective evidence linking fatness and outcome may be irrelevant for future predictions.

The conclusion is that for all these reasons, child cutoff points for BMI based on risk are currently not useful. Whether this will remain so in the future is not clear.

National BMI Cutoff Point

The obvious alternative to a risk-based cutoff point is a cutoff relying on BMI centiles. This is population based to ensure that a fixed percentage of the reference population lies above the cutoff point at all ages (e.g., 5% above the 95th centile). Though this is simple and convenient (so long as a suitable BMI centile chart exists), it makes the unlikely assumption that the degree of overweight/obesity is the same at all ages. In practice, this assumption is untestable, as no gold standard exists to measure the prevalence of obesity at each age. In the continuing absence of such a gold standard the simpler definition must suffice.

But even this decision does not solve all the problems. We still have to decide what centile to use for the cutoff point. Bearing in mind that the choice of centile defines the prevalence of obesity (i.e., 5% for the 95th centile), the decision is immediately seen to be as much political as clinical. Barlow and Dietz (25) have provided a clear lead in the United States for the use of the 85th and 95th centiles for overweight and obesity, respectively, but their recommendation has been far from universally accepted. A wide range of centiles has been proposed for obesity, overweight, or risk of overweight (e.g., the 85th, 91st, 95th, 97th, 97.5th, and 98th centiles). These provide a sevenfold difference in overweight/obesity prevalence, from 2% to 15%, an enormous range. So long as child obesity studies use their own centile cutoff points and their own BMI reference charts, the prevalences they report will not be comparable. Any statements about the prevalence of overweight or obesity in particular groups are meaningless unless they are accompanied by a description of the definition used.

International BMI Centile Chart

The lack of standardization in the definition of childhood overweight and obesity has been a serious obstacle to obesity research in recent years. As a simple example, the section on child obesity in the WHO obesity report (26) started with the admission that there was no agreed definition of child obesity, which undermined everything else that followed. The problem with establishing a standardized definition is that it must be seen to be international in scope. In the past this has not been a problem: the WHO international growth reference, for example, based on American data, has been widely used over the last 20 years (27). However, the political climate has now changed, and a single-country reference like this would no longer be acceptable in the same way.

An international BMI centile chart could be achieved by pooling reference data from several countries, which would avoid the single-country problem. But this raises other problems of its own: how would the countries be chosen, and would their inclusion imply that they were healthier in some way than other countries? The choice of countries would define the level of obesity that was acceptable—higher for countries from the developed world than from the developing world.

But even if the source of the reference data could be agreed, there would still be the problem of what cutoff point to use. Here again, past experience may no longer be relevant, and a different approach is needed. A workshop held in 1997 by the International Obesity Task Force addressed just this question and came up with a novel proposal that has been widely welcomed (28). It links the child BMI centile cutoff points to the cutoff points used in adults—that is, 25 kg/m^2 for overweight and 30 kg/m^2 for obesity—which are universally recognized. It also creates this link using the LMS method, as described earlier, to construct the centile chart.

Figure 3 illustrates the process with the British 1990 reference. The LMS method allows any centile curves to be drawn, once the individual L, M, and S curves have been derived (Fig. 1). A particular centile is set by the choice of the normal equivalent deviate z_α in the formula ([1] and [2]). To obtain the value of z_α for a centile curve passing through, say, 25 kg/m^2 at 18 years, we substitute $Anth = 25$ into formula [3], and this gives the z score (Z), which is the required value of z_α in formula [2]. Substituting it into formula [2], we get values of the corresponding centile curve over the whole age range, which by definition passes through BMI 25 at 18 years. Figure 3 shows the resulting curves for cutoff points 25 and 30 at 18 years in British children, corresponding roughly to the 90th and 99th centiles, respectively.

This same process can be carried out on other datasets for which LMS curves exist, and they each lead to a pair of centile curves like those for British boys and girls

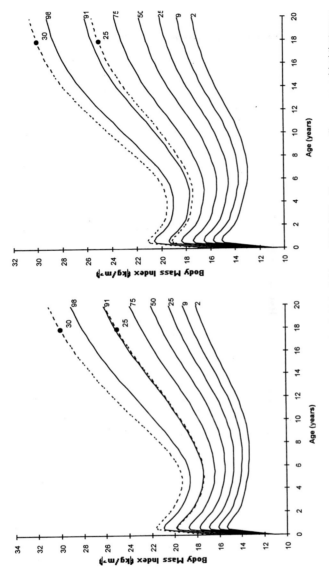

FIG. 3. Body mass index centile curves by sex for British children 1990 (23) with extra centile curves added that pass through the adult cutoff points of 25 and 30 kg/m² at 18 years.

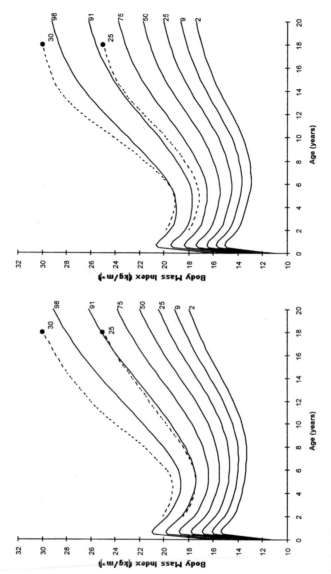

FIG. 4. Body mass index centile curves by sex for British children 1990 (23), with the IOTF overweight and obesity cut-off points (28) superimposed, that pass through the adult cutoff points of 25 and 30 kg/m² at 18 years.

in Fig. 3. Cole *et al.* (28) applied the process to six large nationally representative child BMI surveys from Brazil, Britain, Hong Kong, the Netherlands, Singapore, and the United States. The six country overweight centile curves (all passing through BMI 25 at 18 years) and the six country obesity curves (BMI 30 similarly) were then averaged at each age to give two composite centile curves by sex, and they are shown in Fig. 4 superimposed on the British 1990 reference. Comparison with Fig. 3 shows that the cutoff points are similar to those for British children (not surprisingly, as Britain is one of the six countries), though the International Obesity Task Force (IOTF) cutoff points are slightly higher during puberty.

The cutoff points are defined between the ages of 2 and 18 years and are known as the IOTF overweight and obesity cutoffs. (See the *British Medical Journal* website version of reference 28 for a table of the cutoff points by age and sex.) At the time of writing these cutoff points are relatively novel, so that few studies have made use of them so far.

One example is from Chinn and Rona (29), who have used the IOTF cutoff points to track changes in overweight and obesity from 1974 to 1994 in English and Scottish children of primary school age (4 to 11 years). From 1974 to 1984 the prevalence rates in England fell slightly, while those in Scotland rose slightly. From 1984 to 1994 there were steep rises in both countries, reaching 6% to 9% in the 9- to 11-year-olds. The prevalence of overweight in 1994 was 9% and 14% in boys and girls, respectively, and for obesity it was 2% and 3%. In the future, other studies should show the degree to which these prevalences vary by time and place over the world.

No Cutoff Point at All

So far we have been talking about the need for cutoff points. However, it is worth emphasizing that cutoff points are not always necessary and that the whole BMI distribution can provide useful information about obesity in the population. Mean BMI, for example, tends to be raised in populations where the rate of obesity is high, whatever cutoff is used to define obesity. Similarly, the standard deviation of BMI is increased in fat populations, because BMI in the fattest children tends to outstrip the mean and increases the overall variability. Cutoff points are an inefficient way of comparing population distributions (9).

A simple way to test for changes in the mean and SD of BMI is to convert them to z scores, using a convenient LMS-based reference. The mean and SD ought to be 0 and 1, respectively, so that if either is materially increased, then it provides evidence of a trend to increasing obesity. Bundred *et al.* (30) demonstrated clear trends to increasing BMI over 10 years in 3- to 4-year-old British children in this way: they converted BMI to z scores using the British 1990 reference, and the mean z score increased by 0.4 units over the 10 years, whereas the z score for height did not change. Unfortunately, the paper did not report the corresponding SDs over time.

CONCLUSIONS

BMI is a simple though imperfect measure of overweight in childhood. Reference standards for BMI are important both for clinical and population use in the study of child obesity, to monitor the prevalence and incidence of overweight and obesity. However, there are serious difficulties with nationally based references for making international comparisons, and a different approach is needed to provide a politically acceptable definition.

REFERENCES

1. Cole TJ. Weight–stature indices to measure underweight, overweight and obesity. In: Himes JH, ed. *Anthropometric assessment of nutritional status.* New York: Alan R Liss, 1991: 83–111.
2. Garrow JS, Webster J. Quetelet's index (W/H^2) as a measure of fatness. *Int J Obes* 1985; 9: 147–53.
3. Keys A, Fidanza F, Karvonen MJ, *et al.* Indices of relative weight and obesity. *J Chron Dis* 1972; 25: 329–43.
4. Waterlow JC. Classification and definition of protein–calorie malnutrition. *BMJ* 1972; iii: 566–9.
5. Baldwin BT. Weight-height-age standards in metric units for American-born children. *Am J Phys Anthropol* 1925; 8: 1–10.
6. Rolland-Cachera MF, Sempé M, Guilloud-Bataille M, *et al.* Adiposity indices in children. *Am J Clin Nutr* 1982; 36: 178–84.
7. Cole TJ. A method for assessing age-standardized weight-for-height in children seen cross-sectionally. *Ann Hum Biol* 1979; 6: 249–68.
8. Cole TJ. Weight/height^p compared to weight/height^2 for assessing adiposity in childhood: influence of age and bone age on p during puberty. *Ann Hum Biol* 1986; 13: 433–51.
9. Flegal KM. Defining obesity in children and adolescents: epidemiologic approaches. *Crit Rev Food Sci Nutr* 1993; 33: 307–12.
10. Tanner JM, Whitehouse RH, Takaishi M. Standards from birth to maturity for height, weight, height velocity, and weight velocity: British children, 1965 Parts I and II. *Arch Dis Child* 1966; 41: 454–71, 613–35.
11. Cole TJ. Presenting information on growth distance and conditional velocity in one chart: practical issues of chart design. *Stat Med* 1998; 17: 2697–707.
12. Bailey BJR. Monitoring the heights of prepubertal children by the use of standard charts. *Ann Hum Biol* 1994; 21: 1–11.
13. Cole TJ. Do growth chart centiles need a facelift? *BMJ* 1994; 308: 641–2.
14. Koenker RW, D'Orey V. Computing regression quantiles. *Appl Stat* 1987; 36: 383–93.
15. Healy MJR. Notes on the statistics of growth standards. *Ann Hum Biol* 1974; 1: 41–6.
16. Box GEP, Cox DR. An analysis of transformations. *J R Stat Soc B* 1964; 26: 211–52.
17. Cole TJ. Fitting smoothed centile curves to reference data. *J R Stat Soc A* 1988; 151: 385–418.
18. Cole TJ, Green PJ. Smoothing reference centile curves: the LMS method and penalized likelihood. *Stat Med* 1992; 11: 1305–19.
19. Healy MJR, Rasbash J, Yang M. Distribution-free estimation of age-related centiles. *Ann Hum Biol* 1988; 15: 17–22.
20. Royston P. Estimation, reference ranges and goodness of fit for the 3-parameter lognormal distribution. *Stat Med* 1992; 11: 897–912.
21. Wade AM, Ades AE. Age-related reference ranges: significance tests for models and confidence intervals for centiles. *Stat Med* 1994; 13: 2359–67.
22. Cole TJ, Freeman JV, Preece MA. British 1990 growth reference centiles for weight, height, body mass index and head circumference fitted by maximum penalized likelihood. *Stat Med* 1998; 17: 407–29.
23. Cole TJ, Freeman JV, Preece MA. Body mass index reference curves for the UK, 1990. *Arch Dis Child* 1995; 73: 25–9.
24. Rolland-Cachera MF, Deheeger M, Bellisle F, *et al.* Adiposity rebound in children: a simple indicator for predicting obesity. *Am J Clin Nutr* 1984; 39: 129–35.
25. Barlow SE, Dietz WH. Obesity evaluation and treatment: expert committee recommendations. *Pediatrics* 1998; 102: 29.
26. WHO. *Obesity: preventing and managing the global epidemic.* Report of a WHO consultation Geneva, 3–5 June 1997. WHO/NUT/98.1. Geneva: WHO, 1998.
27. Dibley MJ, Goldsby JB, Staehling NW, *et al.* Development of normalized curves for the international growth reference: historical and technical considerations. *Am J Clin Nutr* 1987; 46: 736–48.
28. Cole TJ, Bellizzi MC, Flegal KM, *et al.* Establishing a standard definition for child overweight and obesity: international survey. *BMJ* 2000; 320: 1240–3.

29. Chinn S, Rona RJ. Prevalence and trends in overweight and obesity in three cross sectional studies of British children, 1974–94. *BMJ* 2001; 322: 24–6.
30. Bundred P, Kitchiner D, Buchan I. Prevalence of overweight and obese children between 1989 and 1998: population-based series of cross-sectional studies. *BMJ* 2001; 322: 326–8.
31. Cole TJ. A chart to link centiles of body mass index, weight and height. *Eur J Clin Nutr* 2002 (in press).

DISCUSSION

Dr. Dietz: I have a comment and a question. My comment is that I did not see persistence of obesity into adulthood among your morbidity criteria. I think there are now sufficient longitudinal studies to allow that to be added as an additional criterion. My question has to do with how one might develop an agenda for defining obesity among Asian children. As you know, in adults the cutoff point appears to be lower, for reasons that are not clear. There is substantial morbidity at lower adult BMIs than is apparently the case in Western societies, which would imply that the cutoff points in, for example, Chinese and Japanese children might well be lower. How would you define the research agenda to explore that issue?

Dr. Cole: Once you accept that the risk in Asian children is greater, then implicitly you are saying that you have got to use a risk-based cutoff. If you are to use a risk-based cutoff, this leads us back to the problem that we don't have a very clear outcome measure that we can use. I think in a sense this just underlines the need for us to try and move forward in this area to clarify our ideas about how to obtain a risk-based cutoff. The other thing we need to remember is that the concept of a "cutoff" is a great oversimplification. We know that the underlying continuum is just as important and that it does not really matter whether you are just below the cutoff point or just above it. This is the danger of cutoffs, and it goes against my statistical philosophy to try to pretend that you have a distribution that is present or absent when we know that that is absolutely not the case. I could probably live with a cutoff that did not have any implications for risk, while accepting that if it were applied to Asian children it would have a different meaning from that in European children—in other words, a given value was likely to be more serious in terms of outcome.

Dr. Uauy: When you approach the change with age, do you take different rates of maturation into account? Children who mature earlier will have a higher BMI during the pubertal period.

Dr. Cole: This is a clinical rather than a population issue. In a population, what matters is the *average* timing of maturation. If they have early maturation, they will show higher rates of overweight at that time in relation to the IOTF cutoff, but once they have passed through puberty the figures will fall back to where they were before. I get nervous when I'm asked this sort of question. It suggests that these cutoff points are wonderfully detailed instruments, but in fact they are about as blunt as you could imagine. They are not designed to give a good answer in individual clinical situations, and maturation is an issue in point. I am sure one could think of lots of others. However, in terms of population studies, and taken broadly over a range of different ages, I think one can get around those difficulties.

Dr. Koletzko: I think it is a big step forward that you have created a global standard for obesity prevalence and changes in incidence. You started your introduction by saying that there is a broad consensus approving the use of the BMI as a standard measurement in children, but now you appear to be questioning that. I wonder whether it is premature to apply the BMI as the standard clinical measure, based on the limited scientific evidence that we have and the various practical limitations. For pediatricians in clinical practice, it is much more inconvenient to calculate the BMI and to look at age- and sex-specific reference values than to use the conventional weight-for-height centiles. I haven't seen any evidence that the use of the BMI in clinical practice is better at identifying children at risk or that it improves the outcome. You indicated—and

I could not agree more—that what we really need is a risk-based approach. Dr. Dietz has already posed the question of standards for a risk-based approach. For example, there are now definite indications that children of low birth weight who develop a high BMI have a much greater risk of metabolic and clinical consequences than infants with the same BMI who had a higher birth weight.

Dr. Cole: Your first point was about the consensus over whether the BMI is a good measure to use in children in clinical practice. I'm not a clinician, but I'm not clear that there is any real alternative to using weight-for-height, and you come back to that at the end. Pediatricians have been working with weight-for-height as a concept since 1966—that is, they have at least 40 years and possibly 50 years of familiarity. However, we know that weight-for-height is not a very good index under certain circumstances. For example, in infancy and adolescence it does not actually work. You'll know that the NCHS weight-for-height chart stopped before you got to adolescence, so for the subject of our meeting here, which mentions adolescence, the NCHS weight-for-height reference would not have been much use. So weight-for-height, which clinicians are very happy to use, didn't actually do the job, while BMI does do the job. So my conclusion is that there is probably clinical support for using it. I accept that it's slightly more difficult to work with because you have to get out your calculator to work it out.

Dr. Koletzko: I'm a friend of the BMI myself. I'm just asking, at this time of evidence-based medicine, whether we are right to tell the world of clinical pediatrics to use the BMI if there is no evidence for any benefit of BMI over weight-for-height. You mentioned adolescence and with the dataset you have you could easily construct a weight-for-height centile for adolescents as well. So the fact that the weight-for-height relation changes in adolescence is not a good argument for using the BMI in my view. I have a question about the application of your standards to German children. When we apply your standards in Germany, then in comparison with our traditional weight-for-height standards it appears that your cutoff point identifies a much lower proportion of children as obese. Do you have an explanation for that?

Dr. Cole: It depends what age you are looking at. As I said, NCHS tried to recognize this difficulty—that if you use weight-for-height in the simple sense in adolescence it really doesn't mean anything. If you try to compare BMI and weight-for-height in adolescence (was this the age range you were referring to?), you will get answers that look very different, and you will have to take it from me—although you may not accept it—that BMI is the more correct of the two answers. If the difference you are referring to are in earlier childhood, then the explanation may simply be that the cutoff points are different, so you will get different apparent rates of obesity. This just underlines the fact that the definition is entirely arbitrary. However, the advantage of the IOTF standard is that it will give the same answer for children of the same size in different countries.

Dr. Birch: I believe these reference data are based on cross-sectional data. It concerns me, from my experience in other areas, that you can get yourself into trouble by drawing inferences about change over time when using cross-sectional data, particularly in an area such as this where there are rapid changes in prevalence, and probably time-of-testing effects. With this in mind, can we really say that crossing centiles is a reasonable way of looking at things, when we are looking at an individual child but comparing that child with cross-sectional group data?

Dr. Cole: Your point is well made. I think it is important to remind people that all charts, from way back, have been based on cross-sectional data, both for weight and height, and yet the concern about centile crossing on those charts tends not to get discussed. I agree you do require longitudinal data to judge the amounts and the significance of centile crossing. We know that the average child is crossing the centiles upward, that charts are getting out of date day by day. This leads on to another debate about whether we should make our charts so that they represent children as they are now, or as they used to be in a halcyon age when everybody was the right fatness. There isn't a simple answer to that, but you do need longitudinal data to assess centile crossing, I agree, and such data are rather sparse.

Dr. Svivastava: You mentioned cutoff points based on risk, but risks may vary from country to country. How do we sort this out and relate risk clearly to obesity?

Dr. Cole: It is a very difficult problem, and it just highlights the difficulty of using any sort of risk-based cutoff. The association between childhood BMI and later outcome is so diffuse and so varied from country to country that it's difficult to pin down the particular outcomes that one wants to focus on, or to come up with such a clear relationship that you are prepared to draw a cutoff on a chart as a result of it. This is why people are not keen to use a risk-based cutoff. There is too much uncertainty.

Dr. Bar-Or: As physiologists, we pride ourselves in our ability to assess the percentage of body fat much more precisely than you can by using BMI or skinfold techniques. Even so, when we arrive at a value for percentage of body fat, we don't really know what it means as far as cutoff points are concerned. In your various datasets, have you encountered subsets that could allow you to correlate the BMI with a more precise measurement of body fat, so that we can make sense of our own data?

Dr. Cole: I think you put your finger on it when you said that we don't know what *percent body fat* means. The bottom line is that we want to come up with some anthropometric indicator of outcome. If that anthropometric indicator happens to be a refined estimate of percent body fat, then so be it. But it might not actually relate to percent body fat particularly well at all. The important thing is that it predicts outcome. So there is a lot of work to do. What we need is an indicator of what is going to happen in the future, so the percent body fat issue is almost a red herring. It might be the solution, but we actually want something that is going to be useful in the long term, and the big difficulty is that we cannot get long-term data other than by hanging around a long time.

Dr. Uauy: I'd like to make a point that the WHO standard was a "guestimate" for risk for a Caucasian population. I don't think it is a valid end point for children until we know the risks associated with given BMIs. In fact, I would for now avoid calling it a "standard"; it would be preferable to call it a reference. I don't think it has been validated, either in terms of body composition or in terms of risk. Both for populations and for individuals we need a standard that is related to risk and to body fat.

Dr. Cole: I agree with that.

Obesity in Childhood and Adolescence, edited by Chunming Chen and William H. Dietz. Nestlé Nutrition Workshop Series, Pediatric Program, Vol. 49. Nestec Ltd., Vevey/Lippincott Williams & Wilkins, Philadelphia © 2002.

Prevalence of Childhood and Adolescent Overweight and Obesity in Asian and European Countries

Mary C. Bellizzi, *Graham W. Horgan, †Michèlle Guillaume, and ‡William H. Dietz

*Health Promotions, Aberdeen, Scotland, UK; *Biomathematics and Statistics Scotland, Rowett Research Institute, Aberdeen, Scotland, UK; †Département Prévention-Santé, Directrice de l'Observatoire et des Centres de Santé, Chaussée d'Houffalize, Bastogne, Luxembourg; ‡Division of Nutrition and Physical Activity, Centers for Disease Control and Prevention, Atlanta, Georgia, USA*

Obesity in children, which is increasingly recognized as a major public health problem worldwide (1), is linked to adult obesity and its related morbidity (2). Childhood obesity is also associated with health risks that can strike young people, including dyslipidemia, hyperinsulinemia, hypertension, and psychosocial problems (3,4). To address this issue, action is needed at local, national, and international levels, with well-documented evidence of the global prevalence of overweight and obesity in children required to develop appropriate health policies.

Obesity is defined as an excess of body fat, but in adults the body mass index (BMI; weight [kg]/height [m^2]) and not adiposity has been accepted internationally as a standard for assessing obesity (1). In children, factors such as growth make definitions of obesity difficult. Not surprisingly, various standards are used to calculate the prevalence of childhood obesity internationally (5). Some studies have used a standard methodology to report the prevalence of overweight in preschool children in developing countries to allow comparisons between countries (6,7), but international comparisons of the prevalence of overweight in older children remain lacking.

Some years ago the working group on childhood obesity of the International Obesity Task Force (IOTF) set out to study the prevalence of overweight and obesity in older children worldwide. Because of the varying standards, it became evident that comparing published prevalence data on overweight and obesity would be difficult. Indeed, the prevalence of overweight children in a country could differ by a factor of 3 when the same dataset is analyzed by different standards (5).

Thus the first task was to identify a suitable international standard. Following recommendations from a workshop on childhood obesity (8), the IOTF's children's group developed a standard defined by the average centiles estimated to pass through

BMI 25 (overweight) and 30 (obesity), respectively, at age 18 years (9). The BMIs of a reference population made up of six nationally representative datasets in children were used to derive the cutoff points in children (2 to 18 years). The countries represented were Brazil, the United Kingdom, Hong Kong, the Netherlands, Singapore, and the United States.

The primary aim of the present study was thus to determine the prevalence of overweight and obesity in 10- and 15-year-old children using the IOTF standard for overweight and obesity developed by Cole *et al.* (9). We looked at all the Asian data available to us and compared prevalence rates with those in some European countries.

At the country level, having as much information as possible about the levels of overweight and obesity is useful for targeting interventions. To illustrate this, the data from Singapore were analyzed by the different ethnic groups. Regional variation in overweight and obesity within a country is demonstrated by using three datasets from Germany.

MATERIALS AND METHODS

Cross-sectional primary anthropometric data for boys and girls were obtained from various surveys with the datasets obtained through several sources, including the IOTF's web site (*www.iotf.org*), the authors' personal networks, and IOTF members. Because of the limited availability of national anthropometric data, countries without national datasets were still encouraged to submit weights and heights to determine the prevalence of overweight children in as many populations as possible.

Sample sizes of 100 or more in each sex were considered acceptable, a choice based on the assumption that with an overweight prevalence of 5%, at least 100 would be necessary to give a standard error of 2% or less. Even so, we included some datasets with less than 100, supplementing them with data from the previous or following year. Cutoff points at ages 10 and 15 years (Table 1) were applied to determine the prevalence of overweight and obese children. Children above or below four standard deviations (SD) for height or 6 SD for weight or BMI were excluded. All the datasets used had fewer than 1% outliers, several fewer than 0.1% (Table 2).

TABLE 1. *Body mass index cutoff points used to determine the prevalence of overweight and obese boys and girls*

Sex	Age (years)	Overweight	Obese
Boys	10	20.20	24.57
	15	23.60	28.60
Girls	10	20.29	24.77
	15	24.17	29.29

Note: Based on the IOTF standard defining total overweight and obesity as BMI ≥ age-specific BMI cutoff points corresponding to BMIs of 25 and 30 at age 18 years, respectively (9).

TABLE 2. *Datasets included in this study*

Country	Survey years	Area	% Outliers	Reference
Germany	1995–96	Dresden	0.080	(10)
Germany	1996	Jena	0.422	(11)
Germany	1995–96	Munich	0.074	(10)
Hong Kong	1993	Countrywide	0.017	(12)
Hungary	1993–94	Pècs	0.176	(13)
Italy	1999	Verona and Brindisi	0.090	(14)
Japan	1997	Osaka	0.075	(15)
Netherlands	1980	Countrywide	0.072	(16)
Singapore	1993	Countrywide	0.070	(17)
Taiwan	1995–96	Taipei	None	(18)
UK	1978–93	Countrywide	0.025	(19)

Internationally, the term *at risk of overweight* is sometimes used for children between the 85th and 95th centiles, and *overweight* is used for children in the 95th centile and beyond. The first of these terms is equivalent to the term *overweight* used by Cole *et al.* (9) to define children with an age-specific BMI corresponding to a BMI of 25 to less than 30. The second is equivalent to the term *obese* used by the same group for children with an age-specific BMI corresponding to a BMI of 30 or more. Because we used the cutoff points of Cole *et al.* in this study, we retained the terminology used in their paper. We also use the term *total overweight* to indicate "either overweight or obese."

Surveys generally used standard procedures for measuring weight and height, which are described in survey reports and referenced in Table 2. Anthropometric data from four countries in Asia (Hong Kong, Singapore, Taiwan, and Japan) and five in Europe (Germany, the United Kingdom, Hungary, Italy, and the Netherlands) are discussed in this paper. The data from Singapore were further analyzed with reference to the nation's three main ethnic groups—Chinese, Malays, and Indians. The German data represented children from Munich, Dresden, and Jena.

The datasets from Singapore, Hong Kong, Italy, the United Kingdom, Hungary, and the Netherlands had weights and heights for both the 10-year-olds and the 15-year-olds. Japan also had 10-year-olds but stopped at 14 years. For Taiwan the dataset included only 15-year-olds, and for Germany, only 10-year-olds.

The datasets spanned the late 1980s to the late 1990s, with the exception of the Netherlands (1980) and part of the United Kingdom dataset (1978).

RESULTS

Total Overweight in 10-Year-Old Children

The prevalence of total overweight among 10-year-olds ranged from less than 5% for boys from the Netherlands to nearly 30% in Italian boys. Similarly, rates ranged broadly among girls, with only 7% of those in the Netherlands being overweight or obese but more than 30% of Italian girls in these classifications.

TABLE 3. *Prevalence of overweight and obesity in 10-year-old boys*

	Sample	Total overweight[a] (%)	Overweight[b] (%)	Obese[c] (%)
Italy	334	29.6	22.2	7.5
Japan	392	27.8	21.7	6.1
Singapore	1,660	25.5	19.4	6.1
Germany (Munich)	314	22.9	19.4	3.5
Hungary	117	20.5	15.4	5.1
Hong Kong	661	20.3	15.6	4.7
Germany (Dresden)	415	15.4	12.0	3.4
Germany (Jena)	114	10.5	7.9	2.6
UK	1,222	9.5	8.1	1.4
Netherlands	847	4.5	4.5	0.0

[a] Based on the IOTF standard that defines total overweight as BMI ≥ age-specific BMI cutoff points corresponding to a BMI of 25 at 18 years of age (9).
[b] Based on the IOTF standard that defines overweight as BMI ≥ age-specific BMI cutoff points corresponding to BMIs of 25 to 30 at 18 years of age (9).
[c] Based on the IOTF standard that defines obesity as BMI ≥ age-specific BMI cutoff points corresponding to a BMI 30 at 18 years of age (9).

Overall, total overweight was more common in boys than in girls. Italy, Japan, Singapore, Germany (Munich), Hungary, and Hong Kong had rates of 20% or more for 10-year-old boys (Table 3), but only Italy and Munich were 20% or more for girls. Rates for girls in the other countries ranged from 8% to less than 20% (Table 4).

In all the Asian countries 10-year-old boys were more likely than their female counterparts to be overweight or obese, with rates for boys being 8 to 10 percentage points higher.

TABLE 4. *Prevalence of overweight and obesity in 10-year-old girls*

	Sample	Total overweight[a] (%)	Overweight[b] (%)	Obese[c] (%)
Italy	344	31.4	23.3	8.1
Germany (Munich)	309	25.9	20.4	5.5
Japan	384	18.5	17.4	1.0
Germany (Dresden)	369	17.6	15.7	1.9
Singapore	1,584	17.6	14.6	3.0
UK	1,113	14.4	13.0	1.3
Germany (Jena)	122	13.9	12.3	1.6
Hungary	115	13.9	9.6	4.3
Hong Kong	623	10.1	8.3	1.8
Netherlands	897	6.7	6.1	0.6

[a] Based on the IOTF standard that defines total overweight as BMI ≥ age-specific BMI cutoff points corresponding to a BMI of 25 at 18 years of age (9).
[b] Based on the IOTF standard that defines overweight as BMI ≥ age-specific BMI cutoff points corresponding to BMIs of 25 to 30 at 18 years of age (9).
[c] Based on the IOTF standard that defines obesity as BMI ≥ age-specific BMI cutoff points corresponding to a BMI of 30 at 18 years of age (9).

Obese 10-Year-Olds

The prevalence of obesity among 10-year-old boys ranged from 0 in the Netherlands to 7.5% in Italy, with Japan and Singapore at 6.1%. Among girls, the rates were lowest in the Netherlands (0.6%), highest in Italy (8.1%), and next highest (5.5%) in Germany (Munich).

As expected, the prevalence of obesity often differed substantially between boys and girls. As was the case for total overweight, 10-year-old boys from Japan, Hong Kong, and Singapore were more likely to be obese than their female peers.

Total Overweight Among 15-Year-Olds

Among 15-year-old boys, the prevalence of total overweight (Table 5) was lowest in the Netherlands (5.8%) and highest in Taiwan (30.5%). In girls this rate ranged from 6.3% in Hong Kong to 21.1% in Taiwan (Table 6).

As with the 10-year-olds, the most notable finding among the Asian 15-year-olds was that total overweight was much more common among boys than among girls.

Obesity in 15-Year-Olds

Obesity rates for 15-year-old boys were highest in Taiwan (7.3%) and lowest in the Netherlands (0.2%). In girls, rates were highest in Hungary (4.7%) and lowest in the United Kingdom (0).

TABLE 5. *Prevalence of overweight and obesity in 15-year-old boys*

	Sample	Total overweight[a] (%)	Overweight[b] (%)	Obese[c] (%)
Taiwan[d]	302	30.5	23.2	7.3
Italy	224	22.8	18.8	4.0
Japan[e]	385	20.0	14.3	5.7
Singapore	1,160	15.3	11.4	3.9
Hungary	106	15.1	12.3	2.8
Hong Kong	456	10.3	7.0	3.3
UK	287	7.0	6.3	0.7
Netherlands	844	5.8	5.6	0.2

[a] Based on the IOTF standard that defines total overweight as BMI ≥ age-specific BMI cutoff points corresponding to a BMI of 25 at 18 years of age (9).

[b] Based on the IOTF standard that defines overweight as BMI ≥ age-specific BMI cutoff points corresponding to BMIs of 25 to 30 at 18 years of age (9).

[c] Based on the IOTF standard that defines obesity as BMI ≥ age-specific BMI cutoff points corresponding to a BMI of 30 at 18 years of age (9).

[d] Because the sample size for Taiwan boys aged 15 years was small ($N = 64$), data for 14-year-olds were added to give a larger sample size ($N = 302$).

[e] Because the dataset for Japan stopped at 14 years, data for 14-year-olds were used in the analyses for 15-year-olds.

TABLE 6. *Prevalence of overweight and obesity in 15-year-old girls*

	Sample	Total overweight[a] (%)	Overweight[b] (%)	Obese[c] (%)
Taiwan[d]	308	21.1	17.9	3.2
Hungary	106	17.9	13.2	4.7
Japan[e]	332	15.7	13.9	1.8
Italy	326	16.3	14.1	2.1
Singapore	946	11.4	8.6	2.9
Netherlands	812	8.6	8.1	0.5
UK	408	7.6	7.6	0.0
Hong Kong	510	6.3	5.3	1.0

[a] Based on the IOTF standard that defines total overweight as BMI $\geq$ age-specific BMI cutoff points corresponding to a BMI of 25 at 18 years of age (9).
[b] Based on the IOTF standard that defines overweight as BMI $\geq$ age-specific BMI cutoff points corresponding to BMIs of 25 to 30 at 18 years of age (9).
[c] Based on the IOTF standard that defines obesity as BMI $\geq$ age-specific BMI cutoff points corresponding to a BMI of 30 at 18 years of age (9).
[d] Because the sample size for Taiwanese girls aged 15 years was small ($N = 71$), data for 14-year-olds were added to give a larger sample size ($n = 308$).
[e] Because the dataset for Japan stopped at 14 years, data for the 14-year-olds were used in the analyses for 15-year-olds.

TABLE 7. *Ethnic differences in the prevalence of overweight and obesity in Singapore*

	Sample	Total overweight[a] (%)	Overweight[b] (%)	Obese[c] (%)
10-year-old boys				
Singapore (all)	1660	25.5	19.4	6.1
Chinese	1274	27.2	20.6	6.5
Malay	204	20.6	15.7	4.9
Indian	182	19.8	14.8	4.9
10-year-old girls				
Singapore (all)	1584	17.6	14.6	3.0
Chinese	1228	17.2	15.0	2.2
Malay	207	20.8	15.0	4.5
Indian	149	16.1	10.7	5.4
15-year-old boys				
Singapore (all)	1160	15.3	11.4	3.9
Chinese	911	15.8	12.1	3.7
Malay	169	12.4	8.3	4.1
Indian	80	15.0	10.0	5.0
15-year-old girls				
Singapore (all)	946	11.4	8.6	2.9
Chinese	676	10.8	8.3	2.5
Malay	162	15.4	9.9	5.6
Indian	108	9.3	8.3	0.9

[a] Based on the IOTF standard that defines total overweight as BMI $\geq$ age-specific BMI cutoff points corresponding to a BMI of 25 at 18 years of age (9).
[b] Based on the IOTF standard that defines overweight as BMI $\geq$ age-specific BMI cutoff points corresponding to BMIs of 25 to 30 at 18 years of age (9).
[c] Based on the IOTF standard that defines obesity as BMI $\geq$ age-specific BMI cutoff points corresponding to a BMI of 30 at 18 years of age (9).

Regional and Ethnic Differences

In Germany, the prevalence (boys and girls combined) of total overweight among 10-year-olds in Munich (24%) was double that in Jena (12%), with Dresden (16%) in between (Tables 3 and 4).

Among both 10- and 15-year-olds in Singapore, boys of Chinese origin were more likely to be overweight or obese than those from the Malay or Indian ethnic groups (Table 7). The order was different for the girls, with the rate of total overweight highest in ethnic Malays, followed by girls of Chinese and Indian origin.

DISCUSSION

Concern has often been expressed at national and international levels about the high but still increasing rates of overweight and obesity in children (1). As we plan future initiatives, we should be mindful that this concern is based on findings from national studies and comparisons that have used different standards of assessment (5).

This study presents for the first time analyses of overweight and obesity in 10- and 15-year-old children from four Asian and five European countries using the same IOTF standard and cutoff points to define overweight and obesity. BMI correlates well with body fat when measured by dual energy x-ray absorptiometry (20,21), but the newly developed IOTF BMI cutoff points for children still require validation with morbidity and other ancillary measurements (e.g., blood pressure, cholesterol, and plasma insulin concentrations) (8).

In an analysis of data from the Bogalusa Heart Study, BMI cutoff points for *at risk of overweight* and *overweight,* based on American population studies, were used to examine the relation of overweight in children (defined as a BMI between the 85th and the 95th centile and more than the 95th centile, respectively) to levels of adverse risk factors (22). The investigators found that the prevalence of several risk factors, including adverse lipid and insulin concentrations and blood pressure, increased greatly at BMI values above the 85th centile. Similar work needs to be carried out to validate the IOTF BMI standards for overweight and obesity in children, especially because more studies are reanalyzing anthropometric data using these cutoff points (23–26).

Studies from developing countries that used a standard definition for *overweight* and *obesity* have shown that overweight is also present in very young children. In Latin America, the prevalence of overweight (>1 SD above mean weight for height) in children aged 1 to 5 years ranged from 6% in Haiti to 24% in Peru in a study of 13 countries (7). Overweight was more common in urban areas and in households of higher socioeconomic status. Another study, of 94 developing countries, showed that nations with the highest prevalence of overweight (weight for height >2 SD from the US National Center for Health Statistics international reference median) were located mainly in the Middle East, North Africa, and Latin America (6). Trend data showed an increase in the prevalence of overweight preschool children in 16 of 38 countries. Similar patterns in developing countries were found in a study of 5-year-olds from 25 countries using the IOTF standards for 5-year-olds. There rates of total overweight (including obesity) ranged from 3% in Namibia to 26% in Peru (Horgan GW, Bellizzi MC, Dietz WH, James WPT, unpublished data).

Our study confirms the notion that overweight in older children is no longer confined to Western countries. Populations in Asia are now victims of this scourge, with prevalence rates of overweight and obesity in 15-year-old boys from Taipei in Taiwan exceeding 30%.

In China, Hesketh and Ding found that the rates of total overweight among 13- to 16-year-olds are twice as high in urban areas as in rural ones (25). This study used the IOTF BMI standard for children in reporting a total overweight rate of 9.8% in boys living in the urban area of the province of Zhejiang but only a 1.7% rate in a rural area of the same province.

Continents other than Asia are also reporting increases in overweight among older children and adolescents. A study of rural South African adolescents reported increased prevalence in overweight in girls, particularly before the growth spurt, up to age 10 or 11 years and after 14 years (27). A study of healthy Nigerian children concluded that, with improvement in living standards, childhood obesity may become a medical problem in Nigeria (28). Using the US definition for overweight, this study estimated that 18% of those studied were obese. A study of Saudi Arabian schoolboys recorded a high prevalence of overweight and obesity, especially in Riyadh, the capital, but a much lower prevalence in Sabea, which is in the southern region of the country (29).

In addition to the widespread high prevalence of overweight and obesity worldwide, the rapid increase in the prevalence of overweight in children concerns many observers in the fields of public health and obesity. In the United Kingdom, reanalysis of anthropometric data using the IOTF BMI cutoffs (9) showed that from 1974 to 1994 the rate of overweight increased steadily in boys and girls aged 4 to 11 years (23). An increase of seven percentage points was recorded in Scottish girls, rising from 8.8% in 1974 to 15.8% in 1994.

In our study, 10-year-old Asian boys and girls had higher rates of overweight and obesity than their 15-year-old counterparts (Tables 3 to 6). These results are not readily explained by maturational differences, but this is an area that ought to be explored when looking at differences in reported rates across or within countries, particularly when there are wide differences in income.

Sex differences in total overweight within both age groups were also observed in our study. In the European countries, except Hungary, the prevalence of total overweight in 10-year-olds was higher in girls than in boys. This contrasted with the Asian countries (Hong Kong, Japan, and Singapore), where the prevalence in boys in both age groups was much higher than that in girls. Similar sex differences have been reported in Chinese children (25). Such patterns may reflect different cultural habits and attitudes toward factors such as body weight, nutrition, and physical activity.

The establishment of ethnic-specific cutoff points defining overweight and obesity in children needs to be explored. A study of adult Chinese, Malays, and Indians in Singapore found that the relation between body fat percentage (calculated using the compartment model) and BMI differs between Singaporeans and whites, and between the three ethnic groups in Singapore (30). The investigators concluded that if obesity is regarded as an excess in body fat and not as excessive weight (increased BMI), the cutoff points for obesity in Singapore that use the BMI would need to be lowered, possibly to a BMI value of 27 instead of 30.

More evidence presented at expert meetings organized by IOTF and others (31) supports the notion that lower BMI cutoff points may need to be set for Asian populations, owing to their predisposition to deposit fat around the waist. In these countries metabolic disease tends to occur at lower BMI values. Conversely, populations from the Pacific Islands tend to get disease at higher BMI values. In children, the risks associated with overweight and obesity defined by BMI differ between whites and blacks and by age (22).

If a lower cutoff point is used to define obesity in adult Asians and the methodology outlined by Cole *et al.* is used (9) to establish cutoff points for Asian children, reported rates of childhood overweight and obesity would rise in Asian countries. We should note that the reference population underlying the BMI cutoff points for children probably reflects Western populations adequately but lacks representation from other parts of the world. The development and validation of ethnic-specific cutoff points with biological indicators thus becomes even more crucial.

Methodologic constraints associated with making cross-national comparisons include the likelihood that equipment and measurement techniques were not standardized between the different studies. Nevertheless, ours is still a valid attempt at applying the same definition for overweight and obesity across the studies, thus giving more meaningful comparisons.

Another limitation of cross-national comparisons is shown by our finding that a country may have great variation by region, as highlighted in Germany, where Munich had twice the rates of overweight and obesity as Jena. Ethnic differences are also masked in these analyses, with the Singapore study clearly showing how important it is to examine data by ethnic group.

Overweight and obesity in childhood are concerns for many reasons. We know that overweight in childhood is associated with raised blood pressure, diabetes, respiratory disease, and orthopedic and psychosocial disorders (3,4). Furthermore, the tracking of obesity from childhood to adulthood (2) and its contribution to obesity-related morbidity and mortality of adults is a major concern (1).

CONCLUSIONS

Tackling the problems of overweight and obesity poses an enormous challenge. Addressing this public health problem requires intervention at international, national, and local levels. The variation in prevalence by age, sex, ethnicity, and geography means that these factors need to be considered when interventions are designed. Novel approaches to preventing and managing overweight and obesity in children must be developed (32,33). Such interventions would require an examination of regional, ethnic, and sex differences in physical activity and nutrition, including breastfeeding, and how these relate to obesity.

With the already high rates of overweight and obesity in children, intervention is also needed at the clinical level. Clear guidelines, such as those published in the United States (34) but perhaps in a more generic form, could be useful at the international level for managing overweight and obesity.

ACKNOWLEDGMENTS

We thank Katrin Kromeyer-Hauschild (Jena, Germany), Sophie Leung (Hong Kong), Ilona Dober (Hungary), Margherita Caroli (Italy), Yuji Matsuzawa (Japan), Machteld Roede (the Netherlands), Uma Rajan (Singapore), Nain-Feng Chu (Taiwan), and Tim Cole (United Kingdom) for allowing us access to their data. We also thank Angela Liese for her role in making the connection between the IOTF project and the ISAAC study in Germany (Munich and Dresden data).

REFERENCES

1. World Health Organisation. *Obesity: preventing and managing the global epidemic.* Report of a WHO consultation. (Technical Report Series.) Geneva: WHO, 2000.
2. Guo SS, Chumlea WC. Tracking of body mass index in children in relation to overweight in adulthood. *Am J Clin Nutr* 1999; 70 : 145–8.
3. Dietz WH. Health consequences of obesity in youth: childhood predictors of adult disease. *Pediatrics* 1998; 101: 518–5.
4. Power C, Lake JK, Cole TJ. Measurement and long-term health risks of child and adolescent fatness. *Int J Obes Relat Metab Disord* 1997; 21: 507–6.
5. Guillaume M. Defining obesity in childhood: current practice. *Am J Clin Nutr* 1999; 70: 126–30.
6. De Onis M, Blössner M. Prevalence and trends of overweight among preschool children in developing countries. *Am J Clin Nutr* 2000; 72: 1032–9.
7. Martorell R, Khan LK, Hughes ML, *et al.* Obesity in Latin American women and children. *J Nutr* 1998; 128: 1464–73.
8. Bellizzi MC, Dietz WH. Workshop on childhood obesity: summary of the discussion. *Am J Clin Nutr* 1999; 70: 173–5.
9. Cole TJ, Bellizzi MC, Flegal KM, *et al.* Establishing a standard definition for child overweight and obesity worldwide: international survey. *BMJ* 2000; 320: 1270–3.
10. Weiland SK, von Mutius E, Hirsch T, *et al.* Prevalence of respiratory and atopic disorders among children in the East and West of Germany five years after unification. *Eur Resp J* 1999; 14: 862–70.
11. Kromeyer-Hauschild K, Zellner K, Jaeger U, *et al.* Prevalence of overweight and obesity among school children (Germany). *Int J Obes Relat Metab Disord* 1999; 23: 1143–50.
12. Leung SSF, Cole TJ, Tse LY, *et al.* Body mass index reference curves for Chinese children. *Ann Hum Biol* 1998; 25: 169–74.
13. Dober I. The prevalence of childhood obesity among school children of Pécs. *Népegészségugy* 1987; 68: 90–3. [In Hungarian with English summary.]
14. Caroli M, Luciano A, Mastro F, Scianaro L. Personal communications. Verona University and Brindisi University, 2000.
15. Matsuzawa Y. Personal communications. Department of Internal Medicine, Osaka University Medical School, Japan, 1997.
16. Cole TJ, Roede MJ. Centiles of body mass index for Dutch children aged 0–20 years in 1980: a baseline to assess recent trends in obesity. *Ann Hum Biol* 1999; 26: 303–8.
17. Rajan U. Obesity among Singapore students. *Int J Obes* 1994; 18: 27.
18. Nain-Feng C, Rimm EB, Wang DJ, *et al.* Clustering of cardiovascular disease risk factors among obese schoolchildren: the Taipei Children Heart Study. *Am J Clin Nutr* 1998; 67: 1141–6.
19. Cole TJ, Freeman JV, Preece MA. British 1990 growth reference centiles for weight, height, body mass index and head circumference fitted by maximum penalized likelihood. *Stat Med* 1998; 17: 407–29.
20. Goran MI, Driscoll P, Johnson R, *et al.* Cross-calibration of body-composition techniques against dual-energy X-ray absorptiometry in young children. *Am J Clin Nutr* 1996; 63: 299–305.

21. Gutin B, Litaker M, Islam S, *et al.* Body composition measurement in 9–11-year-old children by dual-energy X-ray absorptiometry, skinfold thickness measurements, and bioimpedance analysis. *Am J Clin Nutr* 1996; 63: 287–92.
22. Freedman DS, Dietz WH, Srinivasan SR, *et al.* The relation of overweight to cardiovascular risk factors among children and adolescents: the Bogalusa Heart Study. *Pediatrics* 1999; 103: 1175–82.
23. Chinn S, Rona RJ. Prevalence and trends in overweight and obesity in three cross-sectional studies of British children, 1974–94. *BMJ* 2001; 322: 24–6.
24. Wang Y, Wang JQ. Standard definition of child overweight and obesity worldwide. Authors' standard compares well with WHO standard. *BMJ* 2000; 321: 1158.
25. Hesketh T, Ding QJ. Standard definition of child overweight and obesity worldwide. *BMJ* 2000; 321: 1158–9.
26. Kinra S. Standard definition of child overweight and obesity worldwide. *BMJ* 2000; 321: 1159.
27. Cameron N, Getz B. Sex differences in the prevalence of obesity in rural African adolescents. *Int J Obes Relat Metab Disord* 1997; 9: 775–82.
28. Owa JA, Adejuyigbe O. Fat mass, fat mass percentage, body mass index, and mid-upper arm circumference in a healthy population of Nigerian children. *J Trop Pediatr* 1997; 43: 13–9.
29. Al-Nuaim AR, Bamgboye EA, al-Herbish A. The pattern of growth and obesity in Saudi Arabian male school children. *Int J Obes Relat Metab Disord* 1996; 11: 1000–5.
30. Deurenberg-Yap M, Schmidt G, van Staveren WA, *et al.* The paradox of low body mass index and high fat percentage among Chinese, Malays, and Indians in Singapore. *Int J Obes Relat Metab Disord* 2000; 24: 1011–7.
31. WHO/IASO/IOTF. The Asia-Pacific perspective: redefining obesity and its treatment. February 2000. Full document available from: http: //www.idi.org.au/obesity_report.htm.
32. Robinson TN. Reducing children's television viewing to prevent obesity: a randomized controlled trial. *JAMA* 1999; 282: 1561–7.
33. Epstein LH, Goldfield GS. Physical activity in the treatment of childhood overweight and obesity: current evidence and research issues. *Med Sci Sports Exerc* 1999; 31: 553–9.
34. Barlow SE, Dietz WH. Obesity evaluation and treatment: Expert Committee recommendations. The Maternal and Child Health Bureau, Health Resources and Services Administration and the Department of Health and Human Services. *Pediatrics* 1998; 102: electronic pages (www.pediatrics.org/cgi/content/full/102/3/e29).

DISCUSSION

Dr. Bar-Or: Your review certainly shows that overweight is not a problem of developed countries only, but I do wonder about some of the data you showed. Somebody from the media may well come up with a headline that Peruvian preschool children are more overweight than American children! That isn't very likely, knowing the nutritional situation in Peru. Similar inferences may be made about Chilean adolescent girls being as overweight as American girls. I wonder whether this has something to do with the BMI failing to take body proportions into account. Perhaps we need completely different criteria for, say, American Indian children, because of their different body proportions. Do you have any comment on that?

Dr. Bellizzi: It is of course important to remember that undernutrition remains a nutritional problem in many developing countries and that the emerging problem of overweight goes hand in hand with the continuing problem of underweight. I agree that it would be interesting to look at the use of the BMI in relation to body proportions and how this might affect the prevalence rates.

Dr. Steinbeck: I found the sex differences fascinating. You said right at the end that these sex differences need to be clarified, so I wonder if you would expand a little on that. Are we looking at cultural influences, genetic influences, biology?

Dr. Bellizzi: This is something that I hoped would be discussed at this meeting. It is not my area of research. Perhaps some of the delegates here can discuss this more widely.

Dr. Sung: We have done some studies on self-image of children in Hong Kong. We found that girls were more concerned about their self-image than boys. This may reflect the parents' attitudes. In Asian countries, parents put more emphasis on their sons' academic performance than that of their daughters. Their approach to the girls may well be to restrict their diet because they perceive them as "too fat," but if a boy studies well in school that is fine in itself and they are not concerned if he is fat.

Dr. Bellizzi: That is interesting. Such insights may be very useful when designing interventions. It is important to begin to address the reasons for such differences in overweight between boys and girls.

Dr. Rütishauser: I was astonished at the differences between the sexes in some of the South American countries, in particular Chile and Brazil. Is there a cultural explanation for that?

Dr. Bellizzi: Maybe Dr. Uauy would like to expand a little on that?

Dr. Uauy: There are differences in activity levels, dietary patterns, and how the parents bring their children up. In most Latin countries women tend to be less active, unless of course you are in Brazil, where everyone is very active!

Dr. Gortmaker: I have a comment about the issue of countries with high rates of obesity versus the leaner countries. I know that the UK population looked rather lean, but the data were from 1978 to 1980, and as you showed, there has been a very large increase in obesity prevalence there since that time. In the United States, the data were from around 1988 to 1992, and since then there have also been large increases in obesity in the United States. These secular trends need to be considered and I hope taken into account in any discussion of differences between countries.

Dr. Bellizzi: I agree. When we were doing this study, we had cutoff points in terms of how long we searched for and collected the data. For some countries we managed to get up-to-date information, but for others it is unavoidably older—for instance, the Netherlands data are among the oldest that we have. I am aware that they now have more recent studies, but at the time of our research they were not available to us. When we publish the information, there will be a table showing not just the dates when the studies were carried out, but also the areas represented by the studies.

Dr. Srivastava: When talking of prevalence, I think sampling is very important. In India, for example, there are differences between rural and urban children, and within urban children there are differences between the rich and the poor. In New Delhi, if you take private schools, the prevalence of obesity will be 4% to 5%, but in the same city in government schools it will be around 1%. Thus when you talk about a country or a region as a whole, there could be internal differences that you have to take into account.

Dr. Cai: I have a comment about the prevalence of obesity in Shanghai. In the early 1980s we found that it was only 3% to 4%, based on weight-for-height. Using the same criteria, by the beginning of the 1990s the prevalence had increased to 6% to 8%, whereas in 2000 it had increased to almost 10%. This is similar to the European experience. Did you use BMI or weight-for-height in making your comparisons?

Dr. Bellizzi: Most of the figures were derived from BMI for age. Where this information was not available—for example, in preschool children in Egypt—we used 2 SD above the median weight-for-height to define overweight.

Dr. Cai: We found that if we used the WHO standard BMI cutoff points of 25 or 30 for overweight and obesity in children, those values seem very low for the Shanghai population.

Dr. Bellizzi: Yes, that could be expected. You may remember that early on in my presentation I compared the prevalence rates within the same population of Argentinian children using two different references, 125% of the weight-for-height and the BMI. There was double the prevalence of overweight when using BMI for age cutoff points.

Dr. Cole: The problem we had when we wrote our paper was that we did not spell out what we meant by "prevalence of overweight"—whether we meant above the BMI cutoff of 25, which would include everyone who is overweight, or whether we meant between the cutoff of 25 (defining overweight) and the cutoff of 30 (defining obesity). You used the term *total overweight* in your presentation to mean both overweight and obesity. I thought it might be worthwhile spelling out that minor problem.

Dr. Bellizzi: That's right. Total overweight included all BMI values above 25.

Obesity in Childhood and Adolescence, edited by
Chunming Chen and William H. Dietz. Nestlé
Nutrition Workshop Series, Pediatric Program,
Vol. 49. Nestec Ltd., Vevey/Lippincott
Williams & Wilkins, Philadelphia © 2002.

The Growth Pattern of Chinese Children

Chunming Chen

Chinese Center for Disease Control and Prevention, Beijing, China

Children are very sensitive to their nutritional situation, especially during early childhood, and the nutritional status of the young child has consequences for mental development and disease risk, as well as for work capacity in adult life. Optimal growth during childhood is likely to improve immunologic defense mechanisms, resulting in a
decrease in severe infections and a reduction in case fatality rate and child mortality. Over
the longer term, adequately grown children will perform better than poorly grown children during adolescence, and their work capacity will be enhanced, leading to increased
productivity in situations of moderate to heavy workload. There is evidence that linear
growth during early childhood is especially important in achieving these targets. Changes
in linear growth velocity and in attained height are more predictable indicators of child
mortality at a population level than weight gain during nutritional interventions (1).

Surveillance and monitoring of growth in weight and height of young children to
identify their growth patterns during periods of economic development and environmental change are critical components of any intervention strategy. Very often height
lost because of growth faltering during early life cannot be regained later during
school age and adolescence, and so the opportunity for catch-up growth will be lost
(2). A report from India indicated that the height at age 5 years is the key factor in
adult body size (3). A study of the changes in the growth patterns of preschool children that are linked to China's rapid economic development will have an important
impact on the Chinese population, as will the identification of factors related to
growth faltering and the choice of appropriate interventions.

IMPROVEMENT IN NUTRITION STATUS OF CHILDREN UNDER 5 IN CHINA

Since 1990, the Chinese Academy of Preventive Medicine, with the support of
UNICEF, has collaborated with the State Statistics Bureau in establishing a food and
nutrition surveillance system (FNSS) in China and has carried out four rounds of surveillance (in 1990, 1995, 1998, and 2000). In 1990 and 1995, data were collected
from a pilot sample of around 4,000 children under 6 years of age. After these initial
studies, a formal national sample system involving 16,000 children under 6 years of
age was established in 1997 and data were collected in 1998 and 2000.

TABLE 1. *Nutritional status of children under 5 from 1990 to 2000*

| | WAZ < −2 | | | HAZ < −2 | | | WHZ > 2 | |
	Urban	Rural	National	Urban	Rural	National	Urban	Rural
1990	8.6	22.6	19.6	9.4	41.4	34.8	3.5	1.1
1995	4.6	17.8	15.6	8.9	39.1	34.3	6.9	12.6
1998	2.7	12.6	10.0	4.1	22.2	16.7	5.4	3.8
2000	3.0	13.8	11.4	2.9	20.3	16.0	3.6	2.1

Data analysis was carried out, based on the four rounds of surveillance. Dramatic improvements in the nutrition status of Chinese children in the past decade were shown (Table 1). Growth data were related to the WHO standards for children, using z scores.

In the urban population (Table 1), the prevalence of underweight (weight-for-age z score) [WAZ] of (−2 or less) was 3.0% and the prevalence of stunting (height-for-age z score) [HAZ] of (−2 or less) was 2.9% in the year 2000. The highest prevalence of stunting (between 3.8% and 4.1%) occurred between 12 and 23 months of age (Table 2), which is usually the peak age for both underweight and stunting. The prevalence of underweight among children aged 4 to 5 years was 4.3%. If a weight-for-height z score (WHZ) of more than 2 is defined as "overweight," the prevalence of overweight was 3.6% in the urban population.

In rural areas (Table 3), the prevalence of underweight was 10.1% and of stunting, 14.8%. Body weight of infants under 6 months of age was normal, but the prevalence of stunting was 4.7% even at this young age. Prevalences of both underweight and stunting increased rapidly thereafter, reaching 14% and 22.6%, respectively, at 18 months of age. In the first 6 months, the prevalence of overweight was 10.2% as a result of the length deficit.

Comparison of data from the four rounds showed a substantial improvement in nutrition over the past decade. The prevalence of underweight fell by 48% from 1990 to 1998, though it did not change significantly from 1998 to 2000. The prevalence of stunting, which changed little during 1990 to 1995, fell by 51% from 1995 to 1998 (from 34.3% to 16.7%).

TABLE 2. *Nutrition status of children by age group in urban China, 2000*

| Age (months) | WAZ < −2 | | | HAZ < −2 | | |
	Boys	Girls	Total	Boys	Girls	Total
0–	0	0.4	0.2	0.3	1.2	0.7
6–	1.0	0.9	1.0	1.8	2.0	1.9
12–	3.6	2.8	3.2	3.9	4.4	4.1
18–	4.5	2.1	3.5	4.2	3.4	3.8
24–	4.1	3.3	3.7	2.8	3.2	3.0
36–	3.1	4.0	3.5	2.7	2.0	2.4
48–<60	4.2	4.4	4.3	4.2	3.3	3.8
Total	3.1	2.9	3.0	3.0	2.8	2.9

Abbreviations: HAZ, height-for-age z score; WAZ, weight-for-age z score.

TABLE 3. *Nutrition status of children by age group in rural China, 2000*

Age (months)	WAZ < −2			HAZ < −2		
	Boys	Girls	Total	Boys	Girls	Total
0–	1.4	1.0	1.2	5.4	3.8	4.7
6–	5.4	7.0	6.3	9.8	11.1	10.4
12–	14.8	14.1	14.5	17.2	16.5	17.9
18–	15.5	11.7	14.0	23.1	21.8	22.6
24–	9.5	11.0	10.2	11.5	12.5	12.0
36–	7.9	14.2	10.6	14.5	19.4	16.6
48–<60	8.2	13.5	10.6	16.3	16.6	16.4
Total	9.1	11.4	10.1	14.3	15.3	14.8

Note: Data for general rural area, poor rural excluded.
Abbreviations: HAZ, height-for-age z score; WAZ, weight-for-age z score.

Compared with the 1992 national child survey data, the standardized prevalence of underweight in children under 5 years of age in the rural population fell from 19.3% (95% confidence interval, 19.8% to 20.5%) to 12.4% (11.9% to 13.1%), which amounts to a 1.2% reduction annually. The prevalence of stunting fell from 39.1% (39.5% to 40.1%) to 22.2% (21.1% to 22.9%), an annual reduction of around 3% (4).

This apparent improvement in child nutrition is the outcome of rapid socioeconomic development. Our previous study of the major factors involved showed that besides nutrition, factors such as breast-feeding, safe drinking water, reduction in diarrhea, improved maternal education, and better incomes are all relevant to the reduction in childhood stunting in the rural areas (5). These factors have changed greatly since 1990: the prevalence of severe diarrhea in children under 5 years of age fell by 50% in both urban and rural populations; safe drinking water in the rural areas more than doubled; exclusive breast-feeding for 4 to 6 months increased by 40%; the illiteracy rate among mothers fell from 22.5% in 1992 to 7.4% in 1998; and dietary energy intake from animal foods increased from 6.2% to 8.8% from 1992 to 1998 in rural households. However, even though progress in the nutritional welfare of children has been appreciable, in the less developed rural areas children are still suffering from serious malnutrition. In 2000, the prevalences of underweight and stunting in children less than 5 years of age in poor rural areas were 21.0% and 30.7%, respectively.

GROWTH PATTERNS OF CHILDREN DURING CURRENT SOCIOECONOMIC IMPROVEMENT

In general, the weight-for-height z score tends to be near normal and the prevalence of wasting is below 5% in China, which illustrates the parallel growth deficit in weight and height. However, data from 1990 to 2000 showed substantial weight gain as social conditions improved, with a comparable reduction in the prevalence of underweight. During this period, however, there was a large rise in the proportion of children with a WHZ of more than 2 in the rural areas, increasing from 1.1% in 1990 to 12.6% in 1995 (Table 1). This should not be misconstrued as an increase in

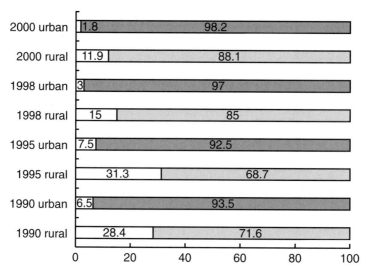

FIG. 1. Percentage of height for age *z* scores <-2 among children with normal weight for age *z* scores in urban and rural areas.

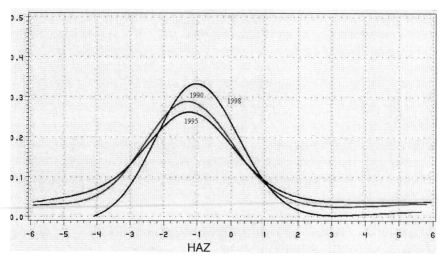

FIG. 2. Distribution of height for age *z* scores (HAZ) in children with weight for age *z* scores better than -2 from 1990 to 1998.

TABLE 4. *Mean height (cm) and height increment of rural children under 6 from 1990 to 1998*

Age (years)	1990	1995	Increment 1990–1995	1998	Increment 1995–1998
0–	64.2	65.0	0.8	66.0	1.0
1–	75.8	78.8	3.0	77.9	−0.9
2–	83.6	85.5	1.9	86.4	0.9
3–	90.1	91.1	1.0	93.8	2.7
4–	97.4	97.3	1.0	100.4	2.9
5–6	102.9	104.5	1.6	106.5	2.0

"overweight," because during that period the prevalence of underweight declined from 22.6% to 17.8% in the rural areas, while stunting prevalence decreased very little (from 41.4% to 39.7%) (6). On further analysis, the proportion of stunted children among those with normal weight-for-age z score was around 30% from 1990 to 1995, but it fell to 15% in 1998 (Fig. 1). Taking this into account, the percentage of children with a WHZ of more than 2 can be normalized to 3.8% in 1998. The HAZ distribution curve shown in Fig. 2 also clearly illustrates the shift in HAZ score during 1998. Analysis of the increments in weight and height in 1990–1995 and 1995–1998 (Tables 4 and 5) also showed that the largest increment in weight was in 1990–1995, diminishing in 1995–1998, whereas the increment in height increased during the latter period, especially in children aged 3 to 6 years of age. This growth pattern is not ethnic, as the growth of children in urban China has followed a different pattern (Fig.1). It is likely that height growth lags behind weight gain by about 3 years in situations where there is a generalized improvement in nutrition.

Evidently, it would be inadvisable and even dangerous to consider the jump in the percentage of WHZ of more than 2 as reflecting "overweight" on account of excess nutrition. A simultaneous check on the prevalence of stunting is essential before conclusions are drawn or actions taken. In view of the biological importance of linear growth during early childhood as an index of mental development, and of the difficulty in regaining lost height growth at a later period in childhood, attention needs to be focused on improvements to linear growth when this type of growth pattern occurs, and interventions must be focused on ways to ensure that height growth matches weight gain. Only in this way can a healthy growth pattern be achieved.

TABLE 5. *Mean weight (kg) and weight increment of rural children under 6 from 1990 to 1998*

	1990	1995	Increment 1990–1995	1998	Increment 1995–1998
0–	7.24	8.01	0.87	7.68	−0.33
1–	9.61	10.98	1.37	10.16	−0.82
2–	11.7	12.58	0.88	12.21	−0.37
3–	13.36	14.04	0.68	14.03	−0.01
4–	14.96	15.64	0.60	15.50	−0.14
5–6	16.39	17.52	1.13	16.96	−0.53

TABLE 6. *Correlation coefficient between food items in complementary foods and HAZ/WAZ of children aged 4–24 months*

Age (months)	HAZ			WAZ		
	Starch	Veg/Fru	E/Fi/Mt	Starch	Veg/Fru	E/Fi/M
4–6	0.20	0.40[a]	0.42[a]	0.05	0.31[b]	0.37[a]
6–12	0.19	0.45[a]	0.47[a]	0.01	0.30[b]	0.35[b]
12–18	0.12	0.25	0.45[a]	−0.06	0.06	0.25
18–24	0.19	0.26	0.47[a]	0.19	0.24	0.40[a]

Abbreviations: Starch, starchy foods; Veg/Fru, vegetables/fruit; E/Fi/M, eggs/fish/meat; HAZ, height-for-age z score; WAZ, weight for age z score.
[a] $p < 0.01$.
[b] $p < 0.05$.

QUALITY OF COMPLEMENTARY FOOD NECESSARY TO IMPROVE LINEAR GROWTH

As the prevalence of stunting peaks at 12 to 18 months and levels off by 5 years of age, it is of critical importance for the growth of children under 5 to improve their nutritional status early on, probably before they are 3. We collected data on complementary feeding in children aged 4 to 24 months in 1998. The correlation analysis given in Table 6 clearly shows that the inclusion of starchy foods is popular but does not affect the degree of stunting. Thus the current intake of starchy foods during complementary feeding is insufficient to ensure adequate growth in height. In the age range of 4 to 12 months, the inclusion of vegetables or fruits is positively correlated with both average HAZ and average WAZ. The use of animal foods (meat/fish/eggs) in complementary feeding in children aged 4 to 24 months is also positively correlated with HAZ and WAZ ($p < 0.01$) (7). Thus increasing the quality of complementary foods by supplementing them with animal foods and with vegetables or fruit should be a priority in attempts to improve the linear growth of children under 2. We strongly recommend action based on improving the quality of complementary foods in children after the age of 4 to 6 months. A campaign to improve complementary feeding should be initiated, as was done for breast-feeding a decade ago.

REFERENCES

1. Martorell R. Promoting healthy growth: rationale and benefits. In: Pinstrup-Andersen P, Pelletier D, Alderman H, eds. *Growth and nutrition in developing countries: priorities for action.* Ithaca, NY: Cornell University Press, 1995: 15–31.
2. Martorell R, Khan LK, Schroeder DG. Reversibility of stunting: epidemiological findings in children in developing countries. *Eur J Clin Nutr* 1994; 48: 45–57.
3. Satyanarayana K, Nadamuni Naidu A, Swanminathan MC, *et al.* Adolescent growth spurt among rural Indian boys in relation to their nutritional status in early childhood. *Ann Hum Biol* 1980; 7: 359–66.
4. Chen CM. Executive summary of food and nutrition surveillance in 1998 and policy recommendations. *J Hyg Res* 2000; 29: 308–12.
5. Fu ZY, Chen CM, Guo BM, *et al.* Multi-factor analysis on malnutrition of children under 5 in rural China. *J Hyg Res* 1996; 26: 87–91.
6. Chang SY, Fu ZY, He W, *et al.* Current situation and trend of child growth in China. *J Hyg Res* 2000; 29: 270–4.
7. Fu ZY, He W, Chen CM. Relationship between growth of young children and complementary feeding. *J Hyg Res* 2000; 29: 279–82.

DISCUSSION

Dr. Bar-Or: These changes are extremely impressive and no doubt they result from an educational campaign to deliver the message to the people. Could you comment on how the population is being taught to use more supplementary foods, to change their breast-feeding habits, for example? What is the educational message and how is it sent?

Dr. Chen: Complementary feeding has not been much stressed in our country up to now. We have put much effort into implementing exclusive breast-feeding. Complementary feeding is mentioned in the child care manual that is provided for Chinese parents, but there has not been much action on promoting it. This is why we want UNICEF to see these data and place more emphasis on complementary feeding.

Dr. Bar-Or: But how do you manage to create such changes over such a short period of time in such a vast population?

Dr. Chen: I have no practical experience with large-scale organization or policy-making. However, from our experience in the field, we have set up intervention trials in certain rural areas. These involve educating people to grow a fruit tree in front of their house and to grow green vegetables in their family garden, which is very well accepted. We also organize parents' classes in the evening for nutrition education, which are quite effective. Chinese housewives are very accepting of nutrition education because by old Chinese tradition nutrition has always been an important part of Chinese medicine. The main bar to improvement comes from the decision makers at community level. Their attitude is that they are poor and nothing can be done. It is their concepts that need to be changed.

Dr. Koletzko: In your fascinating dataset you showed the relation of availability of animal foods—egg, fish, and meat—to height growth. You mentioned that the picture is not so simple if you include milk in the model. Is it your conclusion, then, that it is not so much the animal protein as perhaps other micronutrients that come from animal foods other than milk that are important for height growth?

Dr. Chen: The data are qualitative rather than quantitative, so it's hard to draw inferences on the nutritional requirement. The data just showed that the presence of certain food items was important—animal foods, and vegetables and fruit, and so on. There was no quantitative element to the research. I analyzed the data from the national nutrition survey for 2- to 3-year-old children because we only have data available on individual dietary intakes at that age. We found that low intakes of protein, calcium, and vitamin A were related to stunting in these children.

Dr. Koletzko: But what is the relation between milk intake and length growth?

Dr. Chen: During the survey we did in 1998, we excluded milk from consideration in the category "animal food," because after 4 months many mothers give milk to their children as a substitute for breast milk. This made the equation too complicated, so we excluded milk intake altogether. When we analyzed the year 2000 data, we did consider milk intake, and it is clearly very important. The data have not yet been published, but it seems clear that milk, vegetables, and animal foods are all important for linear growth.

Dr. Freedman: I want to thank you for your explanation of the significance of the weight-for-height z score. This has implications for many other countries. Whenever we use a ratio like the weight-for-height z score or the BMI, we assume that the relation of weight to height in terms of the outcome remains constant. That may not be true in a lot of cases. A heavy child at a medium height might have quite a different risk from a medium weight child who is short. I think this is something important to keep in mind in all the analyses we do.

Dr. Bellizzi: I congratulate you on the 40% increase in exclusive breast-feeding between 4 and 6 months of age. You attributed this partly to baby-friendly hospitals, but from our experience in the UK, that is not enough. Baby-friendly hospitals provide support for the women in the first few days, but to maintain levels of breast-feeding you need to provide support in the community. What is your secret that enabled you to obtain such dramatic increases?

Dr. Chen: Basically, it's just education. The maternal child health department in the Ministry of Health puts a great deal of effort into promoting exclusive breast-feeding. I should explain that "exclusive" breast-feeding in China means breast-feeding with added water. We don't think that water should be excluded.

Dr. Baerlocher: Do you provide any food for children at school, or are they only fed at home?

Dr. Chen: It varies. In urban areas, we have school lunch programs, but in the rural areas this is uncommon. Most take meals at home.

Dr. Ning: I think the improvement is also related to the success of the family planning initiative. Although this has not been so successful in rural areas as in urban areas, families are getting smaller now in rural areas as well, and this contributes to the success of the nutrition program.

Dr. Birch: What are the alternatives to breast-feeding among rural and urban Chinese?

Dr. Chen: Urban children usually get milk and other complementary foods, some of which are prepared at home. Very small numbers of mothers use processed complementary foods. In rural areas, there is a big division according to income group. Some mothers just give plain rice or rice porridge, or something similar. With education they will give some added vegetable or animal foods, including eggs if they have them. All foods will be home-made.

Dr. Campos: Did you study the same groups of children over these 5- or 8-year periods?

Dr. Chen: No, it was not the same group. During the survey, we measure children who are currently in the age range of interest. It's not a follow-up.

Dr. Campos: Did your sample come from the same geographic region? I understand there are height differences in different areas of China?

Dr. Chen: Yes, the children were from the same geographic areas. They are from the areas randomly sampled, and surveillance is carried out at the same sampled countries/cities.

Obesity in Childhood and Adolescence, edited by
Chunming Chen and William H. Dietz. Nestlé
Nutrition Workshop Series, Pediatric Program,
Vol. 49. Nestec Ltd., Vevey/Lippincott
Williams & Wilkins, Philadelphia © 2002.

Obesity Trends in Chilean Children and Adolescents: Basic Determinants

Juliana Kain, Raquel Burrows, and Ricardo Uauy

*Institute of Nutrition and Food Technology (INTA), University of Chile,
Santiago, Chile*

In Chile an epidemiologic transition has been occurring at impressive speed. Chile's biomedical indicators in the 1960s matched those of most Latin American countries—that is, high maternal and infant mortality rates and a high prevalence of infectious diseases and undernutrition. In the late 1990s the Chilean nutrition and health situation looked completely different. The present scenario is an infant mortality rate (IMR) of 10 per 1,000 live births (1), whereas the average in the region is 35.7 (2). Moreover, during this period, noncommunicable chronic diseases have increased from 54% of all deaths in 1970 to 75% in 1998 (1). The main causes of death now are cardiovascular disease, neoplasms, and trauma. Concomitantly, a rapid increase in risk factors for chronic diseases has been noted in several national surveys (3). Among these risk factors is obesity.

A virtual eradication of protein–energy malnutrition and a steady increase in obesity has occurred over the past two decades. Data from a representative sample of the adult population living in Santiago show that in 1992, 11% of men and 24% of women were classified as obese, defined by a body mass index (BMI) of 30 or more, compared with 6% and 14%, respectively, in 1988 (4). In children, there has been an important decline in the prevalence of undernutrition, concomitant with spiraling obesity rates (5). The reasons behind the reduction in childhood malnutrition are most likely related with existing social programs, including food intervention. Greater access to an improved educational system, progress in water and sanitation infrastructure, wide coverage of primary health care interventions, and declining unemployment rates are also major contributors. The improvement in the economic situation and the "modernization" of society have led to an increase in the consumption of energy-dense foods and an alarming increase in sedentary behavior (6). Despite the positive impact of food supplementation programs in preventing undernutrition, these programs may have contributed to the rise in obesity rates, especially among preschool children of low- and middle-income groups.

45

CRITERIA USED TO DEFINE OBESITY IN CHILE

The terms *overweight* and *obesity* are often used interchangeably, despite the fact that they are not identical. *Overweight* is defined as an increased weight (not necessarily excess fat) for a certain height, whereas *obesity* indicates an excess in fat mass (7,8). Although the long-term effect of overweight and obesity on morbidity and mortality in children has not yet been as well documented as in adults, multiple studies have shown that adiposity in childhood is correlated with the rising incidence of diabetes, hypertension, and atherosclerosis observed in this age group (9–13). These harmful consequences of overweight and obesity make it very important to have clear definitions.

In 1992, the Chilean Ministry of Health adopted the World Health Organization (WHO) international reference (NCHS 1977) (14) and the weight-for-height index as the official criteria for evaluating the nutritional status of preschool children, both for undernutrition and overnutrition. The Chilean Ministry of Education, which collects data on weight and height of children in the first and ninth grades, also adopted these criteria for children under 10 years of age, and the body mass index (BMI) compared with the WHO reference (14,15) for adolescents. We are now considering following the international recommendations to use BMI to classify overweight and obese children from the age of 2 (16–20).

No generally accepted reference standards have yet been produced. The WHO (15) and National Center for Health Statistics/Centers for Disease Control (NCHS/CDC) 2000 (21) references are based on the distribution of representative samples of the US population and use statistically based cutoff points to determine the prevalence of overweight and obesity. In contrast, the International Obesity Task Force (IOTF) reference (22) considers BMI cutoff points that are extrapolated from BMI values of 25

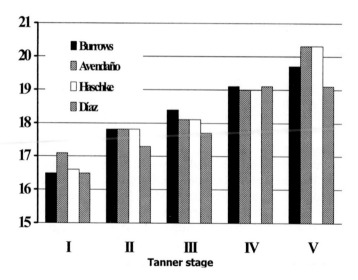

FIG. 1. BMI by Tanner stage (data from 6 studies).

and 30 at age 18. It is assumed that BMI values at those levels in children present an inherent health risk.

Locally, Burrows and Muzzo (23) have provided BMI cutoff points based on a representative sample of schoolchildren of all socioeconomic levels from four regions of Chile, based on anthropometric data collected on 4,531 boys and 5,326 girls between 1985 and 1988. An important contribution by these workers is the suggestion that during adolescence, the BMI should be referred to the Tanner stage of pubertal development rather than to chronologic age. They provided normative data on BMI by Tanner stage for girls aged 10 to 17 years and boys from 11 to 17 years of age. Figure 1 shows that for every one-point change in Tanner stage, there is between a one-half- and one-unit increase in BMI in the 10- to 14-year-old age group, independent of true chronologic age. Similar findings have been observed in other studies in the region (24). However, the specific effect of Tanner staging on adiposity was not evaluated. A critical point for future evaluation will be to compare BMI for age versus BMI for Tanner stage as predictors of adiposity and metabolic alterations in early adolescence.

TRENDS IN OBESITY IN CHILDREN AND ADOLESCENTS

Since 1987 the Ministry of Education has carried out a yearly census among first and ninth graders in state-supported schools. This census includes anthropometric data on children in first and ninth grades, covering approximately 75% and 56% of the country's total population, respectively.

The prevalence of obesity among 6-year-olds who entered first grade in 1987, 1990, 1993, 1996, and 2000 was determined by a cross-sectional analysis and calculated using weight-for-height (WHO 1977), BMI-NCHS/CDC 2000, and BMI-IOTF. First, we used a weight-for-height of greater than +2 SD as an indicator of obesity (13); later, we used BMI-CDC 2000 of more than the 95th centile as the cutoff. Finally, we used BMI-IOTF, determining age-specific cutoff points that project to a BMI of more than 30 at age 18. The prevalence of obesity in 14- to 16-year-old children in the ninth grade was determined for 1993 and 1996, also using BMI and comparing it to three reference datasets—the WHO values (NHANES-I) (15); the revised NCHS/CDC growth charts (21); and the figures provided by IOTF (22). In the first and second categories, children were considered obese if their BMI was beyond the 95th centile; when IOTF was used, the calculations involved cutoff points corresponding to an adult BMI of 30 or more.

Table 1 shows the obesity prevalence in 6-year-old boys and girls using the three criteria described earlier. The prevalence of obesity in boys shows an increase from 6.5% in 1987 to 17% in 2000 when determined by weight-for-height (WHO reference). These figures were slightly lower if BMI-CDC data reference was used, whereas with BMI-IOTF cutoff the values were significantly lower, 1.8% in 1987 and 7.2% in 2000. Over the 13-year period, the increase has been extremely high, at 1.5- to threefold, depending on the reference used. Obesity in girls increased from 7.8% to 18.6% with the first criterion, from 4% to 15.8% with BMI-CDC, and from

TABLE 1. *Prevalence of obesity among 6-year-old Chilean boys and girls defined by three criteria (1987–2000)*

	1987 (%)	1990 (%)	1993 (%)	1996 (%)	2000 (%)
Index and reference to define obesity in boys					
Weight-for-height > 2 SD WHO	6.5	8.9	11.4	13.4	17.0
BMI-CDC ≥ 95th centile	5.1	7.0	10.1	11.8	14.7
IOTF-BMI corresponding to an adult BMI ≥ 30	1.8	2.5	4.3	5.2	7.2
Index and reference to define obesity in girls					
Weight-for-height > 2 SD WHO	7.8	10.1	12.7	15.0	18.6
BMI-CDC ≥ 95th centile	4.0	5.3	8.1	10.0	15.8
BMI-IOTF corresponding to an adult BMI ≥ 30	2.1	2.8	4.6	5.9	7.5

Abbreviations: BMI, body mass index; CDC, Centers for Disease Control; IOTF, International Obesity Taskforce.

2.1% to 7.5% with BMI-IOTF. These increments follow similar trends to those observed for boys. The analysis by sex shows that obesity is more prevalent among girls when determined by weight-for-height and BMI-IOTF.

Obesity prevalence in adolescents, determined in 1993 and 1996 from the census data on schoolchildren in the ninth grade using the stated criteria, show that these rates were low and similar for both sexes. The rate of increase over the 3-year period amounted to 33%. The prevalence in adolescents in 1996 was only one-third to one-fifth of that found in the young children. Muzzo *et al.* (25,26), in a cross-sectional study that included schoolchildren from all socioeconomic levels from several regions of the country, analyzed the nutritional status of boys (12 to 16 years of age) and girls (10 to 16 years of age) in 1986, 1991, 1994, and 1998. Obesity rates (determined using the BMI-CDC data) increased from 1.6% to 9.2% in boys and from 2.3% to 11.8% in girls over this 12-year period.

In summary, obesity in 6-year-olds determined from the school census data and analyzed using three definitions has shown an alarming increase over the past decades. Obesity prevalence determined by weight-for height (NCHS 1977) was greater than that derived from the BMI-CDC reference, whereas the values obtained using the BMI-IOTF data were much lower. Our results confirm the suggestion that in epidemiologic studies of prepubertal children obesity prevalence is substantially underestimated when using BMI-IOTF (27). Presently, no reference to measure childhood obesity has been validated prospectively in terms of predicting the short- and long-term health consequences for given BMI cutoff points.

The difference in obesity prevalence in adolescents compared with prepubertal children may partly be explained by secular trends; obesity is now affecting progressively younger children, whereas historical, older cohorts may have been less affected. This difference would produce a higher prevalence among younger children. We speculate that factors leading to obesity in the population groups undergoing the nutrition transition will have a progressively greater effect on younger children than on adolescents. As income increases, sedentary lifestyles and richer diets become more prevalent at earlier ages. Eventually, as demonstrated by the NHANES-III sample, obesity increases to a point where there are similarly high rates in both young children and adolescents (8). This age-related change may also be explained by the possibility that reference criteria derived from populations in industrialized countries have a reduced sensitivity for detecting obesity in adolescents from developing countries (28). Unfortunately, cross-sectional studies reflect the behavior of different cohorts. This issue can only be resolved by conducting longitudinal follow-up studies where body fat is measured and health effects are determined.

INFLUENCE OF CHANGES IN LINEAR GROWTH ON PREVALENCE OF OBESITY IN DEVELOPING COUNTRIES

The influence of stunting on the prevalence of obesity needs to be considered, given the effect of short stature on BMI and energy balance (29,30). We have observed a fall in stunting rates in Chile concomitant with the rise in obesity. Thus the contribution of stunting to obesity prevalence has decreased over time, suggesting that other factors are responsible for the obesity trends. The prevalence of stunting (height for age z score of less than -2, WHO standard) in 6-year-olds was 10.6% and 7.3% for boys and girls, respectively, in 1987, whereas in 1996 the values declined to 5.8% and 3.4%. During the 10-year period, the average stature of children in this age group increased by 2 cm (31).

In 1987, 6-year-old stunted boys and girls had a higher prevalence of obesity than normally grown children of the same age. In stunted boys, the obesity rate (weight-for-height z score of more than 2, WHO standard) was 10.5%, whereas in boys of normal height it was 6%. In stunted girls, the obesity rate was 12.2%, and in those of normal height, it was 7.4%. In 1996, when the prevalence of stunting had decreased and obesity had increased, stunting was less strongly associated with an increased risk of obesity. The odds ratio for obesity in stunted children in 1987 was 1.83 in boys (95% confidence interval 1.72 to 1.94) and 1.74 in girls (1.62 to 1.86), whereas in 1996, these ratios were 1.34 (1.26 to 1.43) and 1.61 (1.5 to 1.74).

In adolescents, the prevalence of height deficit has also declined considerably. In the study by Burrows *et al.* (25) analyzing cross-sectional samples of adolescents over a 12-year period, stunting (defined as height for age below the 10th centile of the CDC reference) decreased from 44.2% in 1986 to 20.8% in 1998 in boys and from 41.1% to 26.6% in girls. However, the relation between stunting and obesity during adolescence is confounded by the effect of pubertal development, with the obese tending to mature earlier, which affects the interpretation of BMI.

In summary, these data suggest that in countries undergoing the nutrition transition, stunting is associated with an increased risk of obesity, but as stunting decreases, short stature becomes less significant as a risk factor for obesity. In populations of normal height, obesity in children is associated with increased stature (32), most probably secondary to enhanced bone age maturation.

The relation between obesity and stature in adolescents is a particularly difficult problem, as maturational stage will have a significant effect on the BMI. Moreover, the onset of puberty may differ between populations. Sexual maturation during this period affects weight, stature, and body composition (33). Studies published in the 1970s in Chile (34) indicated that in adolescent girls from low socioeconomic groups puberty begins 1 year earlier than in their European counterparts. In 1980, based on assessment of Tanner stage and the reported onset of menses in a representative sample of school girls, the mean age of puberty onset was found to be 12.9 years (35), whereas in 1986, using direct examination and self-reported information of the onset of menses, Burrows *et al.* found the mean age to be 12.6 years (36). More recent data, based on self-reports, showed the mean age to be 12.3 years (37). From these Chilean data, a trend toward earlier menarche is evident. If this trend persists, obesity estimates will be higher in younger prepubertal girls but will have less influence after the menarche. Local data on boys do not show any changes in sexual maturation relative to international standards (34). Because the correction of obesity cutoff points by pubertal stage is difficult to implement in large studies, no population reference takes this issue into account (37).

HEALTH AND NUTRITION PROGRAMS: TRANSITION FROM STUNTING AND UNDERWEIGHT TO OBESITY

Chile is often presented as a paradigm of the success of supplementary feeding programs. There has been a clear correlation between the implementation of these massive interventions and the decline in malnutrition in all age groups. Unfortunately, these programs may be also contributing to the rising prevalence in obesity (5). We have previously published examples of the impact of these assistance programs on the prevalence of obesity. Supplementary feeding programs in Latin America benefit approximately 83 million people of an estimated 414 million in the region (38). The number of malnourished individuals, however, is only !0 million—that is, around 12% of the total number receiving benefit. The explanation for this phenomenon is that nutrition programs have evolved beyond the immediate needs of the malnourished and have become part of the social provision for populations living in poverty. Despite the obvious benefits—namely, the significant reductions in underweight and wasting that have occurred in most countries—these programs have the potential to affect the trends in obesity rates. As stunting remains a problem in most of the developing world, providing food supplements may be beneficial for some individuals while being detrimental for others (39).

We will summarize in the following section the main food supplementation programs for young children and their potential effects on obesity. The Chilean supplementary feeding program, or Programa Nacional de Alimentación Complementaria (PNAC), began in the 1920s as a public milk distribution program for working mothers. It was significantly strengthened in the 1950s with the creation of the National Health Service (NHS), which provides universal health protection and health services for insured workers and the indigent population. Approximately 70% of children aged up to the age of 6 years, pregnant women, and nursing mothers are beneficiaries. The main objectives of the PNAC are to promote normal growth and development in children from conception to 6 years of age by providing food supplements to the mother during pregnancy and lactation, and to the child from birth to 6 years of age; to protect mother's health during pregnancy and lactation; to promote breast-feeding by providing supplements to mothers during pregnancy and lactation; to prevent low birth weight related to maternal malnutrition; to prevent infant and childhood malnutrition among the beneficiaries of the NHS; and to improve coverage of primary health care activities, thus providing an incentive for beneficiaries to attend clinics regularly (40).

Within the activities of the PNAC, the enhanced program was specifically designed for the early control of undernutrition. The energy contribution provided by this program varies from 100% of the requirement for infants of 5 months to 30% for children between 2 and 6 years. The protein contribution is considerably higher, at 180% and 58%, respectively. A controlled evaluation was conducted by Kain and Uauy (41) in a group of infants in whom weight-for-length z score category on entry to the program was compared with the corresponding z score on discharge 12 months later. The results showed that the change in the program beneficiaries in terms of length-for-age was minimal. Moreover, it was similar to that observed in a control group of nonparticipants matched for age and growth indices on entry (42). The benefit of improving mild underweight in 7.5% of the infants was offset by the number of overweight infants, which increased by 10.2%. The evidence from length-for-age z scores suggests that even stunted children gained nothing from the program compared with a control group that did not receive the benefit. The significance of being mildly underweight needs to be reassessed in the light of the emergence of a new paradigm of growth, where more is not necessarily better. What is clear from this evaluation is that if you provide additional food to stunted or normal children, they will mostly gain weight to exceed the median reference value.

A separate example is drawn from the National Nursery Schools Council Program (JUNJI). This was created in 1971 under the Ministry of Education to provide childcare as well as supplementary food for toddlers and preschool children. Coverage is close to 50% of those in need. In 1998 approximately 100,000 children under the age of 5 attended JUNJI. Of these, 95% were preschool children between 2 and 5 years of age, and the rest were infants under 2 years. The food distributed covers 58% or 75% of the children's daily energy needs, depending on whether they attend for a half-day or a full day. The energy contribution is divided by age group as follows: under 12 months, 800 kcal; 12 to 24 months, 950 kcal; 2 to 3 years, 1,000 kcal; 3 to 5 years, 1,150 kcal. If a nutritional deficit is detected, a reinforcement of 150 kcal/day is provided (43). This program seems to have contributed to the notable decrease in stunting observed in the preschool population during the past decade. The percentage of children below -1 SD weight-for-age and height-for-age has fallen significantly, and children who are mildly underweight now account for less than 5% of the total. Concomitantly, a rise in obesity has been observed in the preschool population; in the last decade this has increased from 6% in 1990 to 10.6% in 2000 (weight-for-height > 2 SD, WHO 1977). There has also been a measurable increase in obesity rates on a yearly basis from the time the children start kindergarten to the time they finish their academic year (2). Obesity rates are progressively higher with each age cohort. Observations from a cohort of 8,086 children who attended JUNJI for three consecutive years and were measured every year showed that there was a threefold increase in the number of obese children by the end. During this same period the prevalence of overweight increased by 50% (39). On a more positive note, the program is presently adapting the food provision to the current nutritional profile of the preschool population, and on the basis of doubly labeled water measurements of energy expenditure, the energy content of the food provided has been reduced, and physical activity is being increased. The sugar and saturated fat content of the ration has been lowered, skimmed milk is being provided, and additional fresh fruits and vegetables have been added, favoring the supply of calcium, micronutrients (iron and zinc), and fiber.

TRENDS IN RISK FACTORS FOR OBESITY

Basic Determinants of the Increase in Obesity Prevalence in Chile

To evaluate possible determinants of the rapid increase in obesity in children over the past two decades, we examined indicators that could serve as a proxy for the components of the energy balance equation. As balance equals intake minus expenditure, we hypothesized that both an increase in intake and a decrease in expenditure underlie the rising prevalence of obesity in children and adolescents. We analyzed trends in indicators of components of energy balance over time, and these are depicted in Fig 2. In addition, we explored the relation between these factors and the rising prevalence of obesity in children; univariate correlation coefficients for these are presented in Table 2.

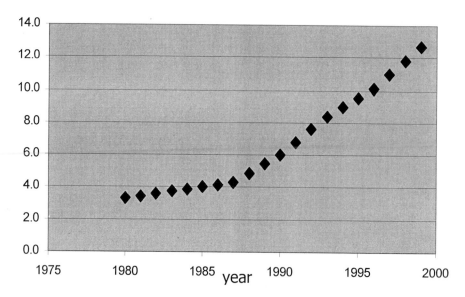

FIG. 2. Obesity percentage prevalence in 6 year olds.

TABLE 2. *Univariate correlations of basic determinants of obesity in children from cross-sectional data, Chile, 1980–2000*

	Obesity, boys (r)	Obesity, girls (r)	Total obesity (r)	Total obesity (R^2)
GNP US $ per person per year	0.98	0.99	0.98	0.97
Indigence, % prevalence	−0.97	−0.97	−0.97	0.942
Poverty, % prevalence	−0.9912	−0.9948	−0.9929	0.98593
Indigence + poverty, % prevalence	−0.9887	−0.9888	−0.9894	0.97892
Energy kcal/person/day	0.835	0.85	0.841	0.708
Protein g/person/day	0.83	0.84	0.84	0.7
Fat g/person/day	0.968	0.973	0.971	0.942
Energy, kcal/poor person/day	0.984	0.991	0.987	0.974
Protein, g/poor person/day	0.984	0.991	0.987	0.975
Fat, g/poor person/day	0.984	0.99	0.986	0.973
Social expenditure, US$/person/year	0.89939	0.91101	0.90294	0.8153
Social expenditure, US$/poor person/year	0.95656	0.96449	0.95926	0.92018
PNAC, kg/person/year	−0.93	−0.93	−0.93	0.861
PNAC, kg/poor person/year	0.7681	0.7682	0.7681	0.5901
Cars per 100 persons	0.97109	0.96647	0.97056	0.94198
Cars per 100 poor persons	0.99108	0.99394	0.99273	0.98551
Infant mortality, o/oo	−0.877	−0.8679	−0.8734	0.7628
Low birthweight, %	−0.8536	−0.8545	−0.8545	0.7302
Late infant mortality, o/oo	−0.9024	−0.89321	−0.89885	0.80793
Death from diarrhea disease per 10^5 persons per year	−0.83	−0.816	−0.824	0.68
Obesity in boys	1	0.999	0.9998	0.9996
Obesity in girls	0.999	1	0.9996	0.9993
Total obesity	0.9998	0.9996	1	1

Note: Correlation coefficient r was calculated using simple linear regression model.

Abbreviations: GNP, gross national product; PNAC, Programa Nacional de Alimentación Complementaría.

Socioeconomic changes may be related to both increased intake and decreased activity, because as income increases, consumption of animal foods and high-fat foods increases, at the same time that physical activity decreases as people use motorized vehicles and other labor-saving devices. We have analyzed the GNP trends in Chile (in 1986 adjusted US$). After 1988 the economy grew at an average of nearly 7% a year for a full decade, income more than doubled, and poverty (defined as percentage of income spent on the basic family food basket) fell considerably. Through the 1980s poverty declined from 50% to around 40%, and during the 1990s it declined still further, to 20%.

As there were no systematic assessments of food intake during this period, we decided to use estimates of food availability, as defined from food balance data collected using FAO standardized methodology. This enabled computation of energy and macronutrient (protein, carbohydrate and fat) availability per capita. Because we were particularly interested in assessing the changes that affected the lower income groups, we also determined the availability per poor person in the country. The assumption that the energy and macronutrients available per poor person serve as an indicator of food availability is an obvious oversimplification. The expression of energy and macronutrient availability per poor person will strengthen the correlation with obesity prevalence; a higher r^2 can be noted in Table 2. As income has more than doubled and poverty has dropped by half during the past two decades, we considered that this oversimplification was necessary for a full assessment of the potential impact of increased food intake. For example, mean daily energy intake per person increased by only 200 kcal over the two decades, but when expressed per poor person, it more than tripled. The changes in dietary fats are particularly pronounced, per capita availability remained stable at around 60 g a day during the 1980s but rose sharply to close to 90 g a day during the 1990s.

This information was validated in part by data from apparent food consumption surveys based on food expenditure according to income group, which have been conducted every 10 years in Chile from 1969 (44). Chilean national food availability data for the last 20 years are consistent with an important increase in the consumption of meat (poultry, +140%; beef, +54%; pork, +200%) and dairy products (+61%), and a stable or decreased intake of cereals and legumes (−10%) (45). A recent analysis of the latest national household food expenditure survey has shown that for the lowest quintile of the income distribution, the highest-ranked items are bread, meat, and soft drinks (46). The mean fat intake as a percentage of total energy is 28%. This is low relative to most industrialized countries yet the prevalence of obesity is rising sharply (1). A food consumption survey carried out in Santiago in 1995 (46) showed that 70% of adults consumed less than two fruits and 59% less than two portions of vegetables a day. This dietary pattern is clearly inadequate to contribute to the prevention of obesity.

Social expenditure, usually targeted to vulnerable low-income groups, is aimed at improving access to food, health, and education. In a country where malnutrition has traditionally been considered the main problem, social expenditure includes direct transfer of food products targeted at pregnant and lactating women, children under 6 years of age, and school-aged children living under conditions of poverty. In terms of US$ per person per year, expenditure on education and health remained more or less constant from 1980 until 1991, when, after the return to democratic rule, it grew steadily, almost doubling over the decade. As the reduction in poverty accelerated during the 1990s and social expenditure increased, expenditure per poor person tripled, assuming that all was spent on the poor. Food distribution programs—taking PNAC for women and children under 6 years as an example—declined by 50% if expressed as the amount given per person per year in the population as a whole, but increased by 20% per beneficiary in the poor population. Data from preschool and school feeding programs were also available but were not included in the analysis, as there have been multiple changes in the selection criteria of the beneficiaries and in the amounts of food provided; nevertheless these programs are reflected in the overall social expenditure.

On the energy output side, we found no systematic survey data on activity patterns of children and adolescents over recent decades, but specific studies support the view that sedentary behavior is very prevalent. This has been assessed by direct observations of children and television viewing. Sedentarism is related to the urbanization process. By 1970, three-quarters of the population lived in urban areas; in 1997 this figure increased to 87%. The number of cars in the country was 363,150 in 1970, increasing to 2,024,510 in 1998. Phone lines increased from 1,818,000 in 1995 to 2,753,000 in 1998, and TV appliances from 12,170 in 1970 to more than 2 million in 1997 (47). In 1988 a survey conducted in Santiago (48) indicated that 55% of men and 77.4% of women were sedentary (performing less than two periods of 15 minutes of exercise a week); these figures had increased to 57.8% in men and 80.1% in women in 1992. In Valparaiso (the second largest city) in 1997, more than 90% of women were inactive in their leisure time, and this figure was even higher (97%) in the lower socioeconomic group (49). Currently, low-income preschool children watch 3 hours of TV daily, increasing to 4 hours during weekends (50). Older schoolchildren also spend a considerable amount of time in sedentary activities. A recent survey conducted in a representative sample of schools of Santiago showed that 90% of school-aged children watched an average of 2 hours of television during weekdays, and 20% watched more than 3 hours daily (51).

Data on the increase in electricity consumption per person over the period are confounded by the inherent increases related to industrial production and economic growth, so we chose the number of cars per 100 persons as a proxy for physical inactivity. This was also expressed after adjustment for the number living in poverty. Both indices remained fairly stable over the 1980s but increased sharply during the 1990s. The slope was steeper when the variable was adjusted by the number of poor people, as the latter decreased over the decade. Because the increase in the number of cars is also closely linked to improved income, the rise in cars per 100 persons will reflect both of the components of the energy balance equation—increased energy intake and decreased activity.

We also considered improvements in health and nutrition in women and children, as these could be construed as indices of improved nutrient utilization, less energy being wasted in responding to infections and diarrheal disease, thus favoring a positive energy balance. Changes were marked over the 1980s, with a fall in infant mortality from 32 per 1,000 live-born infants in 1980 to 16 per 1,000 in 1990; a further fall to 10 per 1,000 occurred over the 1990s. The prevalence of low birth weight fell from 9% to 7% in the 1980s, and further to around 5% over the 1990s. Late infant mortality, which is dominated by deaths from respiratory infections and malnutrition, fell from 15.1 per 1,000 to 8 per 1,000 in the 1980s, and further to around 4 per 1,000 over the 1990s. The marked decline in deaths from diarrheal disease per 10^5 inhabitants, from around 8 in 1980 to close to 1.5 in 1993, has remained stable since, and reflects a significant improvement in environmental sanitation, access to clean water, and appropriate waste disposal. This coincided with an increase in sanitary food control, prohibiting the use of wastewater in the irrigation of vegetables, and intensive educational efforts relating to the consumption of raw vegetables imposed after a cholera scare related to the epidemic that affected Peru and other neighboring countries.

This information was analyzed more specifically for its relation to the rising prevalence of obesity in children entering school. The criteria used to define obesity by

Uauy *et al.* in 1980 (35) (120% of median weight-for-height by sex) were used consistently across the census datasets obtained from 6-year-old children. As these cross-sectional datasets included 1987, 1990, 1993, 1996, and 2000, the prevalence of obesity for the in-between years was derived by interpolation from the two nearest datasets. Simple correlation analyses were conducted and revealed extremely high correlation coefficients. Table 2 summarizes this information, providing correlation coefficients for each sex and for total obesity. It is tempting to speculate on potential causal relations based on the high *r* values, but as most variables are tightly interrelated, we cannot establish causal relations from simple correlation indices. A stepwise multivariate logistic regression analysis was also performed in an attempt to isolate the main determinants. Obesity in the whole population was best explained by including increase in the number of cars per 100 persons, the decrease in deaths from diarrheal disease, and the increase in fat availability per poor person per day. The r^2 value for this analysis was 0.994. To explore possible hierarchies for the main determinants, we forced the exclusion of specified main determinants to examine which variables made an additional contribution to explaining the obesity trends over the decade.

CATEGORIES OF DETERMINANTS FOR OBESITY INCLUDED IN THE ANALYSIS, DEFINITIONS, AND UNITS USED

The following are categories of determinants for obesity:

- *Socioeconomic changes:* Per capita income: gross national product from 1980 to 1999 adjusted to a constant (1986 US$). Data obtained from the Central Bank of Chile.
- *Prevalence of poverty, indigence, and total poverty:* Data for poverty and indigence obtained from the CASEN surveys (socioeconomic characterization of the Chilean population) carried out every 2 years by the Chilean Ministry of Planning since 1987. Data for 1980 were estimated by a regression model that incorporated death from diarrheal disease, low birth weight, and social expenditure (inverse). Data from 1981 to 1986 were obtained from a linear estimate from the 1980 and 1987 figures by the least squares method. This same methodology was applied for the intermediate points from 1987 to 2000.
  Poverty is defined by an income of less than twice the amount necessary to buy a predetermined basic food basket. Indigents are those for whom total income is less than the amount required to buy a food basket; total poverty is the sum of poverty plus indigence.
- *Trends in food availability:* Per capita energy and macronutrient (energy, protein, carbohydrate, fat) availability were obtained from the FAO food balance sheets posted on the Internet. The same indices were computed per poor person in the country, assuming that all food was available for the poor.
- *Social expenditures:* The adjusted 1986 US$ spent on health, education, and housing per person, and the same index per poor person, assuming that all expenditures are concentrated in the poor. Data are provided by the Ministry of Planning.

- *Food distribution programs:* The amount of food supplements provided by PNAC, per person in the country, and the same index per poor person, assuming that all food was provided to the poor. Data from 1980 until 1999 are provided by the Ministry of Health.
- *Increase in sedentarism:* The number of cars per 100 persons, and the same index per poor person, assuming that all cars are available to the poor. Data are available from 1985 until 1999 and are provided by the Ministry of Transport. Data for 1980 to 1984 were estimated by extrapolating from the 1985 to 1990 trend.
- *Improvement in health and nutrition of women and children:* Infant mortality, prevalence of low birth weight, late infant mortality. Data from 1980 until 1998 for the three indices were provided by the Ministry of Health.
- *Improvement in sanitation and decrease in gastrointestinal infections:* Deaths from diarrhea per 10^5 inhabitants. The data for 1980 to 1998 were provided by the Ministry of Health.

CONCLUSIONS

Chile is undergoing a rapid nutritional transition with a progressive increase in the prevalence of obesity in children. The factors responsible for these trends are changes in lifestyle and diet, which are similar to those observed in industrialized societies except for the faster rate of change. We consider that nutrition interventions programs, especially in stunted populations, may aggravate the obesity epidemic. Weight-for-age definition of undernutrition in children without assessment of length will overestimate the dimension of malnutrition and neglect the identification of stunted overweight children. As malnutrition rates fall, the need to prevent overweight and obesity should be considered of equal importance to the eradication of undernutrition.

Based on the observed effect of socioeconomic, dietary, and other environmental factors on the prevalence of obesity between 1980 and 2000, the high correlation coefficients observed, and the multivariate regression analysis, income-related factors explain most of the variance in obesity. However, a decrease in infection and a rise in apparent fat consumption were also significant. The number of cars per 100 persons, especially if adjusted by the decrease in poverty, had the highest relation to the development of obesity in both univariate and multivariate analysis. The contribution of rising income; increased expenditure on social programs, including food supplementation; increase in apparent fat consumption; and rise in indices of sedentary lifestyles in explaining the rise in obesity indicate that the prevalence will continue to rise unless measures are taken to increase physical activity and reduce the consumption of energy-dense foods.

REFERENCES

1. Vio F, Albala C. Nutrition policy in the Chilean transition. *Public Health Nutr* 2000; 3: 49–55.
2. Uauy R, Albala C, Kain J. Obesity trends in Latin America: transiting from under- to overweight. *J Nutr* 2001; 131: 893–9S.
3. Albala C, Vio F. Epidemiological transition in Latin America: the case of Chile. *Public Health* 1995; 109: 431–42.

4. Berríos X. Tendencia temporal de los factores de riesgo de enfermedades crónicas: ¿la antesala silenciosa de una epidemia que viene? *Rev Med Chil* 1997; 125: 1405–7.
5. Kain J, Vio F, Albala C. Childhood nutrition in Chile: from deficit to excess. *Nutr Res* 1998; 18: 1825–35.
6. Albala C, Vio F, Kain J. Obesidad: un desafío pendiente. *Rev Med Chil* 1998: 126: 1001–9.
7. Barlow S, Dietz W. Obesity evaluation and treatment: expert committee recommendations. *Pediatrics* 1998; 102: 29–36.
8. Troiano R, Flegal K. Overweight children and adolescents: description, epidemiology and demographics. *Pediatrics* 1998; 101: 497–504.
9. Power C, Lake J, Cole T. Measurement and long-term health risks of child and adolescent fatness. *Int J Obes* 1997; 21: 507–26.
10. Freedman D, Dietz W, Srinivasan S, Berenson G. The relationship of overweight to cardiovascular risk factors among children and adolescents: the Bogalusa Heart Study. *Pediatrics* 1999; 103: 1175–82.
11. Treviño R, Marshall R, Hale D, *et al.* Diabetes risk factor in low-income Mexican-American children. *Diabetes Care* 1999; 22: 1–6.
12. Berenson G, Srinivasan S, Nicklas T. Atherosclerosis: a nutritional disease of childhood. *Am J Cardiol* 1998; 82: 22–9T.
13. Dietz W. Health consequences of obesity in youth: childhood predictors of adult disease. *Pediatrics* 1998; 101: 518–25.
14. Bulletin of the World Health Organization. *Use and interpretation of anthropometric indicators of nutritional status.* Geneva: WHO, 1986.
15. WHO Expert Committee on Physical Status. *The use and interpretation of anthropometry.* Report of a WHO Expert Committee (Technical Report Series 854). Geneva: WHO, 1995.
16. Dietz W, Bellizzi M. The use of body mass index to assess obesity in children. *Am J Clin Nutr* 1999; 70: 123–5.
17. Pietrobelli A, Faith M, Allison D, Gallagher D, Chiumello G, Heymsfield S. Body mass index as a measure of adiposity among children and adolescents: a validation study. *J Pediatr* 1998; 132: 204–10.
18. Dietz W, Robinson T. Use of body mass index (BMI) as a measure of overweight in children and adolescents. *J Pediatr* 1998; 132: 191–3.
19. Gallagher D, Visser M, Sepulveda D, Pierson R, Harris T, Heymsfield S. How useful is body mass index for comparison of body fatness across age, sex, and ethnic groups? *Am J Epidemiol* 1996; 143: 228–39.
20. Duerenberg P, Weststrate J, Seidell J. Body mass index as a measure of body fatness: age and sex-specific prediction formulas. *Br J Nutr* 1991; 65: 105–14.
21. CDC/NCHS. CDC growth charts: United States. Posted 30 May 2000 on the Internet.
22. Cole T, Bellizzi M, Flegal K, Dietz W. Establishing standard definition for child overweight and obesity worldwide: international survey. *BMJ* 2000; 320: 1–6.
23. Burrows R, Muzzo S. Estándares de crecimiento y desarrollo del escolar chileno. *Rev Chil Nutr* 1999; 1: 26.
24. Díaz E, Burrows R, Muzzo S, Galgani J, Rodríguez R. Evaluación nutricional de adolescentes mediante IMC para etapa puberal. *Rev Chil Pediatr* 1996; 67: 153–8.
25. Burrows R, Cordero J, Ramírez I, Muzzo S. Cambio secular del crecimiento en escolares chilenos de tres regiones del país. *Rev Chil Pediatr* 1999; 70: 390–7.
26. Muzzo S, Cordero J, Burrows R. Cambios en la prevalencia del exceso de peso del escolar chileno en los últimos 8 años. *Rev Chil Nutr* 1999; 26: 311–5.
27. Reilly JJ, Dorosty AR, Emmett PM, the ALSPAC Study Team. Identification of the obese child: adequacy of the body mass index for clinical practice and epidemiology. *Int J Obes* 2000; 24: 1623–7.
28. Wang W, Wang J, Mulligan J, Kinra S. Standard definition of child overweight and obesity worldwide [letter]. *BMJ* 2000; 321: 1158.
29. Schroeder D, Martorell R. Fatness and body mass index from birth to young adulthood in a rural Guatemalan population. *Am J Clin Nutr* 1999; 70: 137–44.
30. Trowbridge FL, Marks JS, Lopez de Romana G, *et al.* Body composition of Peruvian children with short stature and high weight-height. II. Implications for the interpretation for weight for height as an indicator of nutritional status. *Am J Clin Nutr* 1987; 46: 411–18.
31. Kain J, Uauy R, Díaz M, Aburto A. Height increase in school children entering first grade during the last decade. *Rev Med Chil* 1999; 127: 539–46.
32. Bellizzi M, Dietz W. Workshop on childhood obesity: summary of the discussion. *Am J Clin Nutr* 1999; 70: 173–5.

33. Bini V, Celi F, Berioli MG, *et al.* Body mass index in children and adolescents according to age and pubertal stage. *Eur J Clin Nutr* 2000; 54: 214–8.
34. Valenzuela CY. Pubertal origin of sex dimorphism and adult stature of a Chilean population. *Am J Phys Anthropol* 1983; 60: 53–60.
35. Uauy R, Cariaga L, Santana R. Childhood obesity due to nutritional causes. *Rev Chil Nutr* 1984; 12: 7–14
36. Burrows R, Leiva L, Mauricci A, Zvaighaft A, Muzzo S. Características de la pubertad en niñas escolares de la Región Metropolitana. *Rev Chil Pediatr* 1988; 59: 21–5.
37. Burrows R, Muzzo S. Growth and development of Chilean school children. *Rev Chil Nutr* 1999: 26: 95–101.
38. FAO. Targeting for nutrition improvement. Resources for advancing nutritional well-being. FAO. Rome 2001.
39. Rojas J, Uauy R. Need to prevent obesity without neglecting the protection of children at risk of malnutrition. *Rev Chil Nutr* 1999; 26: 35–9.
40. Kain J, Uauy R. Targeting strategies used by the Chilean supplementary feeding program. *Nutr Res* 2001; 21: 677–88.
41. Kain J, Vial I, Muchnik E, Contreras A. An evaluation of the enhanced Chilean supplementary feeding program. *Arch Latinoam Nutr* 1994; 44: 242–50.
42. Kain J, Pizarro F. Effect of an enhanced supplementary feeding program on infant's length. *Arch Latinoam Nutr* 1997; 47: 101–4.
43. Uauy R, Riumalló J. *Work plan in support of guidelines on formulating and implementing nutrition programs (FINP) at the country level. Case study: Chile.* Rome: FAO, 1997.
44. *National surveys on family budget and expenditure* 1969, 1977, 1987, 1997. Santiago: National Institute of Statistics.
45. Espinosa F. SISVAN de Alimentos Indices. Area de Nutrición Pública. INTA, U. de Chile, 2000.
46. Castillo C, Atalah E, Benavides X, Urteaga C. Food patterns in Chilean adults from the metropolitan region. *Rev Med Chil* 1997; 125: 283–9.
47. *Annual summary.* Santiago: National Institute of Statistics.
48. Berríos X. Risk factors for adult chronic disease. An example of epidemiological research. *Bol Esc Med PUC Chile* 1994; 23: 73–89.
49. Jadue L, Vega J, Escobar MC, *et al.* Risk factors for chronic non-communicable diseases: methods and results of CARMEN program basal survey. *Rev Med Chil* 1999; 127: 1004–13.
50. Kain J, Andrade M. Characteristics of the diet and patterns of physical activity in obese Chilean preschoolers. *Nutr Res* 1999; 19: 203–15.
51. Olivares S, Albala C, García F, Jofré I. Television advertisement and food preferences in schoolchildren of Santiago. *Rev Med Chil* 1999; 127: 791–9.

DISCUSSION

Dr. Koletzko: You showed data where you applied different reference standards for defining obesity in your population, so I want to return to the point I made after Dr. Cole's presentation. In applying the IOTF standard you had about a 6% prevalence of children above the upper threshold, and using the traditional standard about 18%—that is, a threefold difference. While we cannot be sure of the consequences of this discrepancy, we ought to question whether it is right to refer to both these outcomes as the "obese population." If we do, we risk confusing the public, not to mention governments and funding agencies. Are we not running a risk that the obesity epidemic may be underestimated?

Dr. Uauy: I agree with your general point, but I think we need to be very careful in our interpretation of Dr. Cole's paper. He does not talk about "standards." He was very careful every time he mentioned the IOTF to use the term *reference.* I hope that everybody here has heard this more than once. It's the IOTF *reference,* not the IOTF standard. We still do not have a risk-based standard, only a population-based standard. You can choose the WHO weight-for-height standard or the latest CDC, and they nearly match. However, the latest CDC standard has obviously recognized the increase in obesity in the US data and has not included current values for children over 6 years of age. Thus I'm not sure whether we can still call the CDC a population-based standard because it's a mixture of a recent survey and an older survey. Eventually, when we have data on BMI versus hyperlipidemia, BMI versus hypertension risk, BMI versus insulin resistance, and so on, then maybe I'll be convinced to use an IOTF risk-based standard. But for now I would use the population-based standard and use the IOTF reference for comparative purposes only.

Dr. Dulloo: When malnourished children are treated it has been known for many decades that fat rather than lean tissue is preferentially recovered. What you are seeing now is surely just an exacerbation of this phenomenon, with our high-fat foods and low levels of activity. Basically, catch-up growth is now catch-up fat. What kind of dietary regimen should we be recommending? It's a very difficult situation.

Dr. Uauy: It's even worse than you say because we know that rapid catch-up growth is not necessarily a good thing if you consider insulin resistance and long-term cardiovascular risk. I think we should redefine what is optimal in terms of recovery from the malnourished state. Gaining fat may be all right if the child is returning to a situation of continued energy deficit. That's what we did in the 1980s when our philosophy was that 1 kg of fat mass would buy 7,500 kcal of deficit later on. But now, as countries are getting better off, there is no point in building up an excess of fat, and we are just setting the children up for an adverse outcome in the future. Another point is that to achieve fat gain, all you need is energy and a little protein. To achieve linear growth, you also need all the micronutrients, so optimizing the micronutrient intake becomes a crucial factor in stunted populations. We need to worry about fetal growth as well, because the cycle starts with malnutrition and stunting *in utero;* this sets the scene for later obesity. There are populations now that are stunted *and* overweight, and the increase in obesity is often clearly related to that. Thus improving the quality of the diet is more than just throwing in calories. Another factor is exercise. Providing exercise is probably important even in early life. Many children in preschool day care centers are given long rest periods when they are told to sit quiet and not move about. We probably should be doing exactly the opposite— this is the time for children to be active. We need to change the generally held view that putting on weight is the most important thing.

Dr. Bar-Or: I'd like to play the devil's advocate for a moment. We are dealing here with populations that for centuries have been undernourished but that now show an improvement in their nutritional status. I wonder if we are not too liberal in our use of the term *obesity.* The BMI and other indicators are mathematical constructs or ratios. You alluded to this yourself— does a disproportionate increase in body fat versus linear growth really make a person obese? Mathematically, yes, but physiologically? I would argue that rather than educating people to reduce their body fat, one should aim to increase their linear growth, at which point they will no longer be obese. I would even go one step further: Is there no danger that, if we jump too early to the conclusion that there is obesity in countries like rural Chile, we will cause the pendulum to swing back in the opposite direction, so that people will again be eating insufficient amounts?

Dr. Uauy: I agree with your overall statement, but when you look at the actual data you find that in most urban centers in developing countries the main causes of death have shifted, as I showed you. It is no longer infectious disease; it is now chronic disease. On a worldwide basis, the burden of disease shifted in 1997 such that there were more deaths from preventable diet-related, chronic, noncommunicable diseases than from malnutrition. I agree with you that the first goal should be to improve height. But you don't need to build obese infants and children to improve their height; you need micronutrients, a better quality of diet overall, and physical activity. And while you are doing that, you will also be preventing obesity. The problem is to get things moving. Governments in particular are too slow to react. In Chile, we have been aware of the problem for a decade, but the government is still giving only three fruits a month in the school feeding program, rather than spending more on fruit and less on calories. We only started to measure linear growth

in 1991; before that, height was not part of routine surveillance, because weight for age was the criterion—anybody under the 50th centile was considered at risk for malnutrition. The result is that we may have overdone it. One needs to put both things into the equation. The first is to improve linear growth, I agree. However, controlling excess weight-for-height is not a contradictory objective; it is complementary. If you do not act to prevent obesity early on, you will end up with the situation that is now occurring in all urban centers in Latin America, where the main cause of death is cardiovascular disease.

Dr. Dulloo: In Europe and the United States, where children and adults become obese without having gone through a period of malnutrition—that is, "normal" obesity—there is an increase not just in fat but also in lean tissue, linear growth, and organ mass. Do you have any data from, say, Chile or Brazil in which organ mass has been assessed in children who are stunted and obese?

Dr. Uauy: I think the best data come from Asia, specifically from Hong Kong, Singapore, and India, where short people develop abdominal obesity predominantly (1). There the metabolic complications of obesity are seen at a lower BMI, so it may not be body fat alone that is the problem but the metabolic response. That's why I would like to define obesity on the basis of risk, not on the amount of adipose tissue per se. This is easier said than done, but I do not think we can talk about a reference standard until we have achieved that.

Dr. Caballero: As you have several decades of good data, have you looked at any effect of early nutritional conditions—for example, birth weight or early growth—on later obesity?

Dr. Uauy: Unfortunately, in Chile the excitement of getting things done has been more than the excitement of getting the evaluations performed. We are now in the process of trying to follow up about 500 of the infants treated in the malnutrition recovery ward to try to answer some of these questions. Unfortunately, while there is money for interventions, there is often none for evaluation.

REFERENCES

1. Obesity: preventing and managing the global epidemic: report of a WHO consultation. WHO Consultation on Obesity 1999. Geneva, Switzerland, 2000.

Obesity in Childhood and Adolescence, edited by
Chunming Chen and William H. Dietz. Nestlé
Nutrition Workshop Series, Pediatric Program,
Vol. 49. Nestec Ltd., Vevey/Lippincott
Williams & Wilkins, Philadelphia © 2002.

The Adult Health Consequences of Childhood Obesity

David S. Freedman, Mary K. Serdula, and Laura Kettel Khan

*Division of Nutrition and Physical Activity, Centers for Disease Control and Prevention,
Atlanta, Georgia, USA*

The short-term complications of severe obesity among children—which include orthopedic complications, pseudotumor cerebri, sleep apnea, gall bladder disease, and polycystic ovary disease—have recently been reviewed (1,2). It is likely, however, that the most common consequences of childhood obesity, including coronary heart disease and the complications of type 2 diabetes mellitus, will not be apparent until adulthood. The recent secular increases in obesity among children, along with the persistence of weight status throughout life, suggest that the impact of childhood obesity on adult morbidity and premature mortality will become increasingly important.

Although overweight children are at increased risk of coronary heart disease and premature mortality, it is uncertain if the associations are independent of adult weight status and depend on the development of obesity during critical periods of growth. Additional information on the natural history and effects of childhood obesity would help guide the development of primary and secondary prevention programs.

In this chapter we will review the adult health consequences of childhood obesity. The data presented are derived largely from the Bogalusa Heart Study (Louisiana), a long-term study of the early natural history of coronary heart disease that involved seven examinations of children and young adults (ages 2 to 38 years) between 1973 and 1993 (3). The panel design of this study, which has data on coronary heart disease risk factors (anthropometry, serum lipids, insulin, blood pressure) from more than 11,500 subjects in a biracial (black/white) community, allows both cross-sectional and longitudinal analyses to be performed.

ASSESSMENT

Childhood Obesity

Childhood obesity has typically been assessed using various combinations of weight and height or by skinfold thickness measurements. Despite the inherent limitations of using weight/height indices to assess excess adipose tissue, they appear to predict various disease outcomes as well as more direct estimates of body fat.

Adolphe Quetelet, a nineteenth-century Belgian mathematician, first noted that the weight of adults was proportional to height squared, and this ratio—the body mass index (BMI, kg/m^2)—is now widely used in studies of children. BMI measurements in childhood, however, vary substantially with age, with the values increasing markedly during the first year of life, slowly decreasing until about 6 years of age, and then increasing by around 40% up to 18 years (4). The correlation with age (r ranges from 0.5 to 0.6) among school-aged children can greatly complicate the interpretation of the BMI. For example, a small difference in the mean age of two groups of children could result in significantly different BMI levels, and a value of 17.6 kg/m^2 among girls in the United States is the 90th centile at age 5 years, the 50th centile at age 11 years, and the 10th centile at 16 years of age.

It is therefore necessary to relate a childhood BMI to values among sex- and age-matched peers, and BMI-for-age centiles have recently been developed from national data collected in the United States between 1963 and 1980 (5). It has been suggested that children with a BMI above the 95th centile of these data are considered to be overweight and that children between the 85th and 95th centiles are "at risk for overweight." The use of these BMI centiles (and terminology) will greatly simplify comparisons across studies.

Although these centiles account for sex and age differences in BMI levels during childhood, other statistical techniques can provide similar results. For example, residuals from regression models that include sex and age (linear and higher-order terms) yield adjusted BMI values that are highly correlated ($r > 0.95$) with external BMI-for-age centiles. It may also be important to account for sexual maturation and ethnicity, in addition to sex and age, when interpreting BMI levels among adolescents. For example, the risk of developing type 2 diabetes among Asians begins to increase at relatively low BMI levels (6,7).

Body Fat Distribution

Systematic methods for describing body shape were first introduced in the 1930s. It was later suggested (8) that the distribution of body fat among adults might be important in various chronic diseases, and a relative excess of body fat in the abdomen, upper body, and trunk is predictive of total mortality, type 2 diabetes, and coronary heart disease. Although the role of intraabdominal visceral fat has often been emphasized, other fat depots may be important (9), and fat distribution has typically been assessed through the measurement of various circumferences (waist girth or waist/hip) or skinfold thicknesses (subscapular/triceps). As these indices of fat distribution are correlated with BMI, careful statistical adjustments are needed to assess the independent effect of fat distribution.

Although the importance of fat distribution in early life is less certain, associations with coronary heart disease risk factors have been observed. Skinfold and circumference measurements among 3,000 children, for example, indicated that a relative excess of abdominal or truncal fat is associated with adverse levels of triglycerides, low-density lipoprotein (LDL) cholesterol, high-density lipoprotein (HDL) cholesterol, and insulin (10). In agreement with results that have emphasized the use of waist circumference (alone) as a measure of visceral fat mass among children (11), waist girth has often shown more consistent associations with levels of lipids and insulin than other measures of fat distribution.

Additional studies of fat patterning among children are needed to examine its tracking into adulthood and its long-term health consequences. It is also possible that the waist circumference may provide useful information on the risk for pediatric type 2 diabetes.

Secular Trends

The prevalence of childhood obesity has increased in many countries, and trends have accelerated since 1980 (3,12–14). For example, data from 5- to 17-year-olds who were examined in the Bogalusa Heart Study (3) indicate that there were substantial increases in mean levels of weight, BMI, and triceps skinfold thickness between 1973 and 1993. These BMI changes, which varied from 1.5 to 2.0 kg/m^2 across ages, are shown in the top panel of Fig. 1.

These secular increases, however, varied substantially across the distribution of BMI (or skinfold thickness) values, with much larger changes occurring at the upper percentiles (Fig. 1, bottom). Whereas the increase in the median BMI level between 1973 and 1993 was around 1 kg/m^2, the 95th centile increased by about 5 kg/m^2, and about 15% of the children examined in 1993 had a BMI that was above the 95th centile of the 1973 data. These BMI changes reflected large increases in weight, with the 95th centile of weight among 11-year-old boys, for example, increasing from 54 to 67 kg over the 20-year period. (About 4% of the 158 11-year-old boys examined in 1993 had a BMI of more than 30 kg/m^2.) National US data over the same time period also indicate that there was a large increase in the positive skewness of the BMI distribution but little change at lower centiles (12).

BMI levels show an exponential relation to several coronary heart disease risk factors, and severely overweight children are more likely to remain obese in adulthood than moderately overweight children. It is therefore possible that future increases in obesity-associated morbidities will be greater than suggested by an analysis of mean BMI levels.

HEALTH CONSEQUENCES

Social Consequences

The stigmatization of obesity begins early in life (1,2), with obese children in the United States characterized as lazy and ugly by their peers. Although obese adolescents tend to have low self-esteem, eating disorders, and a preoccupation with weight, these associations vary greatly across social and ethnic groups. In addition, it is likely that these associations will be influenced by the recent increase in the number of overweight children.

Obesity is inversely associated with socioeconomic status among women in developed countries, and some evidence indicates that obesity may be a cause as well as a

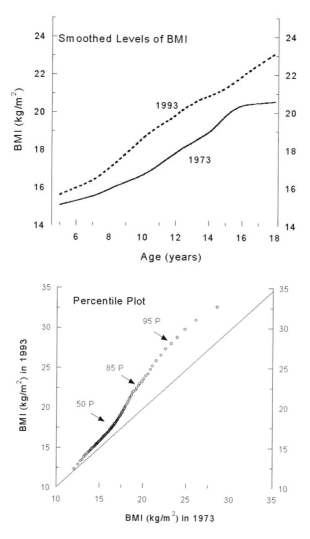

FIG. 1. The top panel shows (lowess) smoothed levels of BMI by age among children in the Bogalusa Heart Study. The bottom panel shows a centile comparison plot for the BMI distributions in 1973 and 1993. The data have been adjusted for sex and age, and the distance above the diagonal line represents the secular increase in BMI at each centile.

consequence of social status. A 7-year follow-up of 16- to 24-year-olds, for example, found that, as compared with women who were of normal weight at baseline, overweight women completed fewer years of education, had lower family incomes, and were less likely to be married (15). These differences could not be explained by family income at baseline, the educational level of the parents, or aptitude test scores. Similar findings have also been observed among overweight girls who subsequently lost weight (16).

Associations between obesity and socioeconomic status in developing and transitional countries are likely to be complex. For example, the relation of income to the prevalence of overweight (BMI 27 kg/m^2) in China is positive in rural areas but negative in cities (17).

Persistence of Obesity

Childhood levels of BMI are predictive of levels in later life, and it has been estimated that around 40% of overweight children will be obese in adulthood (positive predictive value), whereas 15% to 20% of obese adults had been overweight as children (sensitivity) (1,2,4). These estimates, however, have varied markedly across studies, and a wide range of predictive values (26% to 63%) and sensitivities (5% to 44%) has been reported (18). Although these estimates might be expected to be influenced by the length of follow-up, childhood age, and demographic and social characteristics, they are also strongly influenced by the prevalence of obesity. This prevalence is, in turn, partly determined by the categorization of BMI levels.

The influence of these cutoff points can be seen in an analysis of 2,640 2- to 17-year-olds who participated in the Bogalusa Heart Study and who were subsequently reexamined after a mean follow-up of 17 years. Overall, 76% (143) of the 187 children whose BMI was above the 95th centile had an adult BMI 30 kg/m^2 (Table 1), and predictive values differed only slightly between boys (80%) and girls (73%). Of the 586 adults with a BMI $\geq$30 kg/m^2, 24% (sensitivity) had a childhood BMI 95th centile. It is likely that the high predictive value of childhood obesity in this cohort reflected, at least in part, the secular increase in adult obesity during the follow-up period. Of the children with a BMI $\geq$95th centile, one-fourth had an adult BMI 40 kg/m^2, emphasizing the potential consequences of recent secular trends.

These estimates, however, are markedly influenced by the categorization of BMI levels (Table 1). The positive predictive value increased with the childhood BMI cutoff point but decreased with the adult BMI cutoff point, ranging from 53% (childhood BMI $\geq$75th centile and adult BMI $\geq$30 kg/m^2) to 100%. Sensitivity showed the opposite relation to the cutoff points, ranging from 3% (adults with a BMI $\geq$25 kg/m^2 who had a childhood BMI $\geq$99th centile) to 60%. Relative risks increased with the adult BMI cutoff but varied only slightly across childhood cutoffs. The variability of these estimates can make it difficult to compare the results of studies using different BMI cutoff points.

Simple correlation coefficients, which do not depend upon the categorization of BMI levels, provide a measure of BMI tracking that can be more easily compared across studies. Figure 2 shows the association (Spearman $r = 0.61$) between childhood and adult BMI levels among the 2,640 persons. The magnitude of this association varied only slightly (0.57 to 0.65) across race/sex groups but was weaker for children less than 7 years of age than among older children ($r = 0.50$ versus 0.64). In addition, the strength of the association was inversely associated with the length of follow-up, ranging from $r = 0.76$ (less than 10 years of follow-up) to $r = 0.59$ (20 years). In contrast, the tracking of BMI levels among children in China appears to be substantially lower, with a correlation of 0.39 over a 6-year period among 6- to 13-year-olds (19).

Although childhood obesity is the strongest correlate of adult obesity, with multiple r^2 values (after accounting for race, sex, and age) of up to 0.40, other predictors of adult BMI include parental fatness, birth weight, the timing of sexual maturation, socioeconomic status, and physical activity (20). Children with an early adiposity rebound are also at increased risk of adult obesity, but it is possible that similar information can be obtained more easily from the BMI level at 7 years of age (21). Other anthropometric dimensions in childhood, such as height or triceps skinfold thickness, may also improve the prediction of adult BMI, and many of these characteristics can probably be examined in existing datasets.

Type 2 Diabetes Mellitus

In addition to the severity of obesity, the duration of obesity is an independent predictor of type 2 diabetes mellitus among adults (7). At similar levels of obesity, the

TABLE 1. *Positive predictive values, sensitivities, and relative risks using different BMI cutoff points: the Bogalusa Heart Study*

	Adult BMI	
Childhood BMI	≥ 25 kg/m² (N = 1266)	≥ 30 kg/m² (N = 586)
Positive predictive value[a]		
≥ 75 C (N = 670)	83% (555)	53% (354)
≥ 85 C (N = 443)	88% (392)	62% (274)
≥ 95 C (N = 187)	94% (175)	76% (143)
≥ 99 C (N = 32)	100% (32)	91% (29)
Sensitivity[b]		
≥ 75 C (N = 670)	44%	60%
≥ 85 C (N = 443)	31%	47%
≥ 95 C (N = 187)	14%	24%
≥ 99 C (N = 32)	3%	5%
Relative risk[c]		
≥ 75 C (N = 670)	2.3	4.5
≥ 85 C (N = 443)	2.2	4.4
≥ 95 C (N = 187)	2.1	4.2
≥ 99 C (N = 32)	2.1	4.2

Abbreviation: C, centile.

[a] The proportion of children who became overweight/obese adults; the number of true positives is shown in parentheses. For example, 555 of the 670 children with a BMI > 75th centile had an adult BMI ≥ 25 kg/m², yielding a positive predictive value of 83%.

[b] The proportion of overweight/obese adults whose childhood BMI was above the specified centile. Of the 1,266 adults who had a BMI ≥ 25 kg/m², 44% had a childhood BMI > 75th centile.

[c] The probability that a child with a BMI above the specified centile will be overweight/obese in adulthood as compared with that for a child with a lower BMI level.

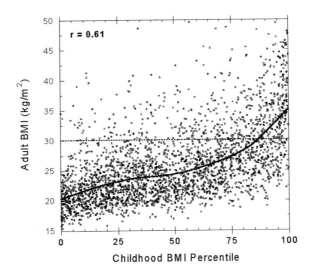

FIG. 2. The relation of childhood BMI centiles (*x* axis) to adult BMI levels over a (mean) 17-year follow-up period among 2,640 participants in the Bogalusa Heart Study. The smoothed line was constructed using the lowess procedure, with levels roughly corresponding to median BMI levels in adulthood. The horizontal line indicates the cutoff point for obesity in adulthood.

diabetes risk among Pima Indian adults is about twice as high among those who had been obese for more than 10 years than among those who had recently become obese (22). Associations with the duration of obesity have also been observed in other ethnic groups (23) and among 15- to 24-year-olds (22). The recent trends in childhood obesity will prolong its duration and probably increase the incidence of type 2 diabetes among adults.

The prevalence of type 2 diabetes among adults in the United States increased by around 40% during the 1980s (24), and an increase in incidence has also been noted. Despite the lack of national data among children, the prevalence of pediatric type 2 diabetes (estimated to be around 0.2%) also appears to be increasing (25,26). The prevalence among American Indian adolescents, for example, increased by around 50% during the 1980s (26), and comparable increases in incidence have been observed among schoolchildren in Tokyo (27). Clinic-based studies support these trends, with the annual number of newly diagnosed cases of type 2 diabetes among adolescents increasing from 2 to 20 (0.7 to 7.2 per 100,000) between 1982 and 1994 in the Cincinnati area (28).

Obesity is very common among newly diagnosed cases of pediatric type 2 diabetes, with mean BMI values ranging from 29 to 38 kg/m^2 in several studies (25), and the high prevalence of diabetes among American Indians, African Americans, and Hispanics may reflect their high rates of obesity. The potential effect of the recent obesity trends is highlighted by a study of Pima Indian adolescents in which a combination of birth weight, weight in childhood, and exposure to diabetes *in utero* accounted for most of the increase in type 2 diabetes since the 1960s (25). Secular increases in type 2 diabetes among schoolchildren in Tokyo have also been accompanied by increases in obesity (27). As the relation of obesity to type 2 diabetes risk among adults is exponential rather than linear, the increased prevalence of very overweight children is of great concern.

Although there are no long-term studies of children with type 2 diabetes, newly diagnosed cases often have microalbuminuria and hypertension, along with raised levels of insulin, C-peptide, and triglycerides (25,26). If the duration of hyperglycemia and hyperinsulinemia is the primary factor in the development of adverse health outcomes, the development of diabetes in early life will probably result in complications at young ages. Poor glycemic control among those with type 2 diabetes (as in type 1 [29]) is predictive of early retinopathy, nephropathy, and vascular disease (6), and high complication rates been observed in the short-term follow-up of children and young adults with type 2 diabetes (6,25). The poor compliance of adolescents with lifestyle modifications and medical treatment is likely to exacerbate these complications.

A better understanding of the natural history of pediatric type 2 diabetes will become increasingly important, as will assessment of the efficacy of various treatments. The possible interaction of childhood obesity with fetal undernutrition (30) in the development of type 2 diabetes should also be explored.

Atherosclerosis

Risk Factors in Childhood

Obesity among children is associated with adverse levels of several coronary heart disease risk factors, the magnitude of the correlations being typically stronger for levels of C-reactive protein, triglycerides, HDL cholesterol, blood pressure, and insulin ($r \sim 0.15$ to 0.30) than for levels of total and LDL cholesterol. Adverse levels of these risk factors are associated with the early stages of atherosclerosis (31) and tend to track into adulthood, but serial correlations are weaker than those for BMI.

Several aspects of the associations with coronary heart disease risk factors should be considered. Many of the relations are nonlinear, with risk factor levels often increasing only at BMI levels above the 75th centile. Furthermore, although most overweight children do not have a specific coronary heart disease risk factor, such as a high plasma triglyceride concentration, most have adverse levels of at least one risk factor (32). Furthermore, children with multiple risk factors may be at particularly high risk for the early stages of atherosclerosis (31), and about three-quarters of these children are overweight.

The standard chemical analysis of lipid levels also may have resulted in underestimating the importance of childhood obesity in dyslipidemia. The major lipoprotein classes—very low density (VLDL), LDL, and HDL—are heterogeneous, with coronary heart disease risk varying by the size of the lipoprotein subclass. The risk is increased by high levels of small LDL and small HDL particles, in contrast to the protective effect of the typically measured HDL cholesterol level, and varies according to the size of VLDL particles (33). Although the relation of lipoprotein subclass levels in childhood to atherosclerosis has not been studied, subclass levels are associated with insulin levels and obesity in childhood.

The relation of BMI and waist circumference to various lipoprotein subclasses among 916 adolescents, determined by nuclear magnetic resonance (NMR) spectroscopy (33), is shown in Table 2. Associations with childhood BMI centiles and waist circumference measurements were generally similar in magnitude, but there were large differences within each lipoprotein class. For example, BMI was related to levels of HDL cholesterol ($r = 0.34$), but the inverse association with large HDL was stronger ($r = 0.50$) and there was a positive association ($r = 0.13$) with levels of small HDL. BMI also showed differing associations with levels of large and small LDL (negative and positive, respectively), and was not associated with levels of small VLDL.

The relation of obesity to various risk factors also varies by race/ethnicity. For example, childhood BMI in the Bogalusa Heart Study is more strongly related to triglyceride levels among whites than among blacks (Fig. 3). Whereas levels of triglyceride among white children differed by about 40 to 60 mg/dl (0.45 to 0.67 mmol/l) across BMI centiles, differences of around 10 mg/dl (0.11 mmol/l) were seen among black girls. Furthermore, overweight black children tended to have triglyceride levels that were similar to those seen among thin white children, a finding that may reflect differences in the activity of lipoprotein lipase. These racial differences, which are also present among young adults, may partly account for the weak relation of obesity to coronary heart disease that has often been seen among black adults.

TABLE 2. *Relation of body mass index (BMI) and waist circumference to levels of lipids and lipoprotein subclasses among 916 10- to 17-year-olds: the Bogalusa Heart Study*

	BMI centile	Waist circumference
Total cholesterol	0.16[a]	0.14
Triglycerides	0.33	0.35
Large VLDL	0.30	0.32
Small VLDL	0.02	0.03
VLDL size[b]	0.24	0.25
LDL cholesterol	0.23	0.22
Large LDL	−0.12	−0.13
Small LDL	0.15	0.13
LDL size[b]	−0.28	−0.28
HDL cholesterol	−0.34	−0.39
Large HDL	−0.50	−0.53
Small HDL	0.13	0.14
HDL size[b]	−0.53	−0.55

Abbreviations: HDL, high-density lipoprotein; LDL, low-density lipoprotein; VLDL, very-low-density lipoprotein.

[a] Values are Spearman correlations that have been adjusted for race, sex, and age. With a sample size of 916, a correlation of 0.08 is statistically significant at the 0.01 level.

[b] The lipoprotein particle sizes, which represent the mass weighted average size of the VLDL, LDL, or HDL particles, are in nanometers. All other lipid measurements are concentrations.

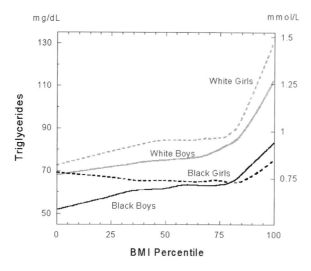

FIG. 3. The relation of childhood BMI centiles to triglyceride levels among children in the Bogalusa Heart Study. Lowess curves were constructed separately for each race/sex group. Black children are shown with black lines, white children with gray lines, boys with solid lines, and girls with dashed lines.

Risk Factors in Adulthood

Obese children have also been found to have adverse levels of lipids, insulin, and blood pressure in adulthood. However, because of the strong tracking of BMI, these associations may reflect the importance of adult rather than childhood weight status. If the development of obesity at specific ages in childhood or adolescence were found to have an independent effect on adult risk factor levels, preventive efforts could focus on these age groups.

These associations were studied among 2,609 people who were initially examined between the ages of 2 and 17 years in the Bogalusa Heart Study and who were followed for an average of 17 years. Childhood BMI was related to adult risk factor levels, with the magnitudes of the correlations ranging from $r = 0.08$ (systolic blood pressure) to $r = 0.26$ (insulin). Mean levels of the examined risk factors in adulthood also differed among those who had a childhood BMI above the 95th centile and those whose childhood BMI was less than the 50th centile, with a 7 mg/dl (0.18 mmol/l) difference seen for levels of HDL cholesterol (Table 3). Within categories of adult BMI (<25 kg/m^2 and 30 kg/m^2), however, risk-factor levels varied only slightly according to childhood weight status. (See the last four columns of Table 3.) Mean concentrations of HDL cholesterol among normal-weight adults, for example, were 54 mg/dl (1.40 mmol/l) for childhood BMI $<$ 50th centile, and 55 mg/dl (1.42 mmol/l) for childhood BMI $\geq$95th centile, and the mean level was 42 mg/dl (1.09 mmol/l) among both subgroups of obese adults. Additional analyses (data not shown) revealed that adult risk factor levels were not influenced by the age of obesity onset (childhood, adolescence, or adulthood).

TABLE 3. *Mean risk factor levels in adulthood by categories of adult body mass index (BMI) and childhood BMI centile (C): the Bogalusa Heart Study*

			Adult BMI (kg/m^2)			
			<25 kg/m^2		>30 kg/m^2	
	Childhood BMI centile		Childhood BMI centile		Childhood BMI centile	
	<50th C	≥ 95th C	<50th C	≥ 95th C	<50th C	≥ 95th C
N	1,317	186	950	12	96	144
Childhood BMI centile	24	97	22	96	28	98
Adult levels						
Age (years)	27	27	27	25	29	27
BMI (kg/m^2)	22.5[a]	34.9[a]	21.1[a]	23.6[a]	33.2[a]	38.1[a]
Triglycerides (mg/dl)[b]	82[a]	108[a]	76[a]	53[a]	130	124
LDL cholesterol (mg/dl)	112[a]	121[a]	107	103	130	126
HDL cholesterol (mg/dl)	52[a]	45[a]	54	55	42	42
Insulin (mU/l)[b]	8[a]	14[a]	7	7	17	17
SBP (mm Hg)	112[a]	117[a]	111	105	117	119
DBP (mm Hg)	72[a]	76[a]	71	68	77	78

Abbreviations: DBP, diastolic blood pressure; HDL, high-density lipoprotein; LDL, low-density lipoprotein; SBP, systolic blood pressure.

[a] $p < 0.05$ for difference in adult levels between persons whose childhood BMI P was < 50th centile or ≥ 95th centile.

[b] Geometric means are shown for levels of triglycerides and insulin.

It should be realized, however, that these results apply to risk factor levels, and childhood obesity may have a long-term cumulative effect on the development of atherosclerosis. The duration of hypercholesterolemia, for example, is strongly correlated with the extent of coronary artery calcification (34), and the duration of obesity may have a similar influence.

Assessment of Atherosclerosis

The initial stages of atherosclerosis begin in the aorta by the age of 3 years, and appear 5 to 10 years later in the coronary arteries, with some of these fatty streaks progressing to more advanced atherosclerotic lesions. Pathology studies of children and young adults who died from external causes indicate that obesity plays a role in the development of these lesions. Among decedents (ages 2 to 39 years) who had participated in the Bogalusa Heart Study (31), previously measured BMI was associated ($r = 0.24$ to 0.41) with both fatty streaks and fibrous plaques. Interestingly, associations with BMI were comparable in magnitude to those with LDL cholesterol levels and were stronger than those with diastolic blood pressure and HDL cholesterol. Another study (35) of young adults (ages 15 to 34 years) found that BMI at death was associated with raised lesions in the coronary arteries among men, but not women.

The role of obesity has also been assessed using noninvasive techniques, such as B-mode ultrasonography and electron beam tomography (EBT), that provide information on the extent of atherosclerosis in the carotid and coronary arteries, respectively (36). Among 384 young adults (mean age 33 years) who had been examined in the Muscatine Heart Study (37), childhood BMI and triceps skinfold thickness were more predictive of EBT-determined coronary artery calcification than were levels of lipids and blood pressure. Somewhat similar associations have also been seen in cross-sectional studies of 28- to 40-year-olds (38), and hypercholesterolemic 11- to 23-year-olds (39).

Associations with intima–media thickness, an early atherosclerotic change that is typically assessed in the carotid artery with B-mode ultrasonography, have been less consistent. Some investigators have found BMI levels to be associated with in-tima–media thickness among children (40) and young adults (41), the magnitude of the correlations being at least as strong as those with lipid levels. However, negative results have also been reported, and the strength of the association varies according to the site at which intima–media thickness is assessed (40).

Despite concerns about disease classification, reproducibility, and specificity (36), these noninvasive techniques would allow serial estimates of the extent of athero-sclerosis to be made in representative cohorts of children. These studies could greatly advance the understanding of the risks associated with childhood obesity and other risk factors. Longitudinal analyses would be able to assess whether the effect of childhood BMI (and body fat distribution) is independent of adult BMI and whether specific ages are critical for the development of obesity.

Adult Morbidity and Mortality

Background

The relation of childhood obesity to adult mortality and morbidity has been examined in several cohort studies (42–48) that have varied in design. Whereas some children have been followed prospectively (46,48), most investigators have identified cohorts in adulthood who had baseline (historical) data previously collected by elementary schools (43,47), by colleges (42), or in preparation for military service (44,45). In ad-dition, some studies of adults (49–51) have been able to examine the relation of BMI at 18 years of age, based on self-reported weight, to morbidity and mortality.

Participation rates in these studies have varied substantially, with around 50% of eligible subjects in some studies not being traced or reexamined (43,47). These sub-stantial losses to follow-up, which are not unexpected over periods of several decades, could greatly increase the potential for bias. The results of the historical co-hort studies, along with those that used self-reported weight at age 18 years, could also be biased if childhood obesity was related to premature mortality that occurred before the formation of the adult cohort.

Other differences among these studies include, first, the classification of normal weight and overweight (typically, the upper fourth or fifth of the BMI distribution, or a value of more than 25 kg/m^2); second, sample sizes that range from 508 (46) to more than 78,000 (45); and third, mean baseline ages that ranged from approximately 8 years (48) to 19 years (42). In addition, few of these studies have information on BMI levels in both childhood and adulthood, precluding the assessment of an inde-pendent effect of childhood BMI on adult disease. Furthermore, in the studies with information on BMI in both adulthood and childhood (43,46) (or at age 18 years [49–51]), one BMI value was always based on self-reported weight.

Effects of Childhood Obesity

Despite the numerous differences in study design, overweight children have consistently been found to be at increased risk of premature mortality, with relative risks (RR) generally ranging from 1.3 to 2.0. This increased mortality is largely attributable to coronary heart disease (RR 1.7 to 2.5). Childhood obesity has also been found to increase the risk for diabetes mellitus, colon cancer, menstrual problems, gestational hypertension, gout, arthritis, and hip fractures in adulthood (2,4). Although information on potential confounders has varied across studies, associations with childhood BMI do not appear to reflect the effects of various socioeconomic characteristics (including number of siblings, education, and social class) (45,48,51), cigarette smoking (46,51), or general health status (45).

The consistency of the findings for the relation of childhood obesity to coronary heart disease and total mortality contrasts with the sometimes weak (or null) results of studies of modest overweight among adults. These differences may be attributable, in part, to the long follow-up periods in studies of childhood obesity, as well as to the lack of confounding by preclinical disease and cigarette smoking. In addition, the relation of adult obesity to mortality, typically assessed with relative risks or rate ratios, is stronger among young adults than among older persons (52), and this interaction with age may extend into adolescence.

However, some differences among these findings should be considered. The effects of modest obesity among adults have often been seen only after a long follow-up, and one study (45) found overweight adolescents to be at increased risk only after the age of 40 years. Other investigators, in contrast, have found the risk among overweight 18- to 19-year-olds to be raised after 5 years of follow-up (44) or highest before 45 years of age (42). It has been suggested that overweight in adolescence is more strongly related to adult disease among boys than to that among girls (46), but the opposite has been found as well (47). It is also possible that associations are J shaped (45,48), with the lowest risks occurring at a childhood BMI between the 25th and 49th centiles (48). The possibility that the effects of childhood obesity may be limited to specific subgroups, such as those who are relatively tall (42) or sedentary, has received little attention.

It should be realized that the typical categorization of childhood BMI levels has resulted in very high BMI levels (e.g., 31 kg/m^2 at age 18 years) being assessed in only one study (44). Studies of the relatively low BMI levels seen among children in the 1920s to 1940s may underestimate the risks associated with the higher BMI levels that are currently seen among children.

Is The Relation Independent of Adult Obesity?

Because of the persistence of weight status throughout life, with overweight children likely to be obese adults, the observed associations could reflect the importance of adult weight status. Although most studies do not have information on BMI levels in both childhood and adulthood, and have therefore been unable to disentangle their effects, results of the Harvard growth study support an independent effect of childhood obesity. Over 55 years of follow-up, multivariable adjustment for adult BMI only slightly reduced the relation of adolescent overweight (BMI more than 75th centile) to mortality from all causes (RR of 2.9 [unadjusted] versus 2.4 [adjusted]) and from coronary heart disease (2.6 versus 1.9) among men (46). Although the adult BMI level was based on self-reported weight at age 53 years from only 61% of the study cohort, it was related to both disease risk and childhood BMI levels (Must A, personal communication).

In contrast to these findings, other results have emphasized the greater importance of adult weight status. For example, although overweight (>20% above average weight) children in Washington County (43) had high adult rates of vascular disease, a cross classification of child and adult weight categories indicated that the risks were highest for thin children who became overweight in adulthood. In addition, multivariable analyses in the Nurses' Health Study indicated that the relation of BMI at age 18 years (based on self-reported weight) to diabetes mellitus (49) and coronary heart disease (50) was attributable to the persistence of obesity. With adjustment for adult BMI, RRs for the upper BMI category at age 18 years decreased from 6.1 to 0.8 (diabetes) and from 1.8 to 1.0 (coronary heart disease). The Harvard Growth Study (46) also found that the relation of adolescent overweight to diabetes in adulthood was mediated by adult weight status.

The possible effects of BMI misclassification in these results, owing to the use of self-reported weight at age 53 years (46) or at 18 years (49–51), should be considered. Although self-reports of previous weights are highly correlated with measured weights ($r > 0.75$), obese adults (particularly women) tend to underestimate earlier weight status by an average of 5 to 8 kg (53). This systemic underreporting by obese persons, along with any nondifferential misclassification, could reduce the strength of the association between BMI and disease. In these studies, the BMI that was calculated from measured weight—whether in childhood (46) or in adulthood (49,50)— has been found to be more strongly related to disease risk than the BMI estimated from self-reported weight.

Weight Gain

Adults with lifelong obesity may have a more favorable distribution of body fat than obese adults who had been normal-weight children (54), and some results suggests that weight gain after childhood is an important predictor of disease. Among overweight adults, those who had been thin in childhood have higher rates of hypertensive vascular disease (43) and diabetes mellitus (55) than those who had been overweight children. It is possible that weight gain after the cessation of growth, which would largely reflect accumulated fat mass, may be more pathologic than weight gain during growth and development (4).

Although it can be difficult to separate the effects of weight gain from attained weight status, other findings have also emphasized the importance of adult weight gain. In the Rancho Bernardo Study (55), the proportional change in weight from age 18 years was a strong predictor of type 2 diabetes. Diabetes risk has also been related to weight gain after puberty among overweight children (56), after age 18 years among women in the Nurses' Health Study (49), and after age 30 to 35 years among Pima Indian men (57). Adult weight gain has also been related to the development of coronary heart disease (50,58), with each 10% increase in weight after age 20 years increasing the risk by 17% (58). Although it has also been reported that adult weight gain is not associated with total mortality (51), its effect on coronary heart disease risk may be largely mediated through an association with diabetes, and with levels of cholesterol, blood pressure, and physical activity.

It should be realized, however, that many of these findings are based on self-reported weight in childhood or at age 18 years (49,50,55,58), and a systematic underreporting of previous weight by obese adults would spuriously increase the magnitudes of the observed associations. In contrast, the importance of weight gain would be underestimated if the confounding effects of cigarette smoking (including its cessation) are not adequately controlled (51,58).

SUMMARY

Overweight children are at increased risk for coronary heart disease and premature mortality in adulthood, and with the recent secular increase in childhood obesity, these long-term consequences will become increasingly evident. It is not certain, however, if these associations reflect the effect of childhood obesity itself, or the persistence of obesity throughout life, with adult weight status being the important factor. Because of the many difficulties involved in following cohorts of children for periods of over 50 years, it would be useful to examine these interrelations using noninvasive techniques, such as ultrasound or electron beam tomography, to quantify the extent of atherosclerosis.

Noninvasive techniques would also be very valuable in assessing the effects of weight gain in adulthood on subsequent coronary heart disease. These cross-sectional and short-term cohort studies would be particularly valuable if recorded information on childhood weights and heights were available. Analyses could then examine the independent effects of childhood and adult weight status, and assess whether the development of obesity at specific ages is particularly detrimental.

It is likely, however, that the first consequence of the recent trends in obesity will be an increase in the incidence of pediatric type 2 diabetes, and a better understanding of its natural history is needed. The difficulties in preventing and reversing obesity, along with the frequent nonadherence of adolescents to lifestyle changes and medical treatment, will complicate treatment and prevention efforts. However, as the long-term complications of diabetes are related to the duration of hyperglycemia, the implications of large numbers of children with type 2 diabetes will be substantial.

REFERENCES

1. Dietz WH. Health consequences of obesity in youth: childhood predictors of adult disease. *Pediatrics* 1998; 101: 518–25.

2. Must A, Strauss RS. Risks and consequences of childhood and adolescent obesity. *Int J Obes Relat Metab Disord* 1999; 23: 2–11.
3. Freedman DS, Srinivasan SR, Valdez RA, Williamson DF, Berenson GS. Secular increases in relative weight and adiposity among children over two decades: the Bogalusa Heart Study. *Pediatrics* 1997; 99: 420–5.
4. Power C, Lake JK, Cole TJ. Measurement and long-term health risks of child and adolescent fatness. *Int J Obes* 1997; 21: 507–26.
5. Kuczmarski RJ, Flegal KM. Criteria for definition of overweight in transition: background and recommendations for the United States. *Am J Clin Nutr* 2000; 72: 1074–81.
6. Yokoyama H, Okudaira M, Otani T, *et al.* Existence of early-onset NIDDM Japanese demonstrating severe diabetic complications. *Diabetes Care* 1997; 20: 844–7.
7. Seidell JC. Obesity, insulin resistance and diabetes—a worldwide epidemic. *Br J Nutr* 2000; 83: 5–8.
8. Vague J. The degree of masculine differentiation of obesities: a factor determining predisposition to diabetes, atherosclerosis, gout, and uric calculous disease. *Am J Clin Nutr* 1956; 4: 20–34.
9. Frayn KN. Visceral fat and insulin resistance—causative or correlative? *Br J Nutr* 2000; 83: 71–7.
10. Freedman DS, Serdula MK, Srinivasan SR, Berenson GS. The relation of circumferences and skinfolds to levels of lipids and insulin: the Bogalusa Heart Study. *Am J Clin Nutr* 1999; 69: 308–17.
11. Daniels SR, Khoury PR, Morrison JA. Utility of different measure of body fat distribution in children and adolescents. *Am J Epidemiol* 2000; 152: 1179–84.
12. Flegal KM, Troiano RP. Changes in the distribution of body mass index of adults and children in the US population. *Int J Obes Relat Metab Disord* 2000; 24: 807–18.
13. Lazarus R, Wake M, Hesketh K, Waters E. Change in body mass index in Australian primary school children, 1985–1997. *Int J Obes Relat Metab Disord* 2000; 24: 679–84.
14. De Onis M, Blossner M. Prevalence and trends of overweight among preschool children in developing countries. *Am J Clin Nutr* 2000; 72: 1032–9.
15. Gortmaker SL, Must A, Perrin JM, Sobol AM, Dietz WH. Social and economic consequences of overweight in adolescence and young adulthood. *N Engl J Med* 1993; 329: 1008–12.
16. Sargent JD, Blanchflower DG. Obesity and stature in adolescence and earnings in young adulthood. Analysis of a British birth cohort. *Arch Pediatr Adolesc Med* 1994; 148: 681–7.
17. Popkin BM, Keyou G, Zhai F, Guo X, Ma H, Zohoori N. The nutrition transition in China: a cross-sectional analysis. *Eur J Clin Nutr* 1993; 47: 333–46.
18. Serdula MK, Ivery D, Coates RJ, Freedman DS, Williamson DF, Byers T. Do obese children become obese adults? A review of the literature. *Prev Med* 1993; 22: 167–77.
19. Wang Y, Ge K, Popkin BM. Tracking of body mass index from childhood to adolescence: a 6-y follow-up study in China. *Am J Clin Nutr* 2000; 72: 1018–24.
20. Parsons TJ, Power C, Logan S, Summerbell CD. Childhood predictors of adult obesity: a systematic review. *Int J Obes Relat Metab Disord* 1999; 23: 1–107.
21. Williams S, Davie G, Lam F. Predicting BMI in young adults from childhood data using two approaches to modelling adiposity rebound. *Int J Obes Relat Metab Disord* 1999; 23: 348–54.
22. Everhart JE, Pettitt DJ, Bennett PH, Knowler WC. Duration of obesity increases the incidence of NIDDM. *Diabetes* 1992; 41: 235–40.
23. Sakurai Y. Duration of obesity and risk of noninsulin-dependent diabetes mellitus. *Biomed Pharmacother* 2000; 54: 80–4.
24. Harris MI, Flegal KM, Cowie CC, *et al.* Prevalence of diabetes, impaired fasting glucose, and impaired glucose tolerance in U.S. adults. The Third National Health and Nutrition Examination Survey, 1988–1994. *Diabetes Care* 1998 ; 21: 518–24.
25. Dabelea D, Pettitt DJ, Jones KL, Arslanian SA. Type 2 diabetes mellitus in minority children and adolescents. An emerging problem. *Endocrinol Metab Clin North Am* 1999; 28: 709–29.
26. Fagot-Campagna A, Pettitt DJ, Engelgau MM, *et al.* Type 2 diabetes among North American children and adolescents: an epidemiologic review and a public health perspective. *J Pediatr* 2000; 136: 664–72.
27. Kitagawa T, Owada M, Urakami T, Tajima N. Epidemiology of type 1 (insulin-dependent) and type 2 (non-insulin-dependent) diabetes mellitus in Japanese children. *Diabetes Res Clin Pract* 1994; 24: 7–13.
28. Pinhas-Hamiel O, Dolan LM, Daniels SR, Standiford D, Khoury PR, Zeitler P. Increased incidence of non-insulin-dependent diabetes mellitus among adolescents. *J Pediatr* 1996; 128: 608–15.
29. DCCT Research Group. The relationship of glycemic exposure (HbA1c) to the risk of development and progression of retinopathy in the diabetes control and complications trial. *Diabetes* 1995; 44: 968–83.

30. Phillips DI. Insulin resistance as a programmed response to fetal undernutrition. *Diabetologia* 1996; 39: 1119–22.
31. Berenson GS, Srinivasan SR, Bao W, Newman WP, Tracy RE, Wattigney WA. Association between multiple cardiovascular risk factors and atherosclerosis in children and young adults. The Bogalusa Heart Study. *N Engl J Med* 1998; 338: 1650–6.
32. Freedman DS, Dietz W, Srinivasan SR, Berenson GS. The relation of overweight to cardiovascular risk factors among children and adolescents: the Bogalusa Heart Study. *Pediatrics* 1999; 103: 1175–82.
33. Freedman DS, Otvos JD, Jeyarajah EJ, Barboriak JJ, Anderson AJ, Walker JA. Relation of lipoprotein subclasses as measured by proton nuclear magnetic resonance spectroscopy to coronary artery disease. *Arterioscler Thromb Vasc Biol* 1998; 18: 1046–53.
34. Schmidt HH, Hill S, Makariou EV, Feuerstein IM, Dugi KA, Hoeg JM. Relation of cholesterol–year score to severity of calcific atherosclerosis and tissue deposition in homozygous familial hypercholesterolemia. *Am J Cardiol* 1996; 77: 575–80.
35. McGill HC, McMahan CA, Zieske AW, *et al.* Associations of coronary heart disease risk factors with the intermediate lesion of atherosclerosis in youth. The Pathobiological Determinants of Atherosclerosis in Youth (PDAY) Research Group. *Arterioscler Thromb Vasc Biol* 2000; 20: 1998–2004.
36. O'Rourke RA, Brundage BH, Froelicher VF, *et al.* American College of Cardiology/American Heart Association Expert Consensus Document on electron-beam computed tomography for the diagnosis and prognosis of coronary artery disease. *J Am Coll Cardiol* 2000; 36: 326–40.
37. Mahoney LT, Burns TL, Stanford W, *et al.* Coronary risk factors measured in childhood and young adult life are associated with coronary artery calcification in young adults: the Muscatine Study. *J Am Coll Cardiol* 1996; 27: 277–84.
38. Bild DE, Folsom AR, Lowe LP, *et al.* Prevalence and correlates of coronary calcification in black and white young adults: The Coronary Artery Risk Development in Young Adults (CARDIA) Study. *Arterioscler Thromb Vasc Biol* 2001; 21: 852–7.
39. Gidding SS, Bookstein LC, Chomka EV. Usefulness of electron beam tomography in adolescents and young adults with heterozygous familial hypercholesterolemia. *Circulation* 1998; 98: 2580–3.
40. Tonstad S, Joakimsen O, Stensland-Bugge E, *et al.* Risk factors related to carotid intima–media thickness and plaque in children with familial hypercholesterolemia and control subjects. *Arterioscler Thromb Vasc Biol* 1996; 16: 984–91.
41. Ciccone M, Maiorano A, De Pergola G, Minenna A, Giorgino R, Rizzon P. Microcirculatory damage of common carotid artery wall in obese and non obese subjects. *Clin Hemorheol Microcirc* 1999; 21: 365–74.
42. Paffenbarger RS, Wing AL. Chronic disease in former college students: the effects of single and multiple characteristics on risk of fatal coronary heart disease. *Am J Epidemiol* 1969; 90: 527–35.
43. Abraham S, Collins G, Nordsieck M. Relationship of childhood weight status to morbidity in adults. *HSMHA Health Rep* 1971; 86: 273–84.
44. Sonne-Holm S, Sorensen TI, Christensen U. Risk of early death in extremely overweight young men. *BMJ* 1983; 287: 795–7.
45. Hoffmans MD, Kromhout D, de Lezenne Coulander C. The impact of body mass index of 78,612 Dutch men on 32-year mortality. *J Clin Epidemiol* 1988; 41: 749–56.
46. Must A, Jacques PF, Dallal GE, Bajema CJ, Dietz WH. Long-term morbidity and mortality of overweight adolescents. A follow-up of the Harvard Growth Study of 1922 to 1935. *N Engl J Med* 1992; 327: 1350–5.
47. Nieto FJ, Szklo M, Comstock GW. Childhood weight and growth rate as predictors of adult mortality. *Am J Epidemiol* 1992; 136: 201–13.
48. Gunnell DJ, Frankel SJ, Nanchahal K, Peters TJ, Davey Smith G. Childhood obesity and adult cardiovascular mortality: a 57-y follow-up study based on the Boyd Orr cohort. *Am J Clin Nutr* 1998; 67: 1111–8.
49. Colditz GA, Willett WC, Stampfer MJ, *et al.* Weight as a risk factor for clinical diabetes in women. *Am J Epidemiol* 1990; 132: 501–13.
50. Willett WC, Manson JE, Stampfer MJ, *et al.* Weight, weight change, and coronary heart disease in women. Risk within the "normal" weight range. *JAMA* 1995; 273: 461–5.
51. Yarnell JW, Patterson CC, Thomas HF, Sweetnam PM. Comparison of weight in middle age, weight at 18 years, and weight change between, in predicting subsequent 14 year mortality and coronary events: Caerphilly prospective study. *J Epidemiol Community Health* 2000; 54: 344–8.
52. Stevens J, Cai J, Juhaeri, Thun MJ, Williamson DF, Wood JL. Consequences of the use of different

measures of effect to determine the impact of age on the association between obesity and mortality. *Am J Epidemiol* 1999; 150: 399–407.

53. Perry GS, Byers TE, Mokdad AH, Serdula MK, Williamson DF. The validity of self-reports of past body weights by US adults. *Epidemiology* 1995; 6: 61–6.
54. Albrink MJ, Meigs JW. Interrelationships between skinfold thickness, serum lipids and blood sugar in normal men. *Am J Clin Nutr* 1964; 15: 255–61.
55. Holbrook TL, Barrett-Connor E, Wingard DL. The association of lifetime weight and weight control patterns with diabetes among men and women in an adult community. *Int J Obes* 1989; 13: 723–9.
56. DiPietro L, Mossberg HO, Stunkard AJ. A 40-year history of overweight children in Stockholm: lifetime overweight, morbidity, and mortality. *Int J Obes* 1994; 18: 585–90.
57. Hanson RL, Narayan KM, McCance DR, *et al.* Rate of weight gain, weight fluctuation, and incidence of NIDDM. *Diabetes* 1995; 44: 261–6.
58. Rosengren A, Wedel H, Wilhelmsen L. Body weight and weight gain during adult life in men in relation to coronary heart disease and mortality. A prospective population study. *Eur Heart J* 1999; 20: 269–77.

DISCUSSION

Dr. Dietz: In response to earlier questions about the predictive validity of the BMI, we can say that these data now represent the second dataset showing that a BMI above the 95th centile is of substantial predictive value for persistence of obesity, the other being the Whitaker dataset (1). With Dr. Freedman's earlier paper on the association of cardiovascular disease risk factors with a BMI over the 95th centile—at least in the US population (2)—these data should allow us to argue that there is some clinical validity using these cutoff points.

Dr. Freedman: One thing to note, though, is that these are continuous variables and where exactly to make the cutoff point can be debated. If the cutoff point was the 94th or the 96th centile, much the same associations will be seen. So although it is true that there is a strong association between childhood obesity and adult obesity, it is not exactly clear where to make the cutoff.

Dr. Endres: You described "pediatric diabetes" starting in the third decade. Isn't that rather out of the frame of pediatrics?

Dr. Freedman: I did show a slide of the development of diabetes before the age of 30, but I used that because there are no cohort studies of pediatric type 2 diabetes. When I was referring to "pediatric" type 2 diabetes, I really meant before the age of 18. Some of the secular trends referred to in the Pima Indians involve 10- to 19-year-olds, and I think that would be accepted as pediatric type 2 diabetes.

Dr. Dulloo: On the issue of ethnicity and the relation of BMI to percentage body fat, I have a question about the Mauritian data, as I originally came from Mauritius. The data you presented from the Dowse study (3,4) were in Mauritian Chinese, in whom for a particular BMI the prevalence of diabetes was increased. However, I'm sure the investigators must also have obtained data from Indian Mauritians, who are also classified as Asians, and from the Africans who inhabit the island. How do they compare with the ethnic Chinese?

Dr. Freedman: In a study by Deurenberg (5) I think the Chinese in Mauritius came fairly close to the median for the Asian populations. Although I hate to admit it, the situation is much more complicated than I presented. For example, different results are found among Chinese in Singapore versus Chinese in Beijing in terms of the relation of BMI to percent body fat. With regard to BMI and diabetes in Mauritian Indians and Africans, I'm afraid I do not recall the findings of the Dowse study.

Dr. Gortmaker: It's a small point, but you say that the data from the nurses' and health professionals' studies imply there is no independent effect of obesity in adolescence on the onset of diabetes in adulthood. However, if obesity in adolescence is seen as a *cause* of obesity in adulthood, then you could say that there is this very strong indirect pathway whereby adolescent obesity does in fact cause diabetes in adult life. At least that's the way I interpret it. Can you comment?

Dr. Freedman: That's true. The question is whether you consider it to be a confounding factor or an intervening factor. If childhood obesity is a cause of adult obesity, which it is, then there is an effect of childhood obesity on adult diabetes, but it's mediated through its association with adult obesity. One can interpret the data, at least in the Nurses' Health Study, to imply that a nonoverweight child who becomes an obese adult will have the same risk of developing diabetes in adulthood as a person who had been obese for their entire life.

Dr. Dulloo: I would like to return to one of your graphs illustrating the tracking of obesity, where you had adult BMI versus childhood BMI. There was a large scatter and a very slow rising curve between the 5th and the 75th centiles, which only became exponential between the 75th and the 95th centiles. Your overall *r* value was 0.6. If you were to eliminate that last bit of the graph between the 75th and 95th centiles, would you still see a correlation?

Dr. Freedman: One should be very careful about interpreting graphs showing BMI centiles. They can be very useful because you don't have to worry about controlling for age and sex in the analysis, but in terms of centiles, a change from, say, the 90th to the 95th centile represents a large change in BMI units, whereas a different 5 percent change, say from the 50th to the 55th centile, represents only a very small change in BMI units. If you were to apply BMI in childhood versus BMI in adulthood and at the same time control for age and sex, you would find it much more linear than on that chart.

Dr. Dulloo: But if we just look at the centiles between 0 and 75, I won't expect any relation between childhood and adult BMI.

Dr. Freedman: To some extent, that is true, but the reason for it is that the change going from the 75th centile of BMI up to the 100th centile is probably much larger than the change going from zero to the 75th centile in terms of actual BMI units. That's in large part the reason for the curvilinearity and why the relation would be much weaker if you were to eliminate the upper 25 percent. But you are right in terms of that chart—the association would be much weaker if you eliminated the top 5 or 10 percent of BMI.

Dr. Cole: The point that you are just making is that it would actually be better to work on a scale of BMI *z* score rather than BMI centiles. If you used BMI *z* score as your *x* axis on that graph, you would avoid the problem of squashing together the high centiles and the low centiles, and you would be working on a scale that is closer to BMI itself.

Dr. Freeman: Thank you. Other people have suggested that to me, and I looked at that. Surprisingly, it was almost exactly the same—it was curvilinear in the same way as the BMI centiles.

Dr. Cole: I'm glad it was the same, but as a general point it is not a good idea to do calculations on the centile scale because it is nonlinear and bounded at the upper and lower ends, unlike the *z* score scale.

Dr. Endres: I know you tried to simplify your analysis of the relation between obesity and disease in later adulthood by limiting the amount of data, but do you have information on correlations between obesity in childhood and other factors related to cardiovascular disease, such as cholesterol, uric acid, or homocysteine? Are such data worthless?

Dr. Freedman: No, they are not worthless at all. There are many strong associations with risk factors for coronary heart disease such as HDL cholesterol, LDL cholesterol and so on, and these have been reported in many cross-sectional studies. What I think is the most interesting now is that people are measuring lipoprotein subclasses, and sometimes there are different associations within each subclass (6,7). For example, childhood obesity is related to the small, dense LDL, but there is really no association with the larger LDL particles. There are some differences as well in the HDL and VLDL subclasses. I should also mention that in these cross-sectional associations there are often ethnic differences in outcomes. For example, there appears to be a weaker association between childhood obesity and triglyceride levels among black children than among white children (8,9).

Dr. Jacob: Have you seen any consequences of childhood obesity on eating disorders in adults?

Dr. Freedman: I'm afraid I'm not familiar with that literature.

REFERENCES

1. Whitaker RC, Wright JA, Pepe MS, *et al.* Predicting obesity in young adulthood from childhood and parental obesity. *N Engl J Med* 1997; 337: 869–73.
2. Freedman DS, Dietz W, Srinivasan SR, *et al.* The relation of overweight to cardiovascular risk factors among children and adolescents: The Bogalusa Heart Study. *Pediatrics* 1999; 103: 1175–82.
3. Dowse GK, Qin H, Collins VR, *et al.* Determinants of estimated insulin resistance and beta-cell function in Indian, Creole and Chinese Mauritians. The Mauritius NCD Study Group. *Diabetes Res Clin Pract* 1990 ; 10: 265–79.
4. Dowse GK. Incidence of NIDDM and the natural history of IGT in Pacific and Indian Ocean populations. *Diabetes Res Clin Pract.* 1996; 34: 45–50.
5. Deurenberg P, Yap M, van Stavern WA. Body mass index and percent body fat: a meta analysis among different ethnic groups. *Int J Obes Relat Metab Disord* 1998; 22: 1164–71.
6. Freedman DS, Otvos JD, Jeyarajah EJ, *et al.* Relation of lipoprotein subclasses as measured by proton nuclear magnetic resonance spectroscopy to coronary artery disease. *Arterioscler Thromb Vasc Biol* 1998; 18: 1046–53.
7. Campos H, Moye LA, Glasser SP, *et al.* Low-density lipoprotein size, pravastatin treatment, and coronary events. *JAMA* 2001; 286: 1468–74.
8. Freedman DS, Bowman BA, Otvos JD, *et al.* Levels and correlates of LDL and VLDL particle sizes among children: the Bogalusa Heart Study. *Atherosclerosis* 2000; 152: 441–9.
9. Freedman DS, Bowman BA, Otvos JD, *et al.* Black/white differences in the relation of obesity to levels of triglycerides and VLDL subclasses among children: the Bogalusa Heart Study. *Am J Clin Nutr* (in press).

Obesity in Childhood and Adolescence, edited by
Chunming Chen and William H. Dietz. Nestlé
Nutrition Workshop Series, Pediatric Program,
Vol. 49. Nestec Ltd., Vevey/Lippincott
Williams & Wilkins, Philadelphia © 2002.

Early Origins of Obesity

Atul Singhal, Julie Lanigan, and Alan Lucas

MRC Childhood Nutrition Research Centre, Institute of Child Health, London, England, UK

The global epidemic of childhood obesity is a major public health issue. Although a positive energy balance is likely to be a final common pathway for obesity, the determinants of this imbalance are much debated. Secular changes in eating behavior and genetic susceptibility are factors that have received a considerable amount of attention recently. However, programming—the process by which factors acting during early life may have a longer-term effect on health—has been suggested as a further potentially important mechanism that could contribute to the development of obesity (1). For instance, adults born during the Dutch famine whose mothers were exposed to poor nutrition in the first and second trimesters were more likely to be obese (and those exposed in the last trimester, leaner) than their unexposed peers (2,3). The greater propensity to obesity in later life seen in children heavier at birth, and an increase in central fat distribution in those with low birth weight, also suggest that fetal life is a critical window for programming later body fatness (4).

The contribution of the early *postnatal* environment, and particularly early nutrition, to the programming of obesity, however, has received relatively little attention. An effect of nutrition is suggested by an association between greater weight gain in infancy and a slightly greater risk of obesity as adults (5), and by the finding that breast-feeding is associated with a lower risk of later obesity (6,7). However, although consistent with the hypothesis that nutrition in infancy may influence the later propensity to obesity, these previous studies have rarely followed subjects beyond the age of 7 years (4), and such observational data could be confounded by factors influencing both early diet and later adiposity (4). Nevertheless, experimental data from animal models support this underlying hypothesis: Rats food-restricted before weaning were permanently lighter, regardless of how much food was available after weaning (8), whereas baboons overfed before weaning developed obesity in adolescence and adult life (9).

Despite the strong epidemiologic data, in humans a causal association between early factors such as poor fetal growth or infant nutrition and later risk of fatness has not been established. Paradoxically, recent evidence suggests that intrauterine growth retardation may program lower lean mass rather than greater body fatness (10–12). Also, the mechanisms that link early factors to later obesity have been inadequately researched, although programming of the hypothalamic–pituitary axis, insulin-like growth factor 1 (IGF-1) concentrations, and, recently, leptin has been suggested to play an important role. In this review we consider the evidence that intrauterine and early postnatal factors influence body composition in later life, discuss the possible mechanisms involved, and suggest possible experimental studies that could help establish a causal association between early factors such as nutrition and later obesity.

FETAL PROGRAMMING OF OBESITY

Fetal Growth

A recent systematic review of the childhood predictors of adult obesity identified 20 reports that suggested an association between greater fetal growth as measured by birth weight and a later index of obesity such as a high body mass index (BMI) (4). More recent reports have confirmed the association between birth weight and BMI (13,14), and this association has now been seen in adults and children, in both developing and developed countries, and appears to be independent of gestation (4).

Birth weight, however, is related to various other factors, such as maternal size, which could explain any association between greater size at birth and later obesity. Studies that attempted to adjust for maternal size have shown inconsistent findings. For example, BMI increased with birth weight only for offspring of mothers with a medium rather than a thin or heavy build (4); and in another study, birth weight of more than 3.5 kg was associated with obesity only in children whose mothers were in the first and second (but not the third or fourth) quartiles for BMI (4). Despite this inconsistency, several studies have now reported an association of birth weight with later BMI that is independent of maternal size. However, as both birth weight and later BMI are likely to share genetic determinants, the critical influence of genetic make-up on the association between birth weight and later obesity remains unresolved.

Socioeconomic status is another factor that could influence both fetal growth and the susceptibility to obesity. Low socioeconomic status is associated with a higher risk of obesity (particularly in women) but with a *low* rather than *high* birth weight. Socioeconomic factors could therefore be expected to confound the association between birth weight and later obesity, although several studies have shown this association to remain positive after adjusting for these factors (4). For example, in 17-year-old adolescents, birth weight was associated with a greater risk of later obesity (odds ratio of 2.2 for BMI of more than the 90th centile) after controlling for maternal age, education level, and social class as measured by area of residence (4).

Although most studies have consistently shown a positive association between birth weight and BMI, relatively few have assessed the influence of birth weight on direct measures of adiposity such as skinfold thickness. Compared with these direct measures of fatness, body mass index may not identify obese subjects accurately because at any given BMI there is a large range of percentage body fat. Methods to determine body composition are available, but these techniques have rarely been used to assess the influence of fetal growth on later obesity. Nevertheless, a high birth weight has been associated with an increase in the sum of triceps, subscapular, and suprailiac skinfolds or of triceps and subscapular skinfolds in children below 5 years of age (4). By contrast, in older subjects and after adjustment for BMI, Barker *et al.* showed a negative association between birth weight and later skinfold thickness, which would oppose the view that a high birth weight programs a greater risk of later obesity (15). Similarly, Okosun *et al.*, using data from the third US National Health and Nutrition Examination Survey, found that birth weight was *negatively* associated with subscapular skinfold thickness in white, black, and Hispanic American children (16). In the same study, birth weight was also negatively related to suprailiac skinfold thickness in blacks and Hispanics, and to the sum of four skinfolds (subscapular, suprailiac, triceps, and biceps) in blacks only (16). These observations, which appear to contradict the hypothesis that a high birth weight programs greater adiposity in later life, have been explained by ethnic differences in the association of birth weight and later fat distribution, or by the possibility that poor fetal growth programs more truncal fat. Consistent with this hypothesis, several studies have shown an association between low birth weight and a high subscapular to triceps skinfold ratio in later life (a measure of truncal fat distribution) in both children and adults (4). The mechanisms underlying these associations are unknown but, as high glucocorticoid concentrations are associated with a truncal fat distribution, programming of a greater sensitivity to glucocorticoids by low birth weight has been suggested as one possibility.

Data on the influence of intrauterine factors on visceral fat mass (an established risk factor for insulin resistance and cardiovascular disease), rather than truncal fat, are less consistent. Significant correlations between birth weight and waist-to-hip ratio have been reported in some but not most populations (4). In one study the association between low birth weight and greater waist-to-hip ratio was a consequence of low birth weight predicting a smaller hip circumference rather than a greater waist circumference (13). Furthermore, in the only study to measure visceral fat directly, using computerized tomography, there was no significant association between birth weight and later visceral obesity (17). These recent observations do not, therefore, support the hypothesis that associations between low birth weight and later cardiovascular risk are mediated by programming of greater visceral adiposity.

Programming of Lean Tissue

The concept that a greater birth weight may program a high BMI, an established cardiovascular risk factor, contradicts the considerable evidence that a high birth weight is associated with a reduced rather than an increased susceptibility to cardiovascular disease and its risk factors (18) (Fig. 1). One explanation for this apparent discrepancy could be the possibility that low birth weight programs greater visceral fat mass (which would increase the metabolic risk of cardiovascular disease), although the evidence for this hypothesis is inconclusive. Alternatively, as BMI correlates strongly with both total lean and total fat mass, positive associations between birth weight and later BMI could represent programming of lean rather than fat tissue. Consequently,

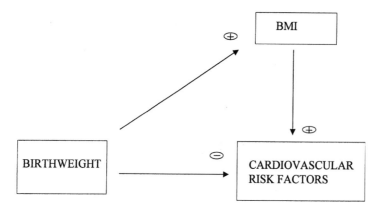

FIG. 1. Associations between birth weight and later cardiovascular risk factors.

as muscle is an important site for glucose uptake in response to insulin, a high birth weight could program increased muscle mass and therefore improved insulin sensitivity and a reduced risk of cardiovascular disease.

Recently, several studies have suggested that a favorable intrauterine environment, as determined by greater fetal growth and birth weight, programs greater lean rather than fat mass (10–12). For example, Hediger et al. compared muscularity (mid-upper-arm circumference and mid-upper-arm muscle area) in children from the third National Health and Nutrition Survey who were born small, appropriate, or large for gestation (11). Children born small for gestation tended to remain smaller throughout childhood, with the discrepancy in weight attributable to differences in lean body mass rather than fat mass. Similarly, adults with low birth weight had lower weight and muscle mass (measured by urinary excretion of creatinine) (10), and birth weight was positively related to thigh muscle and bone area in a study of 192 men aged 17 to 22 years (12). However, although consistent with the hypothesis that a high birth weight programs greater lean mass, these studies were based on regional measures of lean mass (such as the composition of the upper arm or thigh) and not on whole-body composition.

Relatively little is known about the mechanisms underlying the association between birth weight and lean body mass in later life. Barker et al. have suggested that fetal muscle growth may be sacrificed as a consequence of intrauterine stress in order to favor brain development (18). An inadequate nutrient supply in utero would predispose to fetal hypoglycemia and so limit insulin secretion and subsequently increase protein breakdown and decrease protein accretion. Alternatively, genetic factors that predispose to insulin resistance in the fetus could explain associations between low birth weight and insulin resistance (19), and so possibly between low birth weight and lower lean tissue mass in later life. Genetically determined insulin resistance could result in low insulin-mediated fetal growth and therefore a small, thin baby (19). The same genetic factors could lead to insulin resistance in later life and an increased susceptibility to obesity as a consequence of the lower metabolic activity associated with less lean tissue.

In summary, although there is a consistent and positive association between birth weight and later BMI, the concept that fetal growth programs later propensity to obesity rather than body size or lean body mass remains unproven. Genetic factors have a major influence on BMI, and separating these influences from the intrauterine environment has proved difficult up to now. There is some evidence that low birth weight may predispose to a truncal fat distribution, but the evidence suggesting programming of visceral obesity is inconclusive.

Maternal Factors

Associations between several maternal factors known to change the fetal environment and the later propensity to obesity are consistent with the "fetal programming" of obesity hypothesis. As reviewed recently, maternal obesity, diabetes, and pregnancy weight gain have all been linked to an increased susceptibility to obesity in the offspring (20). However, these studies have not been able to isolate the influence of the uterine environment from transmitted genetic factors, which are also likely to have a marked effect on the propensity to obesity.

Suggestive evidence that the intrauterine environment is a critical window for the programming of obesity comes from the Dutch Famine study. Conscripts (aged 19 years) exposed *in utero* to the famine of 1944–45 during the first half of gestation had a prevalence of obesity of 2.8% (defined as body weight for height in excess of 120%), compared with 0.8% in those exposed in the last trimester and 1.8% in non-exposed men (2). At the later follow-up at the age of 50 years, the BMI of women exposed to famine in early gestation was 7.4% greater than in those who were not exposed, but in men the BMI was unaffected by exposure to famine at any stage of gestation (3). Waist circumference was also greater in women exposed to famine, which suggested that these women tended to deposit fat intraabdominally. Interestingly, there were no differences in birth weight between those exposed or not exposed to famine in early pregnancy, which suggests that intrauterine factors other than those affecting fetal growth contributed to the programming of obesity (3).

As discussed previously (20), several factors prevent a causal interpretation of the link between maternal nutritional deprivation and the later risk of obesity identified by the Dutch Famine study. For example, babies exposed to famine who were less prone to obesity may have had a higher mortality. Also, women who conceived during the famine may have been a selected group (although the association of famine exposure and BMI at age 50 years was unaffected by adjustment for maternal characteristics likely to influence fertility) (3). Furthermore, the role of maternal undernutrition in the programming of obesity has not been confirmed in subjects exposed to famine *in utero* during the German siege of Leningrad in 1941–44, or from comparable levels of maternal undernutrition from studies in developing countries (20).

Maternal factors known to influence the fetal environment that are less extreme than famine also support the fetal programming of obesity hypothesis. For instance, maternal diabetes during pregnancy has been associated with a greater risk of obesity in the offspring. This association has been shown in at least 11 studies and appears to be independent of maternal weight or birth weight (20), which is therefore consistent with the hypothesis that the intrauterine environment alters the propensity to obesity independent of genetic factors. The mechanism whereby this occurs remains speculative, but one hypothesis is that chronic hyperinsulinemia or hyperglycemia in the fetus may down-regulate insulin receptors or postinsulin receptor signaling, thereby increasing insulin resistance in the fetus. However, despite these strong associations, a causal link between the intrauterine environment in diabetic mothers and the later risk of obesity in the offspring has not been established. Correcting for maternal weight does not exclude the influence of genes that could affect both the risk of diabetes in the mother and the susceptibility to obesity in the offspring.

Further support for the fetal programming of obesity has emerged from the intriguing association between early cold exposure and an increased susceptibility to obesity (14). Adults who were born in the first half of the year (and therefore exposed to cold *in utero*) had a greater prevalence of obesity (BMI > 30 kg/m^2). The relation between birth weight and adult obesity was also stronger in those born in the first 6 months of the year or following cold winters than in those born in the last 6 months of the year or following mild winters. These observations are consistent with evidence from animal studies indicating that exposure to lower environmental temperatures before or soon after birth promotes the development of obesity in the newborn. The physiologic links between climate and obesity in later life are conjectural, but factors that are sensitive to both temperature and season, such as nutrition, are postulated to be involved.

EARLY DIET AND LATER OBESITY

The hypothesis that diet in infancy (and particularly overfeeding) can program the later risk of obesity has often been considered, but as discussed recently, few studies have addressed the influence of early diet on obesity beyond childhood (4). In one such report, Charney *et al.* showed that 36% of those whose weight exceeded the 90th centile as infants were overweight as adults, compared with 14% of the average and light weight infants (5). The association between a vigorous breast-feeding pattern, which was associated with a higher energy intake, and greater obesity in later life also supports a role for "overfeeding" in infancy and the later susceptibility to obesity (21). Nonetheless, the role of early energy or nutrient intake on the later susceptibility to obesity remains unproven (4).

Research on the programming of body composition by early diet has focused mainly on whether breast-feeding reduces the risk of adult obesity. Formula-fed infants are larger than breast-fed infants, but whether this contributes to obesity in later life is debated. Although comparatively small studies have not shown any association between breast-feeding and the later risk of obesity (4), several larger cohorts have found that breast-fed infants are less predisposed to obesity in later life. For instance, a protective effect of breast-feeding against obesity was shown in cross-sectional studies of adolescents born in the late 1960s (6) and in a recent cohort of over 134,000 children aged 5 and 6 years from Germany (7). In both studies the protective effect of breast-feeding appeared to be independent of confounding factors such as social class, which suggested that properties of breast milk rather than lifestyle factors associated with breast-feeding programmed the lower later risk of obesity. Consistent with this hypothesis, a longer duration of breast-feeding was associated with lower subsequent fatness, even after adjustment for socioeconomic status (6). How breast milk intake protects against subsequent fatness is debated, but one hypothesis is that higher insulin concentrations in infants who are formula-fed could stimulate fetal fat deposition and the early development of adipocytes.

MECHANISMS

Proposed mechanisms for the programming of obesity fall into two broad categories: (a) the influence of genes on the relations between early factors and later risk of obesity, which is strongly supported by data from twins (22), and (b) the effects of the fetal and early postnatal environment. As reviewed previously (23), it has been suggested that environmental influences on the programming of obesity act either at the level of the fat cell or as a consequence of abnormalities of hypothalamic function (3,23).

The fat cell theory, which proposes that overnutrition in late gestation and early postnatal life (e.g., as a consequence of maternal overweight or fetal hyperinsulinemia in the offspring of diabetic mothers) affects either adipose cell number or metabolism, is supported by an extensive animal literature (20,23). As comprehensively reviewed (24), adipose cell development *in utero* is regulated by a complex interaction of maternal endocrine and paracrine influences that could affect the tendency for later obesity. For example, the offspring of pigs with experimentally induced diabetes have been shown to have an increased number and size of lipid-containing adipocytes and a 40-fold increase in fetal adipose tissue lipogenesis. There are, however, few data to support the *in utero* programming of adipocyte number or function in humans (24).

By contrast, there is some preliminary evidence that the intrauterine environment could program hypothalamic function in humans. Fetal undernutrition has been suggested to program higher growth hormone or IGF-1 concentrations in later life (18). This programming of the hypothalamic–pituitary axis could then affect adipocyte cell function. Further, Ravelli *et al.* have proposed that maternal energy deprivation could affect fetal hypothalamic development and impair later appetite regulation (3). Leptin, a key regulator of appetite and body fatness, has been suggested as a potential candidate for this hormonal programming (25).

Programming of Leptin Concentrations

Obesity in humans is associated with a high leptin concentration relative to fat mass, leading to the concept that resistance to the actions of leptin could impair appetite regulation and so predispose to obesity. Associations between low birth weight and higher leptin concentrations relative to fat mass are consistent with the hypothesis that programming of leptin physiology, and specifically greater leptin resistance, is one mechanism for the early origins of obesity (25). Studies in rats that showed that a hypercaloric diet early in postnatal life programmed greater leptin resistance (26), support this hypothesis and suggest that the critical window for the programming of leptin physiology may extend beyond the fetal period.

As being overweight in infancy might increase the later risk of obesity, we tested the hypothesis that a higher nutrient intake in infancy programs greater leptin concentrations relative to fat mass in humans (Singhal A, et al., in press). Also, as breast-feeding rather than formula feeding is associated with a lower susceptibility to obesity, we explored the hypothesis that breast milk consumption is associated with lower leptin concentrations relative to fat mass in adolescence. A cohort of children randomized at birth to a nutrient-enriched or standard diet provided a unique opportunity to test our hypothesis in an experimental study with prospective follow-up (27).

The participants were born preterm in the early 1980s and had been randomized at birth in two trials to a nutrient-enriched preterm formula versus banked donated breast milk, or preterm formula versus standard formula (27) (Fig. 2). A representative subgroup of 216 children was followed up at age 13 to 16 years to assess the impact of early nutrition on cardiovascular risk factors, obesity, and leptin concentrations. Serum leptin concentrations were measured by a radioimmunoassay, and fat mass was estimated by bioelectric impedance analysis ($N = 197$).

Combining trials 1 and 2, as originally planned, we found the ratio of leptin to fat mass was significantly greater in children randomized to nutrient-enriched preterm formula at birth (geometric mean 0.84 µg/l/kg) than in those randomized to standard formula or banked breast milk (0.62 µg/l/kg), the mean difference being 30.8% (95% confidence interval [CI] for difference, 8.4% to 53.2%; $p = 0.007$). Similar observations were obtained for the ratio of leptin to percentage fat mass. The difference between randomized dietary groups remained significant after adjustment for age, sex, Tanner stage, social class, and fat mass. Human milk intake was associated with lower leptin concentrations relative to fat mass in adolescence (regression coefficient), (-0.3% change per 100 ml increase in human milk intake; 95% CI), (-0.6 to -0.04%; $p = 0.023$) (Fig. 3), independent of potential confounding factors. There were, however, no differences in total fat mass between randomized groups.

Given the experimental design, our observations strongly supported an influence of early diet on later leptin concentrations. Leptin concentration relative to fat mass was 30% greater in children randomized to a nutrient-enriched preterm formula at birth than in those randomized to one of the two standard diets, and this difference was independent of population differences at birth or in adolescence. However, unlike previous studies in children born at term, low birth weight in our preterm cohort was not related to relative hyperleptinemia in adolescence, possibly because the programming of leptin concentrations by antenatal factors such as obesity differs according to the timing of the in utero insult. Alternatively, the association between birth weight and later leptin concentrations may be disturbed by relative hyperleptinemia in adolescence, which could also explain the higher leptin concentrations relative to fat mass in our study compared with data from adults.

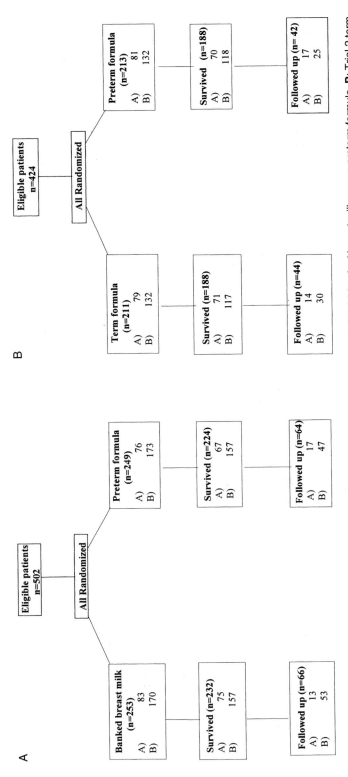

FIG. 2. Follow-up at age 13 to 16 years of children randomized at births to different diets. **A**: Trial 1 banked breast milk versus preterm formula. **B**: Trial 2 term formula versus preterm formula. A, Subjects receiving assigned milk as sole diet; B, Subjects receiving assigned milk as a supplement to mother's expressed breast milk.

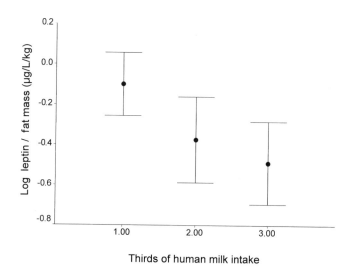

FIG. 3. Geometric mean (95% confidence interval) of leptin concentration relative to fat mass according to thirds of percentage human milk intake (from lowest to highest, 1–3).

We postulate that programming of leptin physiology could be one mechanism that links early nutrition with a later propensity to overweight or obesity. Although adolescents previously fed the nutrient-enriched diet were not fatter at 13 to 16 years of age, the tendency for excess weight gain in some nonobese populations with high leptin concentrations at baseline (25) suggests that they are at higher risk of becoming obese in adult life. Whether they will become so is a key aspect for further follow-up. Nonetheless, it seems likely that factors acting in childhood may promote obesity in early adulthood (4). We postulate that insensitivity to leptin in individuals who received a nutrient-enriched diet could program the commonest onset of obesity, which is that seen in early adult life. Lower leptin resistance in infants fed human milk could also provide one potential mechanism for the long-term benefit of breast-feeding on adiposity.

Possible Mechanisms

We postulate that higher leptin levels associated with greater body fatness early in postnatal life program the leptin-dependent feedback loop, such that the regulation of body fat is less sensitive to leptin in later life. The physiologic mechanisms for this could involve down-regulation of hypothalamic leptin receptors or postreceptor effector mechanisms—analogous in animal studies to the up-regulation of hypothalamic leptin receptors when there is a lack of functioning leptin (28), or to the greater expression of receptors within the hypothalamus of feed-restricted versus well-fed ewes (probably caused by down-regulation of leptin receptors in well-fed ewes) (29). Therefore if exposed to an environment favoring a positive energy balance, these individuals will be more susceptible to greater body fatness, particularly when there is physiologic leptin insensitivity and an increase in body fat, such as at puberty.

FUTURE STUDIES

The Need for Experimental Studies

Previous studies of the early origins of obesity have been based on retrospective and observational data and so could suffer from the problems of confounding and selection bias. These studies have also relied on measures of body size (e.g., BMI) rather than direct measures of fat mass. There is a clear need therefore for interventional studies that use an experimental design to control for potential confounding factors, and for studies that use sophisticated measures of body composition (e.g., the four-component model of body composition). Also, different compartments within the whole-body fat mass should be better identified, (e.g., by using magnetic resonance imaging to measure visceral adiposity directly). Finally, as programming effects may amplify with age and be most marked after puberty, subjects should be followed beyond childhood (4). For instance, in one of the few experimental studies of the programming of obesity, Morley and Lucas found no significant difference in skinfold thicknesses or body mass index in children randomized to a nutrient-enriched or a standard diet (27). However, the lack of any influence of early diet on obesity at age 7 to 8 years in that study is consistent with both animal data (9) and our own data for blood pressure in the same cohort, which suggest that programming effects may not emerge until after puberty.

Studies in Twins

The observation that the BMI of monozygous twins raised apart is strongly correlated despite their markedly different postnatal environments suggests a large genetic component to the development of obesity. Genetic factors are likely therefore to be the major confounder of data that support the early origins of obesity hypothesis. Studies in twins discordant for birth weight could, however, provide a unique approach to test the influence of the fetal environment on later adiposity that is independent of genetic and postnatal environmental factors. In one such study, in monozygous twins discordant for birth weight, the between-pair differences in birth weight correlated with between-pair differences in adult height but not with adult BMI (30). This study therefore did not support the intrauterine environment as critical to the programming of later whole-body adiposity, although programming of specific fat compartments such as visceral fat, which may be relevant to the development of cardiovascular disease, could not be excluded. On the other hand, this study was consistent with the hypothesis that factors acting *in utero* may program lean body mass in later life. Further studies in twins could therefore help elucidate the influence of fetal factors on later body composition.

CONCLUSIONS

Much preliminary evidence suggests that factors acting *in utero* and early in postnatal life program the later susceptibility to obesity. However, a causal association between early factors and later susceptibility to obesity has not been established owing to a lack of experimental data in humans. The influence of early factors on whole-body composition, rather than just BMI, and the relative contribution of environmental and genetic factors to the early origins of obesity also remain unknown.

At present, the contrasting associations between birth weight and the later risk of obesity compared with other cardiovascular risk factors (such as insulin resistance), and our lack of understanding of the physiology of programming of obesity, prevents the implementation of soundly based intervention strategies. However, given the growing evidence that the association between low birth weight and an increased propensity to cardiovascular disease may be most marked in those who become obese (18), further research on the early origins of obesity is now of the highest priority.

REFERENCES

1. Dietz WH. Critical periods in childhood for the development of obesity. *Am J Clin Nutr* 1994; 59: 955–9.
2. Ravelli GP, Stein ZA, Susser MW. Obesity in young men after famine exposure *in utero* and early infancy. *N Engl J Med* 1976; 295: 349–53.
3. Ravelli ACJ, Meulen van der JHP, Osmond C, Barker DJP, Bleker OP. Obesity at the age of 50 y in men and women exposed to famine prenatally. *Am J Clin Nutr* 1999; 70: 811–6.
4. Parsons TJ, Power C, Logan S, Summerbell CD. Childhood predictors of adult obesity: a systematic review. *Int J Obes* 1999; 23: 1–107.
5. Charney E, Goodman HC, McBride M, Lyon B, Pratt R. Childhood antecedents of adult obesity. Do chubby infants become obese adults? *N Engl J Med* 1976; 295: 6–9.
6. Kramer MS. Do breast-feeding and delayed introduction of solid foods protect against subsequent obesity? *J Pediatr* 1981; 98: 883–7.
7. Von Kries R, Koletzko B, Sauerwald T, *et al.* Breast feeding and obesity; cross sectional study. *BMJ* 1999; 319: 147–50.
8. McCance RA, Widdowson EM. The determinants of growth and form. *Pro R Soc Lond B Biol Sci* 1974; 185: 1–17.
9. Lewis DS, Bertrand HA, McMahan CA, McGill HC, Carey KD, Masoro EJ. Preweaning food intake influences the adiposity of young adult baboons. *J Clin Invest* 1986; 78: 899–905.
10. Phillips DIW. Relation of fetal growth to adult muscle mass and glucose tolerance. *Diabetic Med* 1995; 12: 686–90.
11. Hediger ML, Overpeck MD, Kuczmarski RJ, McGlynn A, Maurer KR, Davis WW. Muscularity and fatness of infants and young children born small- or large for gestational- age. *Pediatrics* 1998; 102: E60.
12. Kahn HS, Narayan KMV, Williamson DF, Valdez R. Relation of birth weight to lean and fat thigh tissue in young men. *Int J Obes* 2000; 24: 667–72.
13. Byberg L, McKeigue PM, Zethelius B, Lithell HO. Birth weight and the insulin resistance syndrome: association of low birth weight with truncal obesity and raised plasminogen activator inhibitor-1 but not with abdominal obesity or plasma lipid disturbances. *Diabetologia* 2000; 43: 54–60.
14. Phillips DIW, Young JB. Birth weight, climate at birth and the risk of obesity in adult life. *Int J Obes* 2000; 24: 281–7.
15. Barker M, Robinson S, Osmond C, Barker DJP. Birth weight and body fat distribution in adolescent girls. *Arch Dis Child* 1997; 77: 381–3.
16. Okosun IS, Liao Y, Rotimi CN, Dever GEA, Cooper RS. Impact of birth weight on ethnic variations in subcutaneous and central adiposity in American children aged 5–11 years. A study from the Third National Health and Nutrition Examination Survey. *Int J Obes* 2000; 24: 479–84.
17. Choi CS, Kim CH, Lee WJ, *et al.* Association between birth weight and insulin sensitivity in healthy young men in Korea: role of visceral adiposity. *Diabetes Res* 2000; 49: 53–9.
18. Barker DJP, Gluckman PD, Godfrey KM, Harding JE, Owen JA, Robinson JS. Fetal nutrition and cardiovascular disease in adult life. *Lancet* 1993; 341: 938–41.
19. Hattersley AT, Tooke JE. The fetal insulin hypothesis: an alternative explanation of the association of low birthweight with diabetes and vascular disease. *Lancet* 1999; 353: 1789–92.

20. Whitaker RC, Dietz WH. Role of the prenatal environment in the development of obesity. *J Pediatr* 1998; 132: 768–76.
21. Agras WS, Kraemer HC, Berkowitz RI, Hammer LD. Influence of early feeding style on adiposity at 6 years of age. *J Pediatr* 1990; 116: 805–9.
22. Stunkard AJ, Harris JR, Pedersen NL, McClearn GE. The body-mass index of twins who have been reared apart. *N Engl J Med* 1990; 322: 1483–7.
23. Proietto J, Thorburn AW. Animal models of obesity—theories of aetiology. *Baillieres Clin Endocrinol Metab* 1994; 8: 509–25.
24. Martin RJ, Hausman GJ, Hausman DB. Regulation of adipose cell development in utero. *Proc Soc Exp Biol Med* 1998; 219: 200–10.
25. Lissner L, Karlsson C, Lindroos AK, *et al.* Birth weight, adulthood BMI, and subsequent weight gain in relation to leptin levels in Swedish women. *Obes Res* 1999; 7: 150–4.
26. Plagemann A, Harder T, Rake A, *et al.* Observations on the orexigenic hypothalamic neuropeptide Y-system in neonatally overfed weanling rats. *J Neuroendocrinol* 1999; 11: 541–6.
27. Morley R, Lucas A. Randomised diet in the neonatal period and growth performance until 7.5–8 y of age in preterm children. *Am J Clin Nutr* 2000; 71: 822–8.
28. Huang XF, Lin S, Zhang R. Upregulation of leptin receptor mRNA expression in obese mouse brain. *Neuroreport* 1997; 8: 1035–8.
29. Dyer CJ, Simmons JM, Matteri RL, Keisler DH. Leptin receptor mRNA is expressed in the ewe anterior pituitary and adipose tissues and is differentially expressed in hypothalamic regions of well-fed and feed-restricted ewes. *Domest Anim Endocrinol* 1997; 14: 119–28.
30. Allison DB, Paultre F, Heymsfield SB, Pi-Sunyer FX. Is the intra-uterine period really a critical period for the development of adiposity? *Int J Obes* 1995; 19: 397–402.

DISCUSSION

Dr. Dietz: You referred to intrauterine exposure of infants to cold being associated with a higher prevalence of later obesity. My interpretation of those same studies is the opposite, that it is the postnatal exposure to cold that is associated with a greater likelihood of leanness. That would make more sense from a physiologic point of view because of the potential role of programming brown fat in early childhood. In fact, at one point Danforth in the USA was arguing that all infants should be exposed to cold for a week, and if we did that, we would reduce the prevalence of obesity!

Dr. Singhal: The data I was referring to were published by Phillips *et al.* in the *International Journal of Obesity* (1). They showed that children born in the first half of the year—whose mothers were therefore exposed to the cold of the winter—had a higher risk of obesity in later life. They also showed that children who were born heavier in the first half of the year after a cold winter had a stronger association between birth weight and an increased risk of obesity. Thus the effect seemed to be related to cold exposure in pregnancy rather than postnatally.

Dr. Dietz: I also have a comment relating to the earlier discussion about the effects of low birth weight. We need to determine the potential role of reduced birth weight in the complications of obesity at lower BMIs. We must investigate the prevalence of those complications and adjust for birth weight in the target populations, or else exclude individuals with low birth weights from the analyses, so that we can compare the effects of birth weight or subsequent weight gain in *normal-birth-weight populations* on the risk of later complications of obesity. This is an area where we need much more sophistication so that we can begin to separate the prenatal and postnatal influences.

Dr. Singhal: I completely agree. One thing that's often forgotten about the fetal origins of adult disease hypothesis is that it's not just low birth weight that is associated with an increased risk of cardiovascular disease—it's the interaction between low birth weight and "Western" factors, Western diet, increased obesity, and so on. It is the combination of the two that is important. This is a factor that discriminates between the data from developing countries and those from developed countries. Up to now the developing countries have not been much exposed to Western-type adult risk factors.

Dr. Endres: I always have problems with the term *imprinting*. Could you explain it?

Dr. Singhal: I can try. Three terms have been proposed: *imprinting, entrainment*, and *programming*. There has been active debate about which of these is the most appropriate. From my experience as a user rather than a creator of terminology, I don't have a preference. All three mean the same thing to me: what they imply is that factors acting during critical windows may have a long-term influence, and there may be a period when an influence of these factors is not evident.

Dr. Koletzko: Your data on leptin resistance were fascinating. It appeared to me that in the two graphs you showed, the relative effect was about similar between the highest and lowest tertile of human milk consumption and what you called standard diet and high-nutrient diet. Do you have any indication about whether this is primarily an effect of nutrient intake—in other words, high or low energy, protein, and so on—or do you think it is an effect of human milk per se. So if you compare the human milk group to the term formula group, do you see a difference?

Dr. Singhal: The means for human milk and term formula were very similar, but the individuals who received the most human milk on an epidemiologic basis had lower leptin concentrations. It is hard to say whether the effect is related to protein, energy, or some other nutrient because the preterm formula was mainly enriched with protein, but it also had extra energy.

Dr. Koletzko: The different diets would be associated with different rates of growth early on and different times of discharge from hospital. Is it conceivable that those factors could be the primary cause?

Dr. Singhal: We looked at differences in growth and they did not explain the findings. In fact, when we used a regression model to correct for growth, the data stayed quite robust.

Dr. Dulloo: There appears to be some controversy about the effects of low and high birth weight on later obesity. I'm sure it must have crossed your mind that there may be a U-shaped relation between birth weight and later obesity, with two quite different mechanisms. The metabolic complications are certainly quite different, depending on whether obesity was associated with high or low birth weight. What is your opinion on that?

Dr. Singhal: The programming-of-obesity hypothesis is in its really early days. We don't have good data on fat mass as opposed to BMI, which is a real problem. I personally don't believe in a U-shaped distribution effect because the association between low birth weight and an increased risk of central obesity occurs all across the spectrum and does not change between the lowest and highest birth weights. Similarly, the associations between high birth weight and later high BMI have been seen in 20 populations and are always there. One possible explanation for this, though I don't have any data to back it up, is that you are programming lean tissue rather than adipose tissue. That may seem a controversial statement, but fat mass and lean tissue correlate so strongly with each other that you may not actually be programming obesity.

Dr. Dulloo: I'm glad that you mentioned the need for mechanistic studies, and we certainly need mechanistic theories. When we talk about low birth weight and later obesity, there is a big element of catch-up growth in between—catch-up fat growth basically. Widdowson showed that if you restrict food for a short period in normal-birth-weight animals there was not much tendency to develop obesity later, but if you restrict intake for longer periods, then you do see a higher body fat later. It seems that earlier (intrauterine) malnutrition simply exacerbates the catch-up fat growth.

Dr. Singhal: I don't agree with your interpretation of the McCance and Widdowson data. It was not the duration of nutrition restriction that was important, it was the timing (2). If you restrict food intake before weaning, these animals will stay small, however much nutrition you give them afterward. But if you reduce food intake at any time after weaning, then they will catch up when refed. Their data had nothing to do with birth weight or with the duration of restriction; it was the *timing* of the restriction that introduced the concept of critical windows. However, I do agree that it is important to investigate catch-up fat growth.

Dr. Cai: Where a baby is born with a high birth weight, is there any evidence that prolonged breast-feeding could reduce the risk of a high BMI in later life?

Dr. Singhal: I don't know of any evidence that breast-feeding for a prolonged period can influence the later risk of obesity. There is a well-known hypothesis that breast-fed babies regulate their diet better than bottle-fed babies, because of the cultural tendency to insist that a baby finishes the bottle, or because bottles are given whenever the baby cries. To what extent that contributes to long-term BMI I can't say. I'm a strong advocate of breast-feeding irrespective of the obesity data, but could not say whether long-term breast-feeding would reduce later risk of obesity.

Dr. Srivastava: Babies of low birth weight are not a homogeneous group. There are many different causes of low birth weight. Do such babies behave in a uniform way in terms of later risk? In particular, is there a difference between babies born prematurely to normal mothers and those born small because of maternal malnutrition, which is much more common in developing countries?

Dr. Singhal: I think this is a controversy that continues to run in the fetal programming and adult disease hypothesis. Is it low birth weight per se that's important, or is it low birth weight relative to gestation? There have been letters going to and fro in *Lancet*, with people arguing both stances. I personally believe the low birth weight for gestation situation is much more important—in other words, it is the growth-retarded baby who is at increased risk of later cardiovascular disease and complications. That is my personal opinion, and I have data to support that view (3).

REFERENCES

1. Phillips DIW, Young JB. Birth weight, climate at birth and the risk of obesity in adult life. *Int J Obes* 2000; 24: 281–7.
2. McCance RA, Widdowson EM. The determinants of growth and form. *Proc Roy Soc Biol* 1974; 185: 1–17.
3. Singhal A, Kattenhorn M, Cole TJ, *et al.* Preterm birth, vascular function and risk factors for atherosclerosis. *Lancet* 2001; 358; 1159–60.

Obesity in Childhood and Adolescence, edited by
Chunming Chen and William H. Dietz. Nestlé
Nutrition Workshop Series, Pediatric Program,
Vol. 49. Nestec Ltd., Vevey/Lippincott
Williams & Wilkins, Philadelphia © 2002.

The Adiposity Rebound: Its Contribution to Obesity in Children and Adults

M. F. Rolland-Cachera, M. Deheeger, and *F. Bellisle

*National Institute of Health and Medical Research, INSERM Group, Paris, France;
*National Center for Scientific Research, INSERM and Service Nutrition Hôtel Dieu,
Paris, France*

The increasing prevalence of childhood obesity is a major problem affecting both industrialized and developing countries (1). Given the poor prognosis of treatment in
adults, prevention or early intervention are desirable. Most obese children, however,
will not remain fat as adults, and certain children who are not overweight will develop obesity later (2,3). It is therefore important to be able to identify those overweight children who will remain fat and those nonobese children who may become
fat later. Indicators predicting adult adiposity are of great potential value. They are
useful for pediatricians as guides for intervention and are also useful for researchers.
Studying these indicators should allow progress in understanding the origins of obesity.

Body measurements at different ages and their temporal variations are used to predict adult fatness. These include weight, skinfold thickness, and weight and length
gain (2,4,5). The weight/height^2, Quetelet or body mass index (BMI) is now widely
used to assess nutritional status in children.

Changes in the BMI pattern have been proposed as an indicator predicting adult
adiposity (6,7). Dietz suggests that childhood overweight and obesity develop during
critical periods (8)—the prenatal period, during the adiposity rebound, and in adolescence. Available information related to the adiposity rebound and its value in predicting adult obesity will be considered in this chapter.

ADIPOSITY DEVELOPMENT

During childhood, body composition changes substantially. The percentage of body
fat is about 12% at birth, 22% in 9-month-old infants, and 16% at the age of 5 years.
This percentage rises again up to the age of 10 years. It then decreases at adolescence
in boys and continues to increase in girls (9).

Physical development in childhood is generally followed on the basis of weight
and height measurements. Weight-for-age charts are used to assess nutritional status
(10). As weight is strongly associated with height, weight measurements should be

related to height. Weight-for-height charts, however, do not take age into account. Adjustment of weight for both height and age can be achieved using power indices of the form weight/height^n. The selection of indices was based on low correlations with height, and high correlations with weight and body fat. As a rule, weight/height^2 shows the lowest correlation with height, except at adolescence in boys, where weight/height^3 shows lower correlation with height (6). BMI charts have been constructed for all ages throughout childhood (6). As opposed to other measures based on weight and height (weight for age or weight for height), BMI/age changes reflect real changes in the child's body shape during growth. By the age of 1 year, a child whose BMI is in the mean range looks chubby. Over the next few years, the child will slim down and look thin by the age of 6 years, but will later put on fat again. The similarity between the development of the BMI and more direct measures of fatness such as skinfold thickness (11) (Fig. 1) is a major argument supporting BMI over other indices.

When examining individual BMI patterns, it was noted that the nadir of the BMI curves, which on average takes place by the age of 6 years, could occur earlier or later. The point of minimum BMI value was named the "adiposity rebound" (7). The age at adiposity rebound is associated with BMI development. As a rule, the earlier the adiposity rebound, the greater the degree of adult adiposity (3,4,7,12–17).

Changes in weight status can be clearly understood by examining individual BMI patterns (Fig. 2). For example, a fat 1-year-old child may become a normal-weight adult after a late adiposity rebound, whereas a lean 1-year-old child may become a

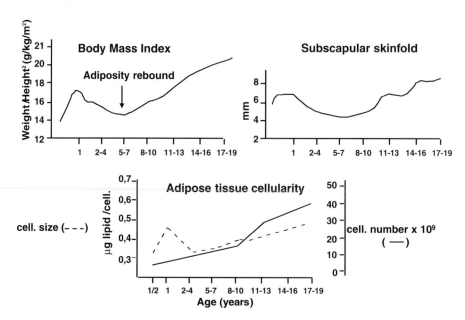

FIG. 1. Development of fatness as assessed by body mass index and subscapular skinfold and changes of adipose tissue cellularity. (Data from Rolland-Cachera *et al.*, 1982 [6]; Sempé *et al.*, 1979 [11]; and Knittle *et al.*, 1979 [19].)

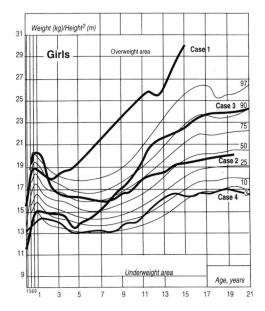

FIG. 2. Four examples of body mass index development. Case 1: fat child at 1 year, remained fat after an early adiposity rebound (2 years). Case 2: fat child at 1 year, did not stay fat after a late adiposity rebound (8 years). Case 3: lean child at 1 year, became fat after an early adiposity rebound (4.5 years). Case 4: lean child at 1 year, remained lean after a late adiposity rebound (8 years). (After Rolland-Cachera *et al.*, 1987 [3].)

fat adult after an early adiposity rebound. These individual BMI patterns explain why, before the adiposity rebound, the child's BMI predicts adult fatness only poorly (2–4). Case 3 in Fig. 2 (a thin child at 4 years becoming overweight after an early adiposity rebound) shows that overweight diagnosed at adolescence actually can have its origin much earlier in life. The onset of obesity can be defined as the time when the BMI overlaps the cutoff centile defining obesity. In those children who are not fat from early childhood, the age of adiposity rebound is generally before that at which obesity is established. It then constitutes useful information for the pediatrician and the researcher.

METHODOLOGY

The age at adiposity rebound corresponds to the point of minimum BMI value, the nadir of the curve preceding the steep increase in the curve. Different methods are used to assess age at adiposity rebound. In some studies (3,7,13,16), BMI curves were drawn for each subject, and the timing of the adiposity rebound was assessed by visual inspection. This involves identifying an upward trend in the BMI after the nadir. In some cases, the descending phase of BMI is followed by a plateau (e.g., case 4 in Fig. 2). In this case, 8 years was considered to be the age of adiposity rebound, because at this age the steep increase in BMI begins. To identify the upward trend in

BMI, Dorosty *et al.* (16) specified that all consecutive measurements of the BMI after the nadir should show an increase and that any increase in the BMI after the nadir
had to equal or exceed 0.1 kg/m². Gasser *et al.* (4) determined the adiposity rebound
from the velocity curve of the BMI. Age at adiposity rebound corresponds to the
point at which the velocity curve becomes positive after the loss of BMI in infancy
and early childhood.

Siervogel *et al.* (12) chose a polynomial model to describe the pattern of change in
BMI. Age at minimum BMI was derived from this model. Other investigators have
used the same approach (14,15,17).

ADIPOSITY REBOUND INVESTIGATIONS

An international growth study was initiated in 1953 (18). In the early 1980s, on the
basis of the French sample, Rolland-Cachera *et al.* described the BMI pattern, emphasizing the ascending and descending phases at different stages of growth (6).
They then established that an early adiposity rebound was associated with a high BMI
at the age of 16 years. This association was observed whatever the BMI at age 1 year
(7). In this study the association between age at adiposity rebound and bone age was
also investigated. The changes in the pattern of BMI and adipose tissue cellularity
(19) during growth were discussed. The increase in BMI during the first year of life
followed by a decrease corresponds to variations in adipocyte *size,* whereas after
the age of 6 years the rise in BMI corresponds to the increase in adipocyte *number*
(Fig. 1). It was suggested that the age at adiposity rebound may reflect the time at
which adipocytes start to increase in number (7,20).

Subsequently, we analyzed the association between adiposity rebound and fatness
development up to the age of 21 years (3) (Fig. 3). Adiposity rebound was significantly associated with both BMI and subscapular skinfold at age 21. We also investigated the association between age at adiposity rebound and previous measurements.

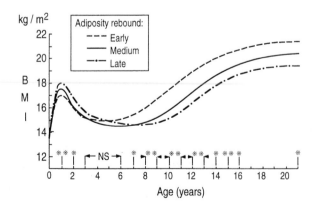

FIG. 3. Mean body mass index curves for three groups of girls classified as early (. . .), average
(——), or late (–.–) adiposity rebound. NS: $p \geq 0.05$; *$p < 0.05$; **$p < 0.01$. (From Rolland-
Cachera *et al.*, 1984, 1987 [3,7].)

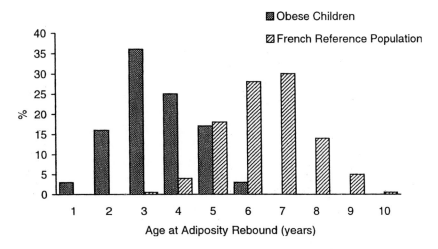

FIG. 4. Distribution of the age at adiposity rebound in the French reference population (*N*, 227; mean age at adiposity rebound, 6.2 ± 1.3 years) and in a sample of children treated for obesity in a department of pediatric endocrinology (*N*, 62; mean age at adiposity rebound, 3.2 ± 1.2 years). In the reference population, age at adiposity rebound was ≤ 6 years in 51% of children; in obese children age at adiposity rebound was ≤ 3 years in 55% of children (3).

An opposite association was found between age at adiposity rebound and BMI at the age of 1 year: The earlier the rebound, the lower the BMI at 1 year. This trend was recorded in both boys and girls, but it reached significance only in girls.

The association between age at adiposity rebound and fatness at adult age emerged even in a sample including mostly normal-weight children. In this sample, mean age at adiposity rebound was 6.2 ± 1.3 years, varying from 3 to 9.5 years (Fig. 4) (3). The discussion of this paper reported unpublished data collected in a department of pediatric endocrinology where children were treated for obesity. Mean age at adiposity rebound was 3.2 ± 1.2 years. Of the 62 children, none had an adiposity rebound later than the age of 6 years. Two children had their adiposity rebound when they were 6 (i.e., average age at adiposity rebound) but more than half of them (55%) had their rebound at or before the age of 3 (Fig. 4). A similar mean age at adiposity rebound recorded in obese children (2.9 years) has been reported elsewhere (21).

On the basis of data recorded in the Fels longitudinal study in children between the ages of 2 and 18 years, Siervogel *et al.* (12) investigated individual changes in body fatness during childhood and adolescence. They reported that both the age when children reach their BMI nadir (the age at adiposity rebound) and BMI level at adiposity rebound were associated with the BMI value at 18 years. Correlations between age at adiposity rebound and adult BMI are negative, as a younger age at adiposity rebound is associated with a greater adult BMI.

In a longitudinal study conducted in Czech children from 1 month to 18 years of age, Prokopec and Bellisle (13) reported similar association between early adiposity rebound and later increased fatness. In that study, most overweight adults (15 of 18 with a BMI of more than 25 kg/m² at 18 years of age) had an early adiposity rebound (before the age of 6 years), and all lean adults had late adiposity rebound (after 6 years).

On the basis of the Zurich sample from the international growth study initiated in 1954 (18), Gasser *et al.* (4) examined the prediction of adult measurements from measurements recorded in infancy and through adolescence. They found that the age at adiposity rebound correlated significantly with adult BMI.

Whitaker *et al.* conducted a retrospective study in adults (14). BMI curves were fitted for each subject between 1.5 and 16 years. Age and BMI level at adiposity rebound were recorded from these curves. The BMI values of parents were also available. Adult obesity was associated with early adiposity rebound, high BMI at adiposity rebound, heavy mothers, and heavy fathers. After adjusting for parent BMI and BMI at adiposity rebound, the odds ratio for adult obesity associated with early versus late adiposity rebound was 6.0 (95% confidence interval, 1.3 to 26.6). Both parent BMI and BMI z score at adiposity rebound were associated with a younger age at rebound. This study showed that an early adiposity rebound was associated with an increased risk of adult obesity independent of parent obesity and the BMI at adiposity rebound.

In a follow-up study conducted in children between the ages of 3 and 18 years, Williams *et al.* (15) reported that BMI in early adulthood was associated with both age at adiposity rebound and BMI at that age. Skeletal maturity was also assessed in that study.

On the basis of a study conducted in the United Kingdom, Dorosty *et al.* (16) investigated the nutritional determinants of early adiposity rebound in children followed from birth to 61 months. Children with very early, early, and later adiposity rebound were compared. There was no evidence of a difference in absolute BMI between the three groups before the adiposity rebound, except in girls with a very early rebound. After the rebound had occurred, BMI was significantly higher in those who had rebounded very early. The association between parental BMI and adiposity rebound was also examined.

On the basis of the Fels longitudinal study, Guo *et al.* (17) examined BMI patterns from early childhood to 35 to 45 years. They showed that changes in childhood BMI were related to adult overweight and adiposity, more so in women than in men. The odds ratios for age at adiposity rebound in relation to adult BMI overweight status (BMI $\geq$ 25 versus BMI $<$ 25) were 0.88 in male subjects and 0.44 in female subjects, showing that an early adiposity rebound was associated with an increased risk of adult obesity in women but not in men.

All the studies described here reported a highly significant association between an early adiposity rebound and the risk of developing obesity at a later age. However, the magnitude of the association varied between studies. In the Fels longitudinal study (12), the correlation between age at adiposity rebound and BMI at 18 years was −0.50. In the study conducted in New Zealand (15), correlations with measurements at 21 years were −0.56 for boys and −0.43 for girls. In the Zurich study (4), correlations between age at adiposity rebound and BMI at adult age were −0.31 for boys and −0.30 for girls.

Some investigators (4,15) noticed that the correlation between the BMI level at the age of 6 or 7 years (mean age at adiposity rebound) and BMI at adult age was similar or higher than the correlation between age at adiposity rebound and BMI at adult age. Williams *et al.* (15) concluded that BMI level recorded by the age at adiposity rebound was a more practical way of predicting BMI in adulthood than assessing age at adiposity rebound. In fact, different aspects must be considered. BMI level by the age at adiposity rebound and the age at adiposity rebound are independent predictors of adult adiposity (12,14). They may give complementary information on the factors initiating the development of fatness. A high BMI at 6 years and an early adiposity rebound correspond to different BMI patterns. BMI at the age of 6 years is significantly associated with later BMI, but also with previous BMI levels. In the Zurich study (4), the correlation between BMI at 6 years and the BMI at adult age was 0.60. It was of the same magnitude ($r = 0.66$) between the BMI at 6 years and the BMI at 1 year. In the French sample of the international growth study, an early adiposity rebound was significantly associated with higher BMI at the age of 21 years, but no such a trend—or even an opposite trend—was observed for the correlations between age at adiposity rebound and measurements at the age of 1 year (Fig. 3). Similarly, Dorosty *et al.* (16) did not find a clear trend of high fatness before an early adiposity rebound. On the basis of the data from a longitudinal study of nutrition and growth (20), we found that both an early adiposity rebound and a high BMI at 6 years predicted a high subsequent BMI level. The association with previous measurements, however, was different for the two indicators. BMI at 6 years was positively and significantly correlated with birth weight ($r = 0.23; p = 0.003$), whereas age at adiposity rebound was not correlated with birth weight ($r = -0.06; p = 0.53$) (Rolland-Cachera MF *et al.*, unpublished data). Consequently, as a rule a fat child at age 6 years is likely always to be fat, whereas a child with an early adiposity rebound develops fatness only from the time of the rebound and is likely to have been thin before rebound (Fig. 3).

An inverse association between BMI level before and after adiposity rebound has been reported in various circumstances (22). For example, comparing different countries, the mean BMI level showed an opposite rank order before and after adiposity rebound. The differences in BMI patterns (permanently high BMI, or low BMI followed by high BMI after adiposity rebound) are probably associated with different obesity-promoting factors. The use of both anthropometric indicators (BMI at 6 years and age at adiposity rebound) may improve the identification of the various determinants of obesity.

FACTORS ASSOCIATED WITH ADIPOSITY REBOUND

Differences Between Studies

Mean age at adiposity rebound varies between studies from 5 to 7 years. As age at adiposity rebound varies according to the method used (15), it is difficult to make valid comparisons between studies. Three studies have used the same method (visual inspection). Two were conducted in France, and one in the Czech Republic. Mean age at adiposity rebound was 6.2 years in children born in 1955 (6) and 5.6 years in those born in 1985 (20). In Czech children, mean age at adiposity rebound was 7 years (13). Three studies used a polynomial model to assess age at adiposity rebound. In American children, mean age at rebound was 5.2 years (12) or 5.5 years (14). In New Zealand it was 6.2 years (15). In a study conducted in China it was 5 years (23). In this last study measurements were recorded until the age of 7 years only. As adiposity rebound may occur up to the age of 10 years, this mean value may be an underestimate.

In addition to differences attributable to the methods used, factors such as the date at measurements, the prevalence of obesity in each sample, and country-specific environmental conditions may affect mean age at adiposity rebound.

Gender

No consistent gender differences emerge from the available data regarding either mean age at adiposity rebound or the association between age at rebound and adult fatness. In the French sample of the international growth study (6,18), age at adiposity rebound was earlier in girls than in boys (6.05 versus 6.26 years). In a study started 30 years later (20), adiposity rebound occurred later in girls than in boys (5.9 versus 5.4 years). In the Fels longitudinal study (12), the rebound took place later in girls (5.34 versus 5.13 years), and in the New Zealand study (15), it was earlier in girls (6.1 versus 6.3 years). In the retrospective cohort conducted in the United States (14), girls tended to reach adiposity rebound earlier than boys (5.4 versus 5.8 years). In the Czech study, no difference was recorded between the sexes (7 years in both boys and girls). The sex differences observed in all these studies are probably not significantly different. A sex difference was observed in the predictive value of the adiposity rebound in the Fels longitudinal study (17). An early adiposity rebound was associated with a greater risk of adult obesity in female subjects but not in male subjects. In other studies no such sex differences appeared (4,7,12–16).

Parental BMI

Two studies have examined the association between parental BMI and age at adiposity rebound. The retrospective study of Whitaker *et al.* (14) showed that parent BMI was associated with a younger age at adiposity rebound. In the study conducted by Dorosty *et al.* (16), mean BMI of parents was significantly higher in children with a very early adiposity rebound. Having at least one obese parent was also associated with both very early and early adiposity rebound.

Skeletal Maturity

Two studies have analyzed the association between age at adiposity rebound and skeletal maturity. An early adiposity rebound was associated with advanced skeletal maturity. In the French longitudinal study (7), a trend for older bone age to be associated with an early adiposity rebound has appeared from the age of 2 years, though this is not yet significant. The trend is clearer between 8 and 13 years of age in girls and between 11 and 15 years in boys. The greatest differences are observed at age 12 years in girls ($p < 0.001$) and at age 15 years in boys ($p < 0.005$). Williams *et al.* (15) also found that an earlier adiposity rebound was associated with more advanced skeletal maturity, but the association was significant for boys only. These observations are consistent with the accelerated growth observed in childhood obesity.

Socioeconomic Status and Parental Education

De Spiegelaere *et al.* (24) found no association between socioeconomic status and adiposity rebound. Dorosty *et al.* (16) reported that there was no evidence of any association between parental education or socioeconomic status and the timing of the adiposity rebound. This is consistent with previous analyses showing that, compared with adult obesity, which is related to lower socioeconomic status, in children such an association is less clear (25).

Physical Activity

In a longitudinal study of nutrition and growth, Deheeger *et al.* (26) investigated the association between physical activity and child development. Physical activity was assessed at the age of 10 years. In spite of a higher energy intake, active children had a lower percentage of fat body mass than nonactive children. A retrospective analysis showed that adiposity rebound occurred later in active children. While physical activity was assessed after the age of adiposity rebound (at 10 years), the higher energy intake and greater lean body mass recorded at all ages in active children, and the results of previous studies showing good tracking of physical activity, suggested that active children at age 10 years were also active at earlier ages. These observations are speculative, but they suggest a role of physical activity on the timing of the adiposity rebound.

Secular Trends

Secular trends have appeared for various measures of growth (27). Children are getting larger, becoming taller (attributable mainly to increased leg length), and reaching maturity more rapidly. A longitudinal growth study was initiated in the early 1950s (6,18). Another longitudinal study, following similar protocol (children recruited in health centers in the Paris area) started 30 years later. Mean age at adiposity rebound was 6.2 ± 1.3 years in children born in 1955 (6) and 5.6 ± 1.9 years in children born in 1985 (20). The trend in age at adiposity rebound is consistent with the secular trend of earlier maturation.

Nutrition

Energy and Nutrient Intakes

In a longitudinal study of nutrition and growth we investigated the nutritional factors associated with age at adiposity rebound (20). Nutritional intakes were assessed at the age of 2 years. Correlations were computed between intakes at 2 years of age at adiposity rebound. No association was found between energy intake, percentage of energy from fat or carbohydrate, and age at adiposity rebound. A negative and significant association was found between the percentage of protein intake and adiposity rebound—that is, the higher the percentage of protein consumed at the age of 2 years, the earlier the adiposity rebound.

More recently, Dorosty *et al.* (16) conducted a similar analysis in a prospective cohort of children followed from birth to 5 years in the United Kingdom. They compared very early (before the age of 3.5 years), early (from 4 to 5 years), and later rebound (after 5 years). They found no evidence of associations between dietary protein or any other dietary variable recorded at the age of 18 months and the timing of the adiposity rebound. They did not confirm the association between protein intake and age at adiposity rebound. They also failed to show any association with either energy or fat intake. A study conducted in Italian children has shown an association between early high protein intake and increased BMI at the time of adiposity rebound (28).

The unexpected results of the French study regarding the association between protein intake and age at adiposity rebound (20) have drawn attention to the inadequate nutrient balance of the infant diet in industrialized countries (29) (Table 1). By the age of 1 year, the infant diet is characterized by high intakes of protein (approximately 4 g/kg body weight or 16% of total energy) and low intakes of fat of about 28%). Protein intake represents about three to four times the protein needs (30). The nutrient imbalance is remarkable because the diet during the first months of life, when human milk is the only food, provides 7% of energy as protein and 54% as fat (9). Paradoxically, the proportion of fat in the infant diet is low at a period of high energy needs. Figure 5 shows the actual nutrient changes from early childhood (20) to adult life (31). The percentage of energy provided by fat increases with age, whereas it should be high in early life and gradually decrease with age.

How would an increased protein intake lead to an early adiposity rebound? Childhood obesity is characterized by accelerated growth and increased stature and lean body mass (19). An early high protein intake may account for these characteristics. These changes in body composition could have occurred through changes in hormonal status (29,32). High plasma, insulin-like growth factor 1 (IGF-1) concentrations and reduced growth hormone secretion (spontaneous or in response to a wide

TABLE 1. *Composition of human milk and nutritional intake in infants from different countries*

Countries	Age in months	Intake			
		Protein g/kg	Protein % energy	Fat % energy	CHO % energy
Human milk			7	54	39
Belgium	12–36	3.8	15.8	29.2	55
Denmark	12	3.3	15.0	28.0	57
France	10	4.3	15.6	27.4	57
Italy	12	5.1	19.5	30.5	50
Spain	9	4.4	15.7	26.4	57.9

From Rolland-Cachera *et al.*, 1999 (29).

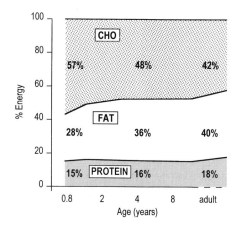

FIG. 5. Actual nutrient changes from early childhood (21) to adulthood (31). The percentage of energy provided by fat increases from infancy to adult age, whereas it should be high in early life and decrease gradually with age.

variety of stimuli) are characteristic features of children with simple obesity (33). Nutritional intake affects hormonal status. Fasting decreases serum IGF-1 concentrations and restoration of IGF-1 is directly associated with the energy and protein content of the diet (34). In protein–energy malnutrition, growth hormone levels are raised and the high growth hormone values are not affected by increasing the energy intake. They fall only when protein is added to the diet (35). These results suggest that protein deprivation acts as a stimulus to growth hormone secretion.

We have previously proposed (32) that the altered hormonal status of obese children (high IGF-1 and reduced growth hormone) could be the mirror image of protein deprivation and thus a consequence of an excess protein intake. Indeed, a high protein intake is often recorded in obese children (36–38). It may increase IGF-1 levels, stimulating protein synthesis and cell proliferation in all body tissues. This could account for the characteristic accelerated growth and increased muscle mass of obese children. As IGF-1 promotes the differentiation of preadipocytes into adipocytes (39), a high protein intake may induce hyperplasia in adipose tissue. The early increase in adipocyte number reported in obese children (19) may be responsible for the early adiposity rebound recorded in the obese. In addition, a high protein intake may, at any age, decrease growth hormone levels, thus decreasing lipolysis and promoting the development and maintenance of high fat stores. A high protein intake may also promote an android type of body fat distribution (40) and hence the development of metabolic complications of obesity such as insulin resistance or cardiovascular disease (41).

Metabolic Adaptation to a Relative Energy Deficit in Infancy

Over the previous few decades, energy and fat intakes have decreased at a population level (42) in children (43), and even in young children (44,45), while the percentage of energy from protein has increased (44).

Energy intake in 1.5- to 2.5-year-old English children declined from 1,264 to 1,045 kcal/day between 1967 and 1993 (44). At the same time, the percentage of energy obtained from protein increased (43,44). The trend to decreased energy intake is the probable consequence of decreasing energy expenditure in older children but is less likely in young children, in whom a reduced energy intake may be related to the composition of the diet. A low fat intake reduces the energy density of the diet and may reduce the total energy intake (46). In addition, a low-fat/high-protein diet can reduce energy intake, as young children prefer flavors associated with high dietary fat (47) and because of the satiating effect of protein (48). Mean energy intakes in infants are generally below estimated requirements (49).

A relative energy deficit could be generated by both a low fat intake and by the increased energy expenditure required for the high protein-associated accelerated growth. The BMI pattern associated with an early adiposity rebound (low fatness in infancy, followed by an early adiposity rebound and subsequent increased fatness) could be explained by the dietary changes with age (Fig. 5); that is, a low-fat/high-protein intake during the first years of life, followed by high-fat intake in later childhood.

The low energy density of the infant's diet could create a relative energy deficit and induce metabolic adaptations (thrifty metabolism). These adaptations may have adverse effects when, at later ages, children eat an adequate or more abundant high-fat diet. Similar patterns of consuming low-fat weaning foods, followed by a more adequate diet, may also occur in developing countries.

The fatness pattern of low BMI followed by increased BMI after the adiposity rebound is consistent with other observations. Low weight for length in early life has been found in men and women with syndrome X (50), and it has been suggested that changes from poor to abundant nutrition could increase the risk of developing diabetes and ischemic heart disease (51). The hypothesis of an association between risk factors and accelerated growth promoted by an excessive early protein intake is also consistent with the association between increased stature, particularly leg length (52), early maturation (2), and health risks. Overweight at adolescence, whatever the weight status by adulthood, is associated with increased risk factors for later diseases (53), showing the importance of the period of growth. Accelerated growth may play a major role in the risks associated with obesity.

CONCLUSIONS

The increasing prevalence of obesity has stimulated interest in the identification of early markers for this condition. Age at adiposity rebound, recorded on individual BMI curves, has been found to be associated with adult weight status. Numerous studies have reported that an early adiposity rebound is associated with an increased risk of obesity.

Some studies have investigated the factors associated with age at adiposity rebound. An early adiposity rebound is associated with advanced skeletal maturity and parental obesity, and there is evidence to suggest an association with a sedentary lifestyle. No association was recorded with socioeconomic status. Studies on nutritional intakes have failed to show any association between energy or fat intake in early childhood and age at adiposity rebound. One study reported an association with a high protein intake at the age of 2 years.

The early adiposity rebound recorded in obese individuals suggests that the determinants act in early life. The results of nutritional studies suggest that infant diets in many industrialized countries are not adapted to the specific needs of children during the different phases of growth.

More research on the factors associated with age at adiposity rebound may help to identify factors promoting overweight and may be useful in preventing the development of obesity at an early stage of life.

SUGGESTIONS FOR FUTURE RESEARCH ACTIVITIES IN THE FIELD

Associations between adiposity rebound and environmental and genetic factors should be investigated. Previous investigations were conducted in populations with homogeneous weight status, feeding practices, and physical activity. The association between adiposity rebound and environmental factors should be conducted in samples that include a broader range of BMI and more varied behaviors.

Mean BMI pattern reflects changes in fatness, but changes in body composition at the time of adiposity rebound may vary according to various factors (e.g., sex, nutrition, genetics, physical activity). Studies on changes in body composition in relation to age at adiposity rebound could be of interest.

An early adiposity rebound and a high BMI by the time of the adiposity rebound relate to different BMI patterns—these two indicators are independent predictors of adult fatness. Comparisons of the association of these indicators with biological markers and long-term health risks should be investigated.

KEY POLICY IMPLICATIONS

Research on adiposity rebound has stressed the role of early determinants of adult obesity and inadequate nutritional intakes in early life.

The combination of decreasing energy intake and increasing prevalence of obesity suggests that rather than energy restriction, improvements in nutrient balance—taking into account the specific needs at the different periods of growth—and promotion of an active lifestyle should be encouraged.

REFERENCES

1. De Onis, Blösner M. Prevalence and trends of overweight among preschool children in developing countries. *Am J Clin Nutr* 2000; 72: 1032–9.
2. Power C, Lake JK, Cole TJ. Measurements and long-term health risks of child and adolescent fatness. *Int J Obes* 1997; 21: 507–26.
3. Rolland-Cachera MF, Deheeger M, Avons P, *et al.* Tracking adiposity patterns from 1 month to adulthood. *Ann Hum Biol* 1987; 14: 219–22.
4. Gasser T, Ziegler P, Seifert B, *et al.* Prediction of adult skinfolds and body mass from infancy through adolescence. *Ann Hum Biol* 1995; 22: 217–33.
5. Ong KKL, Ahmed ML, Emmett PM, Preece MA, Dunger DB, and the Avon Longitudinal Study of Pregnancy and Childhood Study Team. Association between postnatal catch-up growth and obesity in childhood: prospective cohort study. *BMJ* 2000; 320: 967–71.

6. Rolland-Cachera MF, Sempé M, Guilloud-Bataille M, *et al.* Adiposity indices in children. *Am J Clin Nutr* 1982; 36: 178–84.
7. Rolland-Cachera MF, Deheeger M, Bellisle F, *et al.* Adiposity rebound in children: a simple indicator for predicting obesity. *Am J Clin Nutr* 1984; 39: 129–35.
8. Dietz HW. Periods of risk in childhood for the development of adult obesity—what do we need to learn? *J Nutr* 1997; 127: 1884–6S.
9. Poskitt EME. *Practical paediatric nutrition.* London: Butterworth, 1988: 300.
10. WHO expert Committee. Physical status: the use and interpretation of anthropometry. WHO Technical Report Series No 854. Geneva: WHO, 1995: 368–9.
11. Sempé M, Pédron G, Roy-Pernot MP. *Auxologie, méthode et séquences.* Paris: Théraplix, 1979 [in French].
12. Siervogel RM, Roche AF, Guo S, Mukherjee D, Chumlea WC. Patterns of change in weight/stature^2 from 2 to 18 years: findings from long-term serial data for children in the Fels longitudinal growth study. *Int J Obes* 1991; 15: 479–85.
13. Prokopec M, Bellisle F. Adiposity in Czech children followed from one month of age to adulthood: analysis of individual BMI patterns. *Ann Hum Biol* 1993; 20: 517–25.
14. Whitaker R, Pepe MS, Wright JA, Seidel KD, Dietz WH. Early adiposity rebound and the risk of adult obesity. *Pediatrics* 1998; 101: 5.
15. Williams S, Davie G, Lam F. Predicting BMI in young adults from childhood data using two approaches to modeling adiposity rebound. *Int J Obes* 1999; 23: 348–54.
16. Dorosty AR, Emmett PM, Cowin IS, Reilly JJ, and the ALSPAC Study Team. Factors associated with early adiposity rebound. *Pediatrics* 2000; 105: 1115–8.
17. Guo SS, Huang C, Maynard LM, *et al.* Body mass index during childhood, adolescence and young adulthood in relation to adult overweight and adiposity: the Fels longitudinal study. *Int J Obes* 2000; 24: 1628–35.
18. Falkner F, Hindley CB, Graffar M, *et al.* Child development: an international method of study. *Med Probl Pediatr* 1960; 5: 1–237.
19. Knittle JL, Timmers K, Ginsberg-Fellner F, Brown RE, Katz DP. The growth of adipose tissue in children and adolescents. Cross sectional and longitudinal studies of adipose cell number and size. *J Clin Invest* 1979; 63: 239–46.
20. Rolland-Cachera MF, Deheeger M, Akrout M, Bellisle F. Influence of macronutrients on adiposity development: a follow-up study of nutrition and growth from 10 months to 8 years of age. *Int J Obes* 1995; 19: 573–8.
21. Girardet JP, Tounian P, Le Bars MA, Boreux A. Obesité de l'enfant: intérêt des indicateurs cliniques d'évaluation. *Ann Pediatr* 1993; 40: 297–303 [in French].
22. Rolland-Cachera MF. Obesity among children and adolescents: the importance of early nutrition in human growth and development. In: Johnston FE, Zemel B, Eveleth PB, eds. *Human growth in context.* London: Smith Gordon, 1999: 245–58.
23. Ding Z, He Q, Fan Z. National epidemiological study on obesity of children aged 0–7 years in china 1996. *Chin Med J* 1998; 78: 121–3 [in Chinese].
24. De Spiegelaere M, Dramaix M, Hennard P. Socioeconomic status and changes in body mass index from 3 to 5 years. *Arch Dis Child* 1998; 78: 477–8.
25. Sobal J, Stunkard A. Socioeconomic status and obesity: a review of the literature. *Psychol Bull* 1989; 105: 260–75.
26. Deheeger M, Rolland-Cachera MF, Fontvieille AM. Physical activity and body composition in 10-year-old French children: linkages with nutritional intake? *Int J Obes* 1997; 21: 372–9.
27. Cole TJ. Secular trends in growth. *Proc Nutr Soc* 2000; 59: 317–24.
28. Scaglioni S, Agostoni C, DeNotaris R, *et al.* Early macronutrient intake and overweight at 5 years of age. *Int J Obes* 2000; 24: 777–81.
29. Rolland-Cachera MF, Deheeger M, Bellisle F. Increasing prevalence of obesity among 18-year-old males in Sweden: evidence for early determinants. *Acta Paediatr* 1999; 88: 365–7.
30. FAO/WHO/UN University. Energy and protein requirements. Report of a joint expert consultation (WHO technical report series No 274). Geneva: WHO, 1985.
31. Rigaud D, Giachetti I, Deheeger M, *et al.* Enquête française de consommation alimentaire. I. Energie et macronutriments. *Cah Nutr Diet* 1997; 32: 379–89 [in French].
32. Rolland-Cachera MF. Prediction of adult body composition from childhood measurements. In: Davies PSW, Cole TJ, eds. *Body composition techniques in health and diseases.* Cambridge: Cambridge University Press, 1995: 100–45.
33. Loche S, Cappa M, Borrelli A, *et al.* Reduced growth hormone response to growth hormone-releas-

ing hormone in children with simple obesity: evidence for somatomedin-C mediated inhibition. *Clin Endocrinol* 1987; 27: 145–53.

34. Thissen JP, Ketelsleger JM, Underwood LE. Nutritional regulation of the insulin-like growth factors. *Endocr Rev* 1994; 15: 80–101.
35. Pimstone BL, Barbezat G, Hansen JDL, Murray P. Studies on growth hormone secretion in protein-calorie malnutrition. *Am J Clin Nutr* 1968; 21: 482–7.
36. Rolland-Cachera MF, Bellisle F. No correlation between adiposity and food intake: why are working class children fatter? *Am J Clin Nutr* 1986; 44: 779–87.
37. Valoski A, Epstein LH. Nutrient intake of obese children in a family-based behavioral weight control program. *Int J Obes* 1990; 14: 667–77.
38. Ortega RM, Requejo AM, Andres P, *et al.* Relationship between diet composition and body mass index in a group of Spanish adolescents. *BMJ* 1995; 74: 765–73.
39. Ailhaud G, Grimaldi P, Négrel R. A molecular view of adipose tissue. *Int J Obes* 1992; 16: 517–21.
40. Rolland-Cachera MF, Deheeger M, Bellisle F. Nutrient balance and android body fat distribution: why not a role for protein? *Am J Clin Nutr* 1996; 64: 663–4.
41. Vague J. The degree of masculine differentiation of obesities: a factor determining predisposition to diabetes, arteriosclerosis, gout, and uric calculous diseases. *Am J Clin Nutr* 1956; 4: 20–34.
42. Prentice AM, Jebb SA. Obesity in Britain: gluttony or sloth? *BMJ* 1995; 311: 437–9.
43. Nicklas TA, Webber LS, Srinivasan SR, Berenson G. Secular trends in dietary intakes and cardiovascular risk factors of 10 y-old children: the Bogalusa Heart Study (1973–1988). *Am J Clin Nutr* 1993; 57: 930–7.
44. Gregory JR, Collins DL, Davies PSW, Hughes JM, Clarke PC. *National diet and nutrition survey: children aged 1.5 to 4.5 years.* London: HMSO, 1995.
45. Troiano RP, Briefel RR, Carroll MD, Bialostroski K. Energy and fat intakes of children and adolescents in the United States: data from the National Health and Nutrition Examination surveys. *Am J Clin Nutr* 2000; 72: 1343–53S.
46. Michaelsen KF, Jorgensen MH. Dietary fat content and energy density during infancy and childhood; the effect on energy intake and growth. *Eur J Clin Nutr* 1995; 49: 467–83.
47. Johnson SL, McPhee L, Birch LL. Conditioned preferences: young children prefer flavors associated with high dietary fat. *Physiol Behav* 1991; 50: 1245–51.
48. Blundell JE, Tremblay A. Appetite control and energy (fuel) balance. *Nutr Res Rev* 1995; 8: 225–32.
49. Livingstone B. Epidemiology of childhood obesity in Europe. *Eur J Pediatr* 2000; 159: 14–34.
50. Barker DJP, Hales CN, Fall CHD, *et al.* Type 2 (non-insulin-dependent) diabetes mellitus, hypertension and hyperlipidaemia (syndrome X): relation to reduced fetal growth. *Diabetologia* 1993; 36: 62–7.
51. Hales CN, Barker DJP, Clark PMS, *et al.* Fetal and infant growth and impaired glucose tolerance at age 64. *BMJ* 1991; 303: 1019–22.
52. Frankel S, Gunnell DJ, Peters TJ, Maynard M, Smith GD. Childhood energy intake and adult mortality from cancer: the Boyd Orr cohort. *Br J Nutr* 1998; 317: 1350–1.
53. Must A, Jacques PF, Dallal GE, Bajema CJ, Dietz WH. Long term morbidity and mortality of overweight adolescents—a follow-up of the Harvard group study of 1922 to 1935. *N Engl J Med* 1992; 327: 1350–5.

DISCUSSION

Dr. Dulloo: This is a fascinating phenomenon. In relation to protein intake, a correlation coefficient of 0.2—that is, an r^2 value of 0.04—means that protein explains less than 5% of the total variation. Even if that's significant, it's a very weak determinant. What was the correlation coefficient in the other study in which there was also a positive relation, the one by Scaglioni (1)? Was it stronger?

Dr. Rolland-Cachera: Nutrition is just one of many aspects of lifestyle and it is obviously difficult to find associations between nutritional intake and obesity. We have summarized 176 correlations from 34 studies. The main result was that there was no association between nutritional intake and adiposity. I agree that the correlation in your study is very weak; nevertheless, it is still there, and that isn't the case with the other nutrients. It is true that the correlation is too weak to allow us to say that protein increases the risk of obesity, but it does open a window onto a research area.

The study by Scaglioni was not linked to adiposity rebound but to BMI level. The association was weak also.

Dr. Singhal: What is the genetic contribution to the adiposity rebound? Have there been any studies in twins to indicate whether the phenomenon is related to nutrition or to genetics?

Dr. Rolland-Cachera: I don't know of any twin studies, but an association between adiposity rebound and parental BMI suggests that there might be a genetic component, as does the difference between countries.

Dr. Freedman: You showed a slide in which there were eight curves representing different countries. A low BMI at age 2 was associated with an earlier adiposity rebound and then a high BMI at age 18. Would you find the same thing if you were to study individuals? Surely there would not be an inverse association between BMI at age 2 and BMI at age 18, wouldn't there?

Dr. Rolland-Cachera: Yes, children with an early adiposity rebound tend to have a lower BMI before the rebound. To illustrate that, I described the case of a very thin child with an early adiposity rebound who later became fat. What I really wanted to stress was that there may not be only one process of obesity. We should look more carefully at these individual BMI patterns. They might be linked with different determinants—genetic, nutritional, and so on. The U-shaped birth weight curve in relation with risk factors has been mentioned previously. Adiposity rebound may be related to this phenomenon. We should really be looking at the patterns of development that are associated with different risk factors.

Dr. Bellizzi: In your correlations with nutrients, have you ever looked at carbohydrates, and in particular complex carbohydrates?

Dr. Rolland-Cachera: There was no association at all. The association with fat was also nonsignificant, but the trend was in favor of an inverse trend between fat intake in infancy and adiposity at older ages. This is consistent with a beneficial effect of human milk. It is important that advice to decrease fat intake in the population as a whole exclude infants.

Dr. Dulloo: From your graph of adiposity rebound in different countries it seemed that the phenomenon occurs in Senegal and Burundi but not in India. What is your explanation for that?

Dr. Rolland-Cachera: I think the explanation probably lies in the lifelong low intakes of food in the Indian population.

Dr. Cole: I would like to comment on the interpretation of the adiposity rebound, putting it in a different context. I asked myself the question, "Why should an early age at adiposity rebound predict later obesity?" The answer is because at about this age, the median value of the BMI goes down and then goes up again. For this reason, what is in fact an upward centile crossing has the appearance of an early adiposity rebound, and if you are crossing centiles upward, this will predict later obesity. I can illustrate this with two examples [Figs. 6 and 7].

The first example, from Dr. Rolland-Cachera's French study, is that of a child reported to have a late adiposity rebound. BMI centiles are crossed upward until about age 1 year, and then they fall. It's hard to say exactly when the adiposity rebound is but it's certainly late. If you plot that same chart using the BMI z score (right), each centile curve becomes a horizontal straight line, as I explained in an earlier discussion, so it's easier to see what is going on. You can now see that there is upward crossing of the centiles until about 1 year, and then a more or less linear fall until the age of around 10 or 12, so what looks like a late adiposity rebound is simply the downward centile crossing of the BMI.

The second example is that of a child with an extremely early adiposity rebound, at about age 2. If you look on the right hand side of the graph, you can see that the early adiposity rebound is again just simply upward centile crossing. So the child is crossing centiles more or

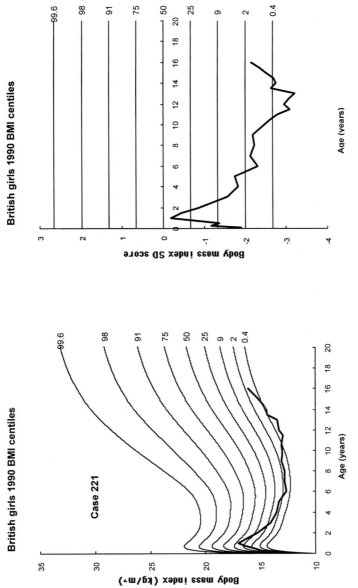

FIG. 6. Late adiposity rebound and centile crossing downward.

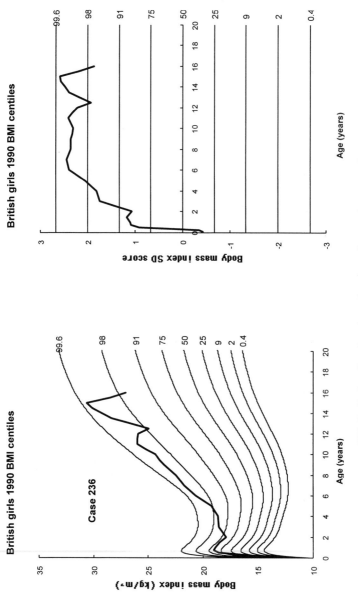

FIG. 7. Early adiposity rebound and centile crossing upward.

less linearly from the age of 1 year to the age of 6 years, after the same centile is maintained.

If you understand that "adiposity rebound" is simply a statement about centile crossing, then three things follow. First, an earlier adiposity rebound will be associated with a low BMI, because you are starting at a low centile and crossing upward. Second, it will be correlated with a high BMI later. Third, whether your BMI is high or low early will correlate with whether your BMI is high or low later.

Dr. Rolland-Cachera: I agree that we should compare data in different ways to gain a better understanding of the phenomenon. Thank you for this additional information.

REFERENCES

1. Scaglioni S, Agostoni C, DeNotaris R, *et al.* Early macronutrient intake and overweight at 5 years of age. *Int J Obes* 2000; 24: 777–81.

Obesity in Childhood and Adolescence, edited by
Chunming Chen and William H. Dietz. Nestlé
Nutrition Workshop Series, Pediatric Program,
Vol. 49. Nestec Ltd., Vevey/Lippincott
Williams & Wilkins, Philadelphia © 2002.

Natural History of Obesity:
A Focus on Adolescence

Linda G. Bandini

Massachusetts Institute of Technology, Cambridge, Massachusetts, USA

Adolescence appears to be a high-risk period for the development of obesity, particularly in girls (1). Adolescent obesity is associated with increased morbidity (2) and is more likely to track into adulthood (1). Additionally, adolescent obesity is often associated with adverse psychosocial well-being (2). Therefore the identification of factors that increase susceptibility to obesity during adolescence is essential in the prevention and treatment of adolescent obesity. This chapter will discuss the normal changes in fatness and body fat distribution that occur throughout the adolescent period, and consider factors that may influence these changes.

MEASUREMENT OF BODY FATNESS

Laboratory Methods

Body fatness can be measured directly by laboratory techniques. These include measures of total body water by isotopic dilution, body density by underwater weighing, potassium content by 40K counting, and fat-free mass by dual-energy x-ray absorptiometry (DEXA). None of these techniques measures body fat directly. All measure fat-free mass based on the assumption that FFM has a constant composition. Once fat-free mass has been estimated, body fat can be calculated by subtracting the fat-free mass from body weight: percentage of body fat = (body weight − fat-free mass)/body weight × 100. Multicompartmental methods to measure different components of body composition will reduce the errors associated with the assumption that FFM has a constant composition, but these methods are limited to research studies. Newer, more sophisticated methods have recently been developed that measure body fat directly. Neutron activation measures total body carbon, which indicates total body fat, but this is a highly specialized method and not available for clinical use.

Bioelectrical impedance (BIA) is not a direct estimate of body composition but provides an estimate of body water. Body fat is then calculated from the difference between body weight and fat-free mass, assuming that the latter is 73% water. Measures of body fatness in children and adolescents derived by BIA are significantly correlated with laboratory measures (3). Measures of change in body fatness measured by BIA are, however, not well established.

Clinical Methods

Measures of skinfold thickness and body mass index (BMI) have been used to identify overweight children and adolescents because of the lack of availability of direct measures of body fatness in a clinical setting. Skinfold thickness provides a measure of subcutaneous fatness. Two assumptions are inherent in the use of skinfolds to measure body fatness. The first is that the skinfold site measured is representative of subcutaneous fat. The second is that subcutaneous fat is representative of total body fat. Because fat distribution changes during childhood and adolescence, the reliance on a single skinfold measure to assess body fatness may be inaccurate.

Body mass index does not measure fatness but is highly correlated with body fat measured by laboratory methods. BMI changes with growth and development in children. Therefore, criteria for identifying overweight will depend on age and sex. Furthermore, body composition changes with growth and development. As discussed by Troiano *et al.* (4), BMI to identify overweight in children should be used cautiously because body composition (e.g., bone mass and the proportion of lean and fat tissues) changes at different times and rates during growth and development.

Many of the reported studies on serial changes of body fatness in children and adolescents are based on measures of skinfold thickness, BMI, and BIA. It is therefore important to keep in mind the limitations of these measurements when interpreting studies. All represent indirect measures of body fatness and it is unclear how well they assess change.

MEASURES OF BODY FAT DISTRIBUTION

Because fat distribution is an independent risk factor associated with the adverse effects of obesity, it is now the subject of many investigations. Increased abdominal fat is often characterized as upper body fatness, increased truncal fatness, or a central body fat distribution. Generally, a central or truncal body fat distribution refers to excess fat in the trunk rather than peripherally—that is, in the arms and legs. Upper body fat distribution is essentially the same as central or truncal body fat, but refers more specifically to an excess of body fat in the upper body.

Many investigators use body circumferences, such as the waist-to-hip ratio or waist circumference, to identify upper-body fat distribution or a central or truncal pattern of distribution. Others use skinfold thickness. Biceps and triceps skinfolds represent peripheral fat stores, whereas abdominal or subscapular skinfold thickness represents truncal fat stores. However, skinfold thickness measures only subcutaneous fat, not intraabdominal adipose tissue.

Intraabdominal adipose tissue appears to be associated with the adverse effects of an upper-body fat distribution (5,6). To differentiate subcutaneous abdominal fat and intraabdominal adipose tissue, magnetic resonance imaging (MRI) or computed tomography (CT) scans are necessary.

Many investigators have studied the relation between anthropometric measurements—such as skinfold thickness and body circumferences—and intraabdominal adipose tissue in children and adolescents. De Ridder *et al.* (7) reported a significant relation between waist circumference and intraabdominal fat in a small sample of girls but no correlation between waist-to-hip ratio and intraabdominal fat. Brambilla *et al.* (8) also did not find a significant relation between waist-to-hip ratio and intraabdominal fat. Goran *et al.* (9) and Fox *et al.* (10) report a stronger relation of trunk skinfold measures than waist-to-hip ratio with intraabdominal adipose tissue. Waist circumference was significantly correlated with intraabdominal adipose tissue in both girls and boys in Fox's initial study (10). However, in their follow-up study (11), waist circumference was not correlated with intraabdominal adipose tissue.

Although it appears that the waist-to-hip ratio may be of value in determining the upper- or lower-body fat distribution of subcutaneous tissues, it is not a useful index of intraabdominal adipose tissue. Trunk skinfold thickness and waist circumference do not give a reliable measure of intraabdominal adipose tissue either, but overall show a better correlation than the waist-to-hip ratio. It also appears that the value of an anthropometric measurement may differ with the stage of sexual maturation.

MEASURES OF MATURATION

Stages of puberty are based on Tanner staging of sexual development (12) and peak height velocity. Tanner staging is somewhat subjective, and the measure of peak height velocity requires serial measurements. Menarche is the only defined time point. Sex hormones may provide direct measures of pubertal status but are often lacking from most studies. Thus studies of the effect of puberty and pubertal stage on obesity may be limited by the measures available to identify periods of maturation.

BODY COMPOSITION THROUGH CHILDHOOD AND ADOLESCENCE

Body fatness changes throughout the period of childhood and adolescence. Twenty-five years ago, Dugdale and Payne (13), using published data on body weight and body composition at various ages, calculated the changes in lean and fat tissue from birth to 17 years of age. They identified periods of lean and fat deposition during childhood and adolescence. Fat deposition predominates in the first year of life, but from then to age 4 years lean tissue deposition predominates. Between 6 and 10 years of age fat deposition increases again. Lean mass deposition increases during adolescence, but by age 17, fat deposition once more predominates. Recent body composition studies have confirmed these cycles of fat deposition and will be reviewed later. I will discuss the period of infancy and prepuberty only briefly and concentrate on the changes during adolescence.

Infancy and Childhood

Recently, body composition in infants through 2 years of age has been studied using a multicomponent model (14). Fat mass as a percentage of body weight increased during the first 6 months and then declined. At 6 and 9 months of age, percentage of body fat was higher in girls than boys.

Differences in body composition in prepubertal boys and girls are small (15). Recently, Taylor *et al.* (16) measured body composition in 3- to 8-year-old children using DEXA. They observed a significantly higher percentage of body fat and smaller amounts of lean tissue in girls in comparison to boys matched for age, height, weight, and BMI. Their data suggest that sexual dimorphism observed in adolescents may begin before puberty. However, only 20 pairs of boys and girls were measured. Further studies on larger numbers of children are needed to verify these findings.

Increases in body fat in both boys and girls begin after 4 to 5 years of age, a period labeled the "adiposity rebound" (17). It has been suggested that an earlier increase in adiposity rebound may be a risk period for the development of obesity (18).

Pubertal Period

During the pubertal period, significant changes in linear growth and body composition occur. These changes differ considerably among boys and girls. While both boys and girls gain lean body mass, boys gain significantly more than girls. Cheek measured total body water in a large cohort of boy and girls of various ages (15). In boys, lean body mass almost doubled from the age of 10 to 15, although there was little change in fat mass. Girls also show large increases in fat-free mass during puberty, although not to the same extent as boys. Girls, however, also gained significant amounts of body fat. This chapter will focus on these changes in body fatness and fat distribution that occur during the adolescent period and the factors that contribute to these changes.

Studies that have examined the change in body composition in girls and boys during puberty have found differences not only in the amount of fat-free mass accretion but also in the rate of accretion. In the Fels longitudinal study (19), girls showed an increase in fat-free mass that slowed over the teenage years, whereas boys showed a continual increase until they reached young adulthood.

Energy Cost of Growth in Adolescence

Many people believe that rapid growth during adolescence increases the energy requirements significantly. However, the extra energy needed to support growth during the adolescent period is relatively small. Approximately 1% to 3% of daily energy expenditure during this period can be attributed to the energy cost of growth.

The cost of excess weight gain is also small. A girl who is at the 50th centile for weight at 9 years of age will be close to the 95th centile of weight for age at 13 if she gains an excess of 4 kg a year. Assuming that this adipose tissue has an energy cost of 7,200 kcal, this would translate to an excess of 80 kcal. Thus growth and excess weight gain do not require large amounts of energy, and the common notion that adolescents need lots of extra energy to support growth is unfounded.

Ethnic Differences in Body Composition

Studies have shown that girls who mature earlier are heavier and fatter than girls who mature later and that early maturation is associated with increased risk of subsequent obesity (20). Morrison *et al.* (21) observed racial differences in sexual maturity and body composition among black and white 9- and 10-year-old girls. They found more black than white girls were pubertal at age 9 and 10, and observed racial differences in body composition among 9- and 10-year-old girls at Tanner stage 2. Thus black girls at this stage had greater weight, height, BMI, and skinfold thickness than white girls. In Morrison's study (21), differences in fatness among black and white girls were observed during puberty but not before puberty, suggesting that puberty is associated with the increase in fatness in black girls. However, in the NHANES III study conducted in the United States between 1988 and 1991, non-Hispanic black girls had a higher prevalence of overweight than white girls during both childhood (6 to 11 years) and adolescence (12 to 17 years) (4).

Longitudinal studies comparing weight changes and body fatness among black and white girls are needed to support the suggestion that during puberty ethnic differences are associated with an increased incidence of obesity in black girls. Data on body fatness among other ethnic groups are limited.

Persistence into Adult Life

It has been proposed that adolescence is a period of increased risk for obesity in girls (1). Among the most concerning consequences of childhood and adolescent obesity is its persistence into adulthood, where it is associated with the morbidity and premature mortality characteristic of adult obesity (2). Furthermore, Must *et al.* (22) have shown that men who were obese as adolescents had an increased risk of all-cause mortality and an increased risk of cardiovascular disease independent of whether they were obese as adults.

In a retrospective longitudinal study, Whitaker *et al.* (23) have shown that the persistence of childhood obesity into adulthood increases with age. An obese adolescent will be more likely to become an obese adult than an obese toddler. Studies that have examined whether persistence is related to gender have produced inconsistent findings. Must and Strauss (2) have reviewed the literature and report that some but not all of the studies show greater persistence in obese adolescent females than in obese adolescent males. Parental obesity and severity of obesity also increase the risk that an obese child will become an obese adult (2,23).

Data are needed to determine whether pubertal changes occurring during adolescence in girls may be related to the increased risk of obesity.

CHANGES IN FAT DISTRIBUTION DURING ADOLESCENCE

Cross-sectional studies have been conducted to examine the change in fat distribution in childhood and adolescence, but few longitudinal data are available.

Changes in the distribution of body fat during puberty from peripheral to central sites are much more pronounced in boys than in girls (24). Obesity in both male and female adolescents has been associated with an increase in truncal fat (25). In a study of obese and nonobese female and male adolescents, using densitometry to measure body fat and skinfold thickness to examine body fat distribution, Hattori *et al.* found that obese adolescents had more truncal fat than nonobese adolescents (25). Obese girls tended to have more truncal fat at the subscapular site, while obese boys had more in the abdominal area. Cowell *et al.* conducted a cross-sectional study of body fatness in individuals from 4 to 35 years of age using DEXA (26). They found that in female subjects there was a tendency for a more central distribution of body fat with increasing adiposity, whereas in male subjects the increase in abdominal fat appeared to be independent of total fat mass.

In the US NHANES I survey, Frisancho and Flegal (27) have shown that early maturation in white children is associated with an increase in body fatness and in the central deposition of body fat. Deutsch and Mueller, however, found that early maturation in boys had an effect on fat distribution but not on fatness, whereas in girls early maturation was associated with fatness but not with fat distribution (28).

Van Lenthe *et al.* (29) conducted a longitudinal study on the changes in skinfold thickness between the ages of 13 and 27 years in males and females as part of the Amsterdam Growth and Health Study (AGHS). They measured four skinfolds and constructed ratios to represent a truncal pattern of fat distribution. Skinfold ratios of girls with early and late menarche differed as follows: Girls with early menarche had significantly higher skinfold ratios than girls with late menarche, suggesting that early maturation is associated with an increase in truncal fat distribution. They did not find an analogous difference in skinfold ratio in relation to maturation in boys as reflected by skeletal age. Given the association of a central fat distribution to increased risk of cardiovascular disease and diabetes, as well as the psychologic impact of early menarche on young girls, it is critical to better understand the interrelationships among these variables.

Factors Associated with a Central Distribution of Body Fat

In girls during early puberty, de Ridder *et al.* have shown that fat distribution is associated with estradiol and testosterone levels (30). Several studies suggest that the endocrine effects on fat distribution may be modified by behavioral factors. Smoking (31), alcohol use (32), and decreased physical activity (32) appear to be associated with a centralized fat distribution in adults, at least in cross-sectional studies. As discussed earlier, Van Lenthe reported an association between early menarche and fat distribution in the AGHS study (29). In another aspect of the AGHS study, Post and Kemper report that early-maturing adolescents were less physically active than slower-maturing adolescents (33). Whether physical activity patterns will alter fat distribution during adolescence needs more study.

There are limited data on the association of diet and changes in body fatness. Findings by Berky *et al.* from a historical cohort of girls suggest that diet and body size are associated with age at peak height velocity and peak growth velocity (34). The age at which girls reached peak growth velocity was younger for girls who were taller before 6 years of age and for those who consumed more animal fat between the ages of 6 and 8. They also suggest that diets higher in protein are associated with earlier menarche. This observation has not been reported elsewhere. Whether macronutrient composition of the diet has an effect on growth and development or fat distribution is unknown.

Intraabdominal Adipose Tissue

Upper-body fatness in adults has been associated with increased risk of cardiovascular disease independent of total body fatness. Using DEXA to estimate regional body fatness, Daniels *et al.* showed that truncal fat distribution in children and adolescents was positively correlated with triglyceride levels, systolic blood pressure, and left ventricular mass, and inversely correlated with high-density lipoprotein (HDL) levels (35). Furthermore, they found that fat distribution was more highly correlated with cardiovascular risk factors than was the percentage of total body fat.

In adults, increases in intraabdominal fat have been associated with increased risk of morbidity and mortality. Caprio *et al.* observed a relation between increased visceral fat and glucose metabolism in obese adolescent girls (5). When they compared girls with similar degrees of obesity but differing amounts of visceral adipose tissue, they found that the group with greater visceral fat deposition had higher insulin levels, both when fasting and in response to glucose stimulation. They also reported that obese adolescent girls with higher levels of visceral adipose tissue had lower HDL cholesterol and higher triacylglycerol levels, both of which are risk factors for cardiovascular disease (6). However, Brambilla *et al.* suggest that the effect of intraabdominal adipose tissue on metabolic risk factors may differ during and after the pubertal period (36). Although the amount of intraabdominal fat did not change over the pubertal period, a significant relation between intraabdominal adipose tissue and glucose metabolism was observed only after puberty (36). Furthermore, intraabdominal adipose tissue was significantly related only to low-density lipoprotein cholesterol before puberty and in the early stages of pubertal development. Four years later the only significant relation among lipoproteins and intraabdominal adipose tissue was a negative one with HDL.

Recently, several studies have measured visceral adipose tissue stores in children and adolescents using MRI scans (8,10,11,38,39). These data provide information on the intraabdominal adipose tissue depots in children and adolescents at various ages. Table 1 summarizes the results of published studies on intraabdominal fat in children and adolescents. Most of the available data are for the early adolescent period. Because many of the studies did not publish the values for intraabdominal subcutaneous fat or the ratio of intraabdominal adipose tissue to total body fat, this information is not provided in the table.

Fox *et al.* reported that the excess fat in 11-year-old girls and boys was deposited more frequently as subcutaneous fat than as visceral fat (10). Leung *et al.* report a

TABLE 1. *Visceral adipose tissue stores in children and adolescents*

Author (ref. no.)	Gender/ethnicity	Age (years)	IAAT fat (cm^2)
Goran (9)	M/F; white; American Indian	6.3 ± 1.2	8.3 ± 5.8
Nagy (37)	M/African American	7.6 ± 1.6	22 ± 23
	F/African American	7.3 ± 1.7	20 ± 17
	M/white	8.2 ± 1.5	24 ± 20
	F/white	7.6 ± 1.4	32 ± 23
Rommenich (38)	M/NA	10.4 ± 0.3	44 ± 5
	F/NA	10.4 ± 0.3	44 ± 5
	M/NA	13.4 ± 0.3	62 ± 6
	F/NA	13.5 ± 0.3	53 ± 5
Fox (10)	M/NA	11.5[a]	17.8 ± 10
	F/NA	11.5[a]	24.8 ± 8.8
Fox (11)	M/NA	13[a]	30.1 ± 11.0
	F/NA	13[a]	38.3 ± 9.9
Leung (39)	M/Chinese	11.4 ± 0.2	30.2 ± 18.9
	F/Chinese	11.4 ± 0.2	20.4 ± 9.0
Brambilla (8)	M/F (obese)	12.8 ± 1.9	49 ± 21
	M/F (non-obese)	12.3 ± 1.9	22 ± 11
de Ridder (7)	F/white	11.5 ± 0.26	24.1 ± 4.1
	F/white	14.0 ± 0.1	25.7 ± 4.1

Abbreviations: IAAT, intraabdominal fat; NA, not available.
[a] Only mean available.

lower ratio of visceral adipose tissue to total abdominal tissue in obese children than in nonobese children (39). This indicates that most of the excess fat in these pubertal children was stored subcutaneously. Brambilla *et al.* examined longitudinal changes in abdominal fat deposition (36). All the subjects (16 obese boys and girls) had become obese before the age of 8. Subjects were studied three times at approximately 2-year intervals. At the time of the first visit (Table 1) subjects were either prepubertal or in the early stages of puberty. At the last visit, the subjects had completed sexual development. Thus the time period over which the subjects were measured represented the pubertal period. Although the BMI and subcutaneous fat tissue had increased on the third compared with the first visit, intraabdominal fat and relative weight at these two time periods was not significantly different. These findings are consistent with those of Fox *et al.* (10), suggesting that excess body fatness before puberty is associated with an increase in subcutaneous fat. They are not, however, consistent with those of Goran *et al.* (9), who presented data only on younger children. Because the increase in the ratio of intraabdominal adipose tissue to total body fat in children from age 4 to 8 years is almost three times that reported in adolescents, Goran *et al.* suggested that the prepubertal period is an important time for the deposition of intraabdominal fat (9). However, the sample size in Goran's study was small ($N = 16$) and the range of intraabdominal adipose tissue large (4 to 21 cm^2). Furthermore, there is a large variation in the amount of intraabdominal fat among subjects in all the studies.

Recently, Fox *et al.* published data on 2-year changes in intraabdominal adipose tissue in the 11-year-old children they previously reported (11). They observed that the increases in abdominal fat for boys during the pubertal period were greater than those for girls. In boys they observed a much greater increase in intraabdominal fat (69%) than in subcutaneous fat (19.1%). However, in girls there was a 48.4% increase in intraabdominal fat, compared with a 78.1% increase in subcutaneous fat over the 2-year period. Their findings suggest that there is sexual dimorphism in intraabdominal adipose tissue deposition during puberty.

The levels of intraabdominal adipose tissue during early adolescence are considerably lower than those reported for adults (117.9 ± 62.1) (40). Although this suggests that late adolescence may be an important period for the deposition of intraabdominal fat, empirical data are lacking. Longitudinal studies that measure intraabdominal adipose tissue and total body fat from puberty through late adolescence are needed for a better understanding of the timing associated with intraabdominal fat deposition.

Because the pubertal period is associated with a change in the distribution of body fat, it may represent a critical time for fat distribution and intraabdominal fat stores. Few data are available on factors that may increase intraabdominal fat in children. Rommenich *et al.* reported an inverse correlation between the energy spent on activity and intraabdominal adipose tissue in boys but no significant interrelationship in girls (41). Because of the association between morbidity and fat distribution, it is important to understand both the timing and the factors that may predispose to a central fat distribution.

SUMMARY

It is clear from published reports that there is sexual dimorphism in the changes in body fatness and body fat distribution during adolescence. Body fatness increases in girls and decreases in boys. The change from a peripheral to a more central pattern of deposition of body fat is more pronounced in boys than in girls. Intraabdominal adipose tissue stores in children and adolescents are small compared with those of adults. However, the factors and time periods associated with an increase in intraabdominal fat in children and adolescents remain unknown. Results of ongoing longitudinal studies of growth and development in children and adolescents will help provide answers to these questions.

REFERENCES

1. Braddon FEM, Rodgers B, Wadworth MEJ. Onset of obesity in a 36 year birth cohort study. *BMJ* 1986; 293: 299–303.
2. Must A, Strauss RS. Risks and consequences of childhood and adolescent obesity. *Int J Obes* 1999; 23 (Suppl): S2–11.
3. Houtkooper LB, Lohman TG, Going SB, Hall MC. Validity of bioelectric impedance for body composition assessment in children. *J Appl Physiol* 1989; 66: 814–21.
4. Troiano RP, Flegal KM, Kuczmarski RJ, Campbell SM, Johnson CL. Overweight prevalence and trends for children and adolescent. *Arch Pediatr Adolesc Med* 1995; 149: 1085–91.
5. Caprio S, Hyman LD, Limb C, *et al.* Central adiposity and its metabolic correlates in obese adolescent girls. *Am J Physiol* 1995; 269: E118–26.
6. Caprio S, Hyman LD, McCarthy S, Lange R, Bronson M, Tamborlane WV. Fat distribution and cardiovascular risk factors in obese adolescent girls: importance of the intra-abdominal depot. *Am J Clin Nutr* 1996; 64: 12–7.

7. De Ridder CM, de Boer RW, Seidell JC, *et al.* Body fat distribution in pubertal girls quantified by magnetic resonance imaging. *Int J Obes* 1992; 16: 443–9.
8. Brambilla P, Manzoni P, Sironi S, *et al.* Peripheral and abdominal adiposity in childhood obesity. *Int J Obes* 1994; 18: 795–800.
9. Goran MI, Kaskoun M, Shuman WP. Intra-abdominal adipose tissue in young children. *Int J Obes Relat Metab Disord* 1995; 19: 279–83.
10. Fox KR, Peters D, Armstrong N, Sharpe P, Bell M. Abdominal fat deposition in 11-year-old children. *Int J Obes* 1993; 17: 11–6.
11. Fox KR, Peters DM, Sharpe P, Bell M. Assessment of abdominal fat development in young adolescents using magnetic resonance imaging. *Int J Obes* 2000; 24: 1653–9.
12. Tanner J. *Growth at adolescence.* Oxford: Blackwell Scientific Publications, 1962.
13. Dugdale AE, Payne RR. Pattern of fat and lean tissue deposition in children. *Nature* 1976; 256: 725–7.
14. Butte NF, Hopkinson JM, Wong W, *et al.* Body composition during the first 2 years of life: an updated reference. *Pediatr Res* 2000; 475: 578–85.
15. Cheek DB. *Human growth.* Philadelphia: Lea and Febiger, 1968.
16. Taylor RW, Gold E, Manning P, Goulding A. Gender differences in body fat content are present well before puberty. *Int J Obes* 1997; 21: 1082–4.
17. Rolland-Cachera MF, Deheeger M, Guilloud-Batalle M. Tracking the development of adiposity from one month of age to adulthood. *Ann Hum Biol* 1987; 14: 219–9.
18. Dietz WH. Periods of risk in childhood for the development of adult obesity—what do we need to learn? *J Nutr* 1997; 127: 1884–6S.
19. Guo SS, Chumlea WC, Roche AF, Siervogel RM. Age- and maturity-related changes in body composition during adolescence into adulthood: the Fels longitudinal study. *Appl Radiat Isot* 1998; 49: 581–5.
20. Garn SM, LaVelle M, Rosenberg KR, Hawthorne VM. Maturational timing as a factor in female fatness and obesity. *Am J Clin Nutr* 1986; 43: 879–83.
21. Morrison JA, Barton B, Biro FM, *et al.* Sexual maturation and obesity in 9- and 10-year-old black and white girls: the National Heart, Lung and Blood Institute Growth and Health Study. *J Pediatr* 1994; 124: 889–95.
22. Must A, Jacques PF, Dallal GE, Bajema CJ, Dietz WH. Long-term morbidity and mortality of overweight adolescents: a follow-up of the Harvard Growth Study 1922 to 1935. *N Engl J Med* 1992; 327: 1350–5.
23. Whitaker RC, Wright JA, Pepe MS, Seidel KD, Dietz WH. Predicting obesity in young adulthood from childhood and parental obesity. *N Engl J Med* 1997; 337: 869–73.
24. Baumgartner RN, Roche AF, Guo S, *et al.* Adipose tissue distribution: the stability of principal components by sex, ethnicity and maturation stage. *Hum Biol* 1986; 58: 719–34.
25. Hattori K, Beque D, Katch VL, Rocchini AP. Fat patterning of adolescents. *Ann Hum Biol* 1987; 14: 23–8.
26. Cowell CT, Briody J, Lloyd-Jones D, *et al.* Fat distribution in children and adolescents—the influence of sex and hormones. *Horm Res* 1997; 48 (Suppl): 93–100.
27. Frisancho R, Flegal PN. Advanced maturation associated with centripetal fat pattern. *Hum Biol* 1982; 54: 717–27.
28. Deutsch MI, Meuller WH. Androgyny in fat patterning is associated with obesity in adolescents and young adults. *Ann Hum Biol* 1985; 12: 275–86.
29. Van Lenthe FJ, Kemper HCG, van Mechelen W, *et al.* Biological maturation and the distribution of subcutaneous fat from adolescence into adulthood: the Amsterdam growth and health study. *Int J Obes* 1996; 20: 121–9.
30. De Ridder CM, Bruning PF, Zonderland, *et al.* Body fat mass, body fat distribution, and plasma hormones in early puberty in females. *J Clin Endocrinol Metab* 1990; 70: 888–93.
31. Barrett-Connor E, Khaw KT. Cigarette smoking and increased central adiposity. *Ann Intern Med* 1989; 111: 783–7.
32. Duncan BB, Chambless LE, Schmidt MI, *et al.* Variation across categories of race, sex, and body mass in the atherosclerosis risk in communities study. *Ann Epidemiol* 1995; 5: 192–200.
33. Post GB, Kemper HCG. Nutrient intake and biological maturation during adolescence. The Amsterdam Growth and Health Study. *Eur J Clin Nutr* 1993; 47: 400–8.
34. Berky CS, Gardner JE, Frazier L, Colditz G. Relation of childhood diet and body size to menarche and adolescent growth in girls. *Am J Epidemiol* 2000; 152: 446–52.
35. Daniels SR, Morrison J, Sprecher DL, Khoury P, Kimball T. Association of body fat distribution and cardiovascular risk factors in children and adolescents. *Circulation* 1999; 99: 541–5.

36. Brambilla P, Manzoni P, Agostini G, *et al*. Persisting obesity starting before puberty is associated with stable intraabdominal fat during adolescence. *Int J Obesity* 1999; 23: 299–303.
37. Nagy TR, Gower BA, Trowbridge CA, *et al*. Effects of gender, ethnicity, body composition, and fat distribution on serum leptin concentrations in children. *J Clin Endocrinol Metab* 1997; 82: 2142–52.
38. Rommenich JN, Clark PA, Berr SS, *et al*. Gender differences in leptin levels during puberty are related to the subcutaneous depot and sex steroids. *Am J Physiol Endocrinol Metab* 1998; 275: E543–51.
39. Leung SSF, Chan YL, Lam CWK, *et al*. Body fatness and serum lipids of 11-year-old Chinese children. *Acta Pediatr* 1998; 87: 363–7.
40. Ross R, Leger L, Morris D, De Guise J, Guardo R. Quantification of adipose tissue by MRI: relationship with anthropometric variables. *J Appl Physiol* 1992; 72: 787–95.
41. Rommenich JN, Clark PA, Walter K, *et al*. Pubertal alterations in growth and body composition. V. Energy expenditure, adiposity, and fat distribution. *Am J Physiol* 2000; 279: E1426–36.

DISCUSSION

Dr. Steinbeck: Was there any difference in the slopes of the BMI before and after menarche, depending on fatness before menarche? In other words, was the slope higher before menarche in the fatter girls?

Dr. Bandini: We did not look at that, mainly because fatness is a continuous variable and separating the subjects in that way would have been very difficult.

Dr. Bar-Or: What is your opinion on the relative roles of the environment and predetermined biologic factors in explaining the patterns you showed, especially in the girls? In other words, are we dealing with factors that we can do very little about, or is this a matter of lifestyle or other variables that can be changed in the girls to prevent them from getting fat?

Dr. Bandini: There are studies in adults suggesting that changes in intraabdominal fat tissue are related to behavioral factors such as smoking, alcohol use, and physical activity [1,2]. We need to do studies in children and adolescents to determine whether such factors influence fat distribution and intraabdominal tissue in early life, and whether modifying them will change the fat distribution pattern.

Dr. Rütishauser: I was interested to hear that there is an overlap in the amount of intraabdominal adipose tissue between obese and nonobese adolescents. Is it known how much is too much?

Dr. Bandini: I don't think it is known how much is too much in adolescence. I believe that in adults 130 cm^2 is associated with adverse effects.

Dr. Dulloo: In the correlation where you showed that testosterone was the main predictor of variation in intraabdominal fat, there was also an increase in fat-free mass. If you adjust for the increase in fat-free mass, how much of the correlation remains significant?

Dr. Bandini: We did not include that in the model, but that is something we could look at.

Dr. Yanovski: Would you care to comment on the racial ethnic differences in changes in body adiposity throughout adolescence?

Dr. Bandini: In general, the increase in fat deposition seems more marked in blacks than in whites. I cannot comment on other ethnic differences at present.

Dr. Gortmaker: Do the differences in body fat distribution by age, sex, and perhaps ethnicity have implications for the kinds of intervention programs we might apply? For example, do you think one might need to do different things for different sexes at different ages?

Dr. Bandini: I think diet and physical activity are the two most important factors in maintaining energy balance and avoiding positive energy balance under all circumstances.

Dr. Gortmaker: But would you think of emphasizing different things at different ages, because of the differences between the sexes at different ages? Might there be optimal times to prevent obesity from developing?

Dr. Bandini: Behaviors developed before the pubertal period are more likely to persist life-long, so that's a good time to establish healthy patterns of activity and food intake.

Dr. Freedman: You showed that girls with an early menarche had a more central fat distribution, which continued up to age 27. Is it possible that some of those differences were present even before menarche? For example, could a central fat distribution be a determinant of menarche?

Dr. Bandini: That is possible. There are published data to suggest that may be the case [3].

Dr. Van Dyk: Have you looked at the effect of growth hormone in the differing growth spurts between boys and girls?

Dr. Bandini: No.

Dr. Uauy: In your hormonal profile, did you also include cortisol? I think that cortisol should be explored in these sorts of studies on central obesity.

Dr. Bandini: No, we did not look at cortisol either. We looked at leptin, the sex hormones, and insulin.

REFERENCES

1. Barret-Connor E, Khaw CT. Cigarette smoking and increased adiposity. *Ann Int Med* 1989; 111: 183–7.
2. Duncan BB, Chambless LE, Schmidt MI, *et al.* Variation across categories of race, sex and body mass in the atherosclerosis risk in communities study. *Ann Epidemiol* 1995; 5: 192–200.
3. Van Lenthe FJ, Kemple HCG, Van Mechelen W, *et al.* Biological maturation and the distribution of subcutaneous fat from adolescence into adulthood: the Amsterdam Growth and Health Study. *Int J Obesity* 1996; 20: 121–9.

Obesity in Childhood and Adolescence, edited by
Chunming Chen and William H. Dietz. Nestlé
Nutrition Workshop Series, Pediatric Program,
Vol. 49. Nestec Ltd., Vevey/Lippincott
Williams & Wilkins, Philadelphia © 2002.

Physiologic Factors Related to the Onset and Persistence of Childhood and Adolescent Obesity

Claudio Maffeis and Luciano Tatò

Department of Pediatrics, University of Verona–Polyclinic, Verona, Italy

Childhood obesity results from failure to modulate environmental pressures affecting the genetic substrate of the individual. The results of genetic and epidemiologic studies suggest that genetic factors are involved in determining susceptibility to fat gain in subjects exposed to a specific environment (1). The influential role played by the environment in the development of obesity in susceptible individuals is strongly supported by evidence that the prevalence of obesity is higher in industrialized countries, where lifestyles and nutritional habits have undergone greater changes over the past few decades (2).

In keeping with the first law of thermodynamics, the various factors involved in the complex genetic–environmental interactions that cause obesity will promote the prolonged positive energy balance that is responsible for fat gain. This process overcomes the efficient self-regulation of energy balance demonstrated in humans. Normally, a kind of homeostatic mechanism seems to promote the maintenance of appropriate body weight and body energy stores from birth to adulthood, and dynamically adjusts body mass and body composition to the varied needs of physical growth and sexual development in the two sexes (3,4). However, the clear evidence of progressively greater worldwide prevalence of childhood obesity suggests a failure of this system to adapt to rapid and profound environmental changes (5,6).

Our purpose in this chapter is to review the physiologic factors related to the development and maintenance of obesity in children, and to suggest future topics for research in this field.

In contrast to adults, children are physiologically in a minimal positive energy balance owing to the additional requirements for growth (energy content of new tissue and energy cost of tissue synthesis). In particular, about 2% of their total energy intake for 1- to 10-year-old children is devoted to growth. The energy cost of growth is about 20% of the total daily energy requirements in 3-month-old infants and about 3% in 6-month-olds (8). During puberty the energy cost of growth is about 5% to 7% of total daily energy requirements (9). This specificity of children does not modify the equation, as growth consists of a physiologic store of energy in new tissues (fat-free mass and fat mass).

ENERGY BALANCE

An average-sized woman may maintain her weight over 10 years by matching approximately 30 million kJ of food intake (intermittent and variable) with the same amount of energy expenditure (continuous and variable). Thus the regulation of this remarkable energy turnover must be very efficient, dynamic, and precise. In an attempt to introduce the concept of time-dependent variability of the components of energy balance, the following equation has been proposed (7):

Rate of energy intake − rate of energy expenditure = rate of change of energy stored[1]

This allows the effect of changing energy stores on energy expenditure to enter into the calculation. In fact, in free-living conditions energy balance is spontaneously achieved by modifications in behavior (appetite and physical activity) over hours and days, and by changes in body weight and composition over weeks and months. Therefore variations in body weight and body composition as a result of a chronic positive (or negative) energy balance tend to promote a compensatory increase (or decrease) in energy expenditure, which opposes further weight gain (or loss) (Fig. 1) (10).

In spite of the self-regulating mechanism of energy balance, the progressively increasing number of obese individuals proves that a minimal mismatch between energy intake and energy expenditure—such that intake exceeds expenditure—may result in a net accumulation of energy stores in the body. A chronic imbalance of just 1% between energy intake and energy expenditure in a 10-year-old normal-weight girl may cause a difference of more than 25,000 kJ/year in her energy balance, which corresponds to around 0.7 kg of fat, or to an increase of approximately 15% of her total fat mass.

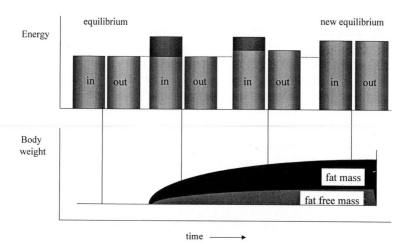

FIG. 1. Relation between energy balance and body weight: increase in fat mass and fat-free mass as a result of a positive energy balance and as a contributor to a new energy balance. From World Health Organization. Report of a WHO consultation on obesity. *Obesity: preventing and managing the global epidemic.* Geneva: WHO, 1997; 113, modified.)

It is important to point out how extremely difficult it is, even with the techniques available today, to assess such a small imbalance between energy intake and energy expenditure in free-living conditions. The evidence that the prevalence of obesity is growing in spite of a progressively lower energy content of children's diet (2,5,6) suggests that a reduction in total energy requirements may be occurring in these populations.

Each of the components of total daily energy expenditure may be responsible for these reduced requirements. Basal metabolic rate (BMR), thermogenesis (T), energy expenditure for growth (EE_G) (negligible except in the first year of life and during puberty), and the energy expenditure for physical activity (EE_{Act}) may all be reduced in preobese children, favoring weight gain and fat gain. Even though the hypothesis that preobese children may have a higher metabolic efficiency requires further investigation, it is not supported by available studies (11). In particular, BMR—which is quantitatively the main component of the total daily energy expenditure—is higher in obese than in nonobese children owing to their greater fat-free mass (i.e., their metabolically active tissue). However, when BMR is adjusted for fat-free mass, no difference is found between obese, postobese, and never obese children (12). Meal-induced thermogenesis, which is the main component of thermogenesis, appears to be slightly lower in obese than in nonobese children (13–15). However, weight loss can eliminate this modest difference, which suggests, by implication, that a reduction in meal-induced thermogenesis is unlikely to be a factor predisposing to obesity in preobese children (16). It follows that most of the relative reduction in energy requirement over energy intake in preobese children reflects a lower EE_{Act}, which is the only discretional component of total daily energy expenditure. This is not surprising, as sedentary behavior is common in today's children and has been identified as a potential predictor of weight gain (17). Indeed, sedentary behavior may precede as well as accompany obesity.

What are the factors that evade the homeostatic control of energy balance and promote the development of obesity, and how do they work? One possible answer to these questions comes from the metabolic characteristics of the principal factors of the energy balance: the nutrients.

NUTRIENT BALANCE

Energy enters the body mainly in the form of three macronutrients: protein, carbohydrates, and fat. The contribution to total energy intake of the two other sources of energy, alcohol and fiber, is negligible, as alcohol is usually not consumed by children, and the energy intake from fiber is far less than 1% of the total energy intake in the typical Western diet (18).

Nutrients may be either oxidized or stored in the body. Thus the energy balance equation may be formulated as the sum of the three nutrient balances (19):

Energy balance = protein balance + carbohydrate balance + fat balance

where each nutrient balance is given by

Rate of nutrient intake − rate of nutrient oxidation
= rate of change of nutrient stored

Theoretically, all three nutrient balances should, like energy balance, be efficiently self-regulated. However, there is convincing evidence that this is the case for protein and carbohydrate balance but not for fat balance. In fact, short-term measurement of the postprandial increase of thermogenesis following the ingestion of equienergetic meals consisting of pure macronutrients has shown that protein and carbohydrate intake stimulates protein and carbohydrate oxidation, whereas fat intake does not stimulate fat oxidation (20). This was clearly demonstrated by Schutz *et al.*, who found only an imperceptible increase in fat oxidation (less than 1%) and total energy expenditure (less than 2%) following ingestion of a large fat supplement (approximately 106 g fat/24 h, or about 35% of total daily energy requirements) (21).

Furthermore, an oxidative "hierarchy" that prefers the oxidation of carbohydrates and protein to that of fat has been identified in the body (22). The efficiency of carbohydrate and protein oxidation reflects the relatively small storage capacity for these nutrients (confined to glycogen, the labile proteins, and the amino acid pool) and the absolute need to maintain circulating glucose levels within strict limits. In contrast, fat storage capacity is not limited. Thus ingested fat is preferentially stored unless it is oxidized, the latter process being independent of fat intake but dependent on the amount of carbohydrate and protein ingested and oxidized. In other words, fat may be considered as the "energetic buffer" of the organism.

Neosynthesis of fat by carbohydrate (*de novo* lipogenesis) has been demonstrated in adipose tissue (23). However, the situations in which *de novo* lipogenesis occurs are far from physiologic, and this process should be regarded as negligible under the dietary conditions prevailing in industrialized countries—in fact, the ingestion of an extremely large amount of simple sugar (500 g of dextrin-maltose, or about 8,500 kJ) resulted in only a few grams of lipid production (24). Moreover, massive carbohydrate overfeeding for several days (with an energy intake of around 21,000 kJ/day, 85% as carbohydrate) resulted in just 150 g/day of lipid synthesis after the saturation of glycogen stores (25). The fact that glucose conversion to fat occurs at negligible rates in adults on mixed diets suggests that, to achieve weight stability, the organism has to oxidize not only protein but also carbohydrate and fat in the same proportions as provided by the diet (19).

FAT INTAKE AND FAT GAIN

The accurate measurement of energy and fat intakes in free-living individuals is difficult and is an important drawback to defining the precise and independent role of food intake in the fat gain process. The validity of food intake reporting must be determined by simultaneous measurements of energy expenditure. This is impossible in epidemiologic studies, so one needs to be cautious about drawing conclusions from such studies (26–28). Energy-balance studies have shown that food intake underreporting is common in obese individuals, as well as in children and adolescents, and underreporting gets progressively more common as energy requirements increase (29–31). Furthermore, a selective underestimation of fat intake has been reported in obese adults (32). Despite these important methodological issues, there is evidence to support the role of fat intake in the development and maintenance of obesity.

A physiologic example of fat gain is to be found in late intrauterine and early extrauterine life. During the first 4 months after birth, the infant's body weight doubles (from about 3,500 g to about 7,000 g) and the fat mass more than triples (from about 500 g to about 1,700 g) (9). During the first months of life, human milk or formula is the only food ingested by infants. The energy content of human milk is around 280 kJ/100 ml, and fat accounts for more than 50% of the total energy. Thus the ingestion of this "high-fat diet" physiologically promotes a positive energy balance as well as a significant fat gain.

Weaning causes a progressive change in diet composition, with an increase in the carbohydrate-to-fat ratio. Simultaneously, body composition changes, with slowing of fat mass growth in favor of the development of muscle and other tissues (9). The fact that a high-fat diet promotes fat gain in infants supports the hypothesis that a high fat intake may favor fat gain in older individuals as well. Studies on prepubertal children and adolescents have confirmed this hypothesis by showing a positive association between fat intake (expressed as energy intake percent) and adiposity (33,34). Moreover, a longitudinal study on a group of prepubertal children showed that fat intake was a risk factor for fat gain in these children (35).

Finally, the results of a long-term dietary manipulation study on adults showed that consuming diets *ad libitum* that looked identical but that had been covertly manipulated to contain 20%, 40%, or 60% fat, respectively, caused a slow fat loss for those on the low-fat diet, a slight fat accumulation for those on the 40% fat diet, and a rapid fat gain with the high-fat diet (36). These results strongly support the role of fat intake in promoting fat gain.

There are several mechanisms whereby fat intake favors fat gain: the higher energy density and palatability of fat-rich foods promote greater food consumption (37); satiation is lower with fat than with carbohydrates and proteins (38); self-compensation of energy intake is less likely after a high-fat meal (39); and meal-induced thermogenesis is lower after fat intake than after carbohydrate or protein intake (19). A recent study of a group of 10-year-old girls showed blunted thermogenesis after a mixed high-fat/low-carbohydrate meal, in comparison to the thermogenesis measured in the same girls after an isoenergetic, isoproteinic meal with a low-fat/high-carbohydrate content (40). The difference was around 30%. Although the impact on total daily energy turnover of the lower thermogenesis induced by a high-fat meal is fairly limited (about 2%), this slight energy saving could be relevant in the long run.

BODY COMPOSITION AND SKELETAL MUSCLE

A direct relation between fat mass and postabsorptive fat oxidation has been reported in both children and adolescents (41,42). An increase in fat stores will increase fatty acid turnover, which increases fasting free fatty acid concentrations and promotes substrate competition between free fatty acids and glucose in the muscles; this in turn enhances insulin resistance (43). Increased insulin levels tend to reduce lipolysis

(44). However, the sensitivity of lipolysis to insulin in the adipose tissue is higher than the sensitivity of fat oxidation to insulin in the muscle. Thus higher levels of circulating insulin are necessary to enhance glucose oxidation and, as a consequence, to reduce fat oxidation. This "mass effect" exerted by adiposity on fat oxidation may be interpreted as a limiting factor in the expansion of fat stores (45,46). Therefore, given a certain energy intake and diet composition, the progressive increase in fat stores promotes a simultaneous increase in fat oxidation, favoring a new fat balance obtained at a higher body weight and body fat content (Fig. 2).

A recent study on a group of 11-year-old children that used the stable isotope technique to differentiate between the postprandial oxidation of fat ingested with a mixed meal and fat of endogenous origin (adipose tissue) showed that around 11% of ingested fat was oxidized (during the nine hours of postprandial respiratory exchange recording), whereas the remaining fat that was oxidized came from the fat stores (47). Expressed as a proportion of the ingested fat, there was less oxidation of endogenous fat as the relative fat mass of the child increased. The relatively blunted oxidation of endogenous fat may be viewed as a protective mechanism to prevent a further increase in fat mass—and hence to maintain fat oxidation at a sufficient rate—when the body is exposed to exogenous fat in a meal.

Skeletal muscle plays an important role in fat balance regulation. The muscles oxidize a large proportion of the fatty acids in the body. Physical activity—especially if done on a regular basis—promotes fat oxidation in the muscles as well as postexercise oxygen consumption (48–50). The fat oxidation rate increased by 20% in a group

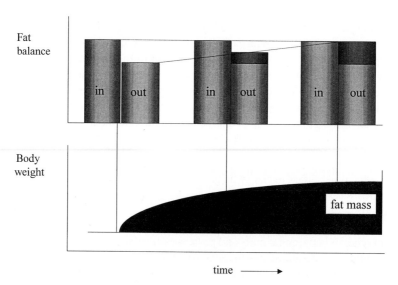

FIG. 2. Fat mass and fat balance. An increase of fat mass as a promoting factor of a new fat balance equation during fat overfeeding.

of adults who took part in a 12-week workout program (51). The kind of exercise (aerobic, anaerobic), its intensity and duration, the training level of the individual, and the environmental conditions (temperature, pressure, humidity) during workouts affect the fat oxidation rate both during and after exercise. Interestingly, the maximum percentage of fat is oxidized during moderate-intensity aerobic exercise (60% VO_{2max}) (52). Thus the fat oxidation caused by skeletal muscle activity may be enhanced by simply modifying one's sedentary lifestyle, so common in the industrialized countries (53).

Finally, the level of physical activity seems to affect food intake. Strenuous exercise retards appetite in adults in the period immediately after an exercise session (54). In children, regular physical activity seems to be accompanied by a trend to self-select a diet with a higher carbohydrate-to-fat ratio (55).

FACTORS AFFECTING FAT INTAKE AND FAT OXIDATION

Several factors affect fat balance by influencing food intake or energy expenditure. One of these is early nutrition. Human milk and formulas have a similar energy content and composition, and the growth of formula-fed infants is little different from that of age-matched breast-fed infants. However, it has been suggested that breast-feeding protects against obesity in older children (56). One possible contributing factor may be the continuous changes in human milk composition and flavor during lactation. Human milk composition changes during feeding and from one feed to the next during the day (57). Moreover, food ingested by the mother affects the flavor of her milk, which thus changes between feeds. The flavor of breast milk may affect milk intake and later food acceptance and consumption (58). Formulas never change in composition or flavor. At present, the potential implications of these differences on later eating habits of the individual are largely unknown.

Finally, modes of feeding may contribute to a higher risk of obesity in later life in formula-fed infants. For instance, a vigorous feeding style—consisting of sucking more rapidly and at higher pressure, with longer suckling sessions and a shorter interval between feeds—has been associated with greater adiposity (59,60).

Early experiences with food, the association of food flavors with the context in which the food is taken, and the consequences of eating may theoretically affect children's food acceptance and food habits. Although the precocious introduction of solid foods into the infant's diet has not been proven to be associated with childhood obesity, further research is necessary to clarify this issue (61,62). Family eating habits, food availability, and access to food in the home affect a child's food preferences (63). A clear association between parental adiposity and fat intake and children's adiposity and fat intake exists (64). Moreover, the parents' encouragement to eat promotes fat gain in their children (65). Another powerful contributor to the development of food preferences and food selection is advertisements for food products and the variety of models and messages about eating that children get through watching television (66,67).

Finally, partitioning of food intake, especially food intake at the time of the evening meal, has recently been associated with adiposity in 7- to 11-year-old children (68). Although this relation requires further experimental investigation, a high food intake at supper—which is not usually followed by physical activity, as breakfast and lunch usually are—could promote efficient energy storage, mainly in the form of fat.

CONCLUSIONS

On the basis of the available studies, some general conclusions may be drawn:

- Net fat storage only occurs when fat intake exceeds fat requirement.
- In the short term, the source of the excess energy (carbohydrate versus fat versus protein) affects the kind and place of storage of the energy excess. A great excess of carbohydrates will be stored primarily as glycogen; in contrast, excess fat will be promptly stored in the adipose tissues, by an extremely efficient process.
- During phases of positive energy balance it is likely that most stored fat comes directly from dietary fat, whereas the suppression of fat oxidation following the ingestion of carbohydrates and protein favors the maintenance of fat that was previously stored.
- Fat intake favors fat gain by means of the high energy density typical of fatty foods and the high palatability of foods rich in fat—both factors promoting food ingestion.
- Meal-induced thermogenesis is lower after a high-fat meal, and this may be a further contributing factor to fat gain.
- Physical activity affects energy expenditure as well as nutrient oxidation; aerobic exercise may be helpful in increasing the overall fat oxidation rate of the organism.
- Other factors, such as early feeding experiences, family eating habits, food availability and accessibility, TV viewing, and food partitioning may contribute to promoting and maintaining obesity in children.

FUTURE CHALLENGES AND POLICY IMPLICATIONS

Although several factors affecting energy and fat balance have been identified, most of the mechanisms regulating fat deposition—especially during late intrauterine and early extrauterine life, but also during puberty and the other growth stages of the child—require further investigation. Moreover, we need more information on skeletal muscle metabolism and the metabolic consequences of physical activity in childhood. Finally, the discovery of more accurate techniques (or the improvement of those already in use) to assess nutrient storage and turnover in free-living conditions would be welcome.

On the basis of the available data, a reasonable approach to the prevention of childhood and adolescent obesity should include interventions at the level of the general population to reduce the energy density and the fat content of the diet. This might help to prevent passive overconsumption but cannot overcome active overconsumption, and it is just one part of a more structured intervention program. As is the case for adults, appropriate lifestyle changes favoring more physical activity should be encouraged. Finally, all interventions designed for children should include the active and collaborative involvement of their parents.

REFERENCES

1. Pérusse L, Bouchard C. Gene–diet interactions in obesity. *Am J Clin Nutr* 2000; 72: 1285–90.
2. World Health Organization. Report of a WHO consultation on obesity. *Obesity: preventing and managing the global epidemic.* Geneva: WHO, 1997.
3. Ravussin E, Schutz Y, Acheson KJ, *et al.* Short-term, mixed diet overfeeding in man: no evidence of "luxuskonsumption." *Am J Physiol* 1985; 249: 470–7.
4. Leibel RL, Rosenbaum M, Hirsch J. Changes in energy expenditure resulting from altered body weight. *N Engl J Med* 1994; 332: 621–8.
5. Freedman DS, Srinivasan SR, Valdez RA, *et al.* Secular increases in relative weight and adiposity among children over two decades: the Bogalusa Heart Study. *Pediatrics* 1997; 99: 420–6.
6. Livingstone MBE. Epidemiology of childhood obesity in Europe. *Eur J Pediatr* 2000; 159: 14–34.
7. Alpert S. Growth, thermogenesis, and hyperphagia. *Am J Clin Nutr* 1990; 52: 784–92.
8. Butte NF, Wong WW, Hopkinson JM, *et al.* Energy requirements derived from total energy expenditure and energy deposition during the first 2 y of life. *Am J Clin Nutr* 2000; 72: 1558–69.
9. Fomon SJ, Haschke F, Ziegler EE, Nelson SE. Body composition of reference children from birth to age 10 years. *Am J Clin Nutr* 1982; 35: 1169–75.
10. Weyer C, Pratley RE, Salbe AD, *et al.* Energy expenditure, fat oxidation, and body weight regulation: a study of metabolic adaptation to long term weight change. *J Clin Endocrinol Metab* 2000; 85: 1087–94.
11. Goran MI, Carpenter WH, Poehlman ET. Total energy expenditure in 4- to 6-year-old children. *Am J Physiol* 1993; 264: 706–11.
12. Maffeis C, Schutz Y, Pinelli L. Effect of weight loss on resting energy expenditure in obese prepubertal children. *Int J Obes* 1992; 16: 41–7.
13. Molnar D, Varga P, Rubecz I, *et al.* Food induced thermogenesis in obese children. *Eur J Pediatr* 1985; 144: 27–31.
14. Tounian P, Girardet JP, Carlier L, *et al.* Resting energy expenditure and food-induced thermogenesis in obese children. *J Pediatr Gastroenterol Nutr* 1993; 16: 451–7.
15. Maffeis C, Schutz Y, Zoccante L, Micciolo R, Pinelli L. Meal-induced thermogenesis in lean and obese prepubertal children. *Am J Clin Nutr* 1993; 578: 481–5.
16. Maffeis C, Schutz Y, Pinelli L. Postprandial thermogenesis in obese children before and after weight reduction. *Eur J Clin Nutr* 1992; 46: 577–83.
17. Berkey CS, Rockett HR, Field AE, *et al.* Activity, dietary intake, and weight changes in a longitudinal study of preadolescent and adolescent boys and girls. *Pediatrics* 2000; 105: 56.
18. Maffeis C. Childhood obesity: the genetic–environmental interface. *Baillieres Best Pract Res Clin Endocrinol Metab* 1999; 13: 31–46.
19. Flatt JP. Importance of nutrient balance in body weight regulation. *Diabetes Metab Rev* 1988; 4: 571–81.
20. Flatt JP, Ravussin E, Acheson KJ, Jéquier E. Effects of dietary fat on postprandial substrate oxidation and on carbohydrate and fat balances. *J Clin Invest* 1985; 76: 1019–24.
21. Schutz Y, Flatt JP, Jéquier E. Failure of dietary fat to promote fat oxidation: a factor favoring the development of obesity. *Am J Clin Nutr* 1989; 50: 307–14.
22. Prentice AM, Poppit SD. Importance of energy density and macronutrients in the regulation of energy intake. *Int J Obes* 1996; 20: 18–23.
23. Chascione C, Elwyn DH, Davila M, *et al.* Effect of carbohydrate intake on *de novo* lipogenesis in human adipose tissue. *Am J Physiol* 1987; 253: 664–9.
24. Acheson KJ, Schutz Y, Bessard T, *et al.* Carbohydrate metabolism and *de novo* lipogenesis in human obesity. *Am J Clin Nutr* 1987; 45: 78–85.
25. Acheson KJ, Schutz Y, Bessard T, *et al.* Glycogen storage capacity and *de novo* lipogenesis during massive overfeeding in man. *Am J Clin Nutr* 1988; 48: 240–7.
26. Bray GA, Popkin BM. Dietary fat intake does affect obesity! *Am J Clin Nutr* 1998; 68: 1157–73.
27. Willet WC. Is dietary fat a major determinant of body fat? *Am J Clin Nutr* 1998; 67: 556–62.
28. Seidell JC. Dietary fat and obesity: an epidemiologic perspective. *Am J Clin Nutr* 1998; 67: 546–50.

29. Bandini LG, Schoeller DA, Cyr HD, *et al.* Validity of reported energy intake in obese and nonobese adolescents. *Am J Clin Nutr* 1990; 52: 421–5.
30. Livingstone MBE, Prentice AM, Coward WA, *et al.* Validation of estimates of energy intake by weighed dietary record and diet history in children and adolescents. *Am J Clin Nutr* 1992; 56: 29–35.
31. Maffeis C, Schutz Y, Zaffanello M, *et al.* Elevated energy expenditure and reduced energy intake in obese prepubertal children: the paradox of poor dietary reliability in obesity? *J Pediatr* 1994; 124: 348–54.
32. Goris AHC, Westerterp-Plantega MS, Westerterp KS. Undereating and underreporting of habitual food intake in obese men: selective underreporting of fat intake. *Am J Clin Nutr* 2000; 71: 130–4.
33. Maffeis C, Pinelli L, Schutz Y. Fat intake and adiposity in 8- to 11-year-old obese children. *Int J Obes* 1996; 20: 170–4.
34. Gazzaniga JM, Burns TL. Relationship between diet composition and body fatness, with adjustment for resting energy expenditure and physical activity, in preadolescent children. *Am J Clin Nutr* 1993; 58: 21–8.
35. Klesges RC, Klesges LM, Eck LH, Shelton ML. A longitudinal analysis of accelerated weight gain in preschool children. *Pediatrics* 1995; 95: 126–30.
36. Stubbs RJ, Harbron CG, Murgatroyd PR, Prentice AM. Covert manipulation of dietary fat and energy density: effect on substrate flux and food intake in men feeding *ad libitum. Am J Clin Nutr* 1995; 62: 316–29.
37. Stubbs RJ, Ritz P, Coward WA, Prentice AM. Covert manipulation of the dietary fat to carbohydrate ratio and energy density: effect on food intake and energy balance in free-living men feeding ad libitum. *Am J Clin Nutr* 1995; 62: 330–7.
38. Rolls BJ, Kim-Harris S, Fischman MW, *et al.* Satiety after preloads with different amounts of fat and carbohydrate: implications for obesity. *Am J Clin Nutr* 1994; 60: 476–87.
39. Blundell J, Burley VJ, Lawton CL. Dietary fat and the control of energy intake: evaluating the effects of fat on meal size and postmeal satiety. *Am J Clin Nutr* 1993; 57: 772–8.
40. Maffeis C, Schutz Y, Grezzani A, *et al.* Meal-induced thermogenesis and obesity: is a fat meal a risk factor for fat gain in children? *J Clin Endocrinol Metab* 2001; 86: 214–19.
41. Maffeis C, Pinelli L, Schutz Y. Increased fat oxidation in prepubertal children: a metabolic defense against further weight gain? *J Pediatr* 1995; 126: 15–20.
42. Molnar D, Schutz Y. Fat oxidation in nonobese and obese adolescents: effect of body composition and pubertal development. *J Pediatr* 1998; 132: 98–104.
43. Randle PJ, Garland PB, Hales CN, Newsholme EA. The glucose fatty-acid cycle. Its role in insulin sensitivity and the metabolic disturbances of diabetes mellitus. *Lancet* 1963; i: 785–9.
44. Golay A, Chen Y-D, Reaven G. Effect of differences in glucose tolerance on insulin's ability to regulate carbohydrate and free fatty acid metabolism in obese individuals. *J Clin Endocrinol Metab* 1986; 62: 1081–8.
45. Schutz Y, Tremblay A, Weinsier RL, Nelson KM. Role of fat oxidation in the long-term stabilization of body weight in obese women. *Am J Clin Nutr* 1992; 55: 670–4.
46. Zurlo F, Lillioja S, Esposito-Del Puente A, *et al.* Low ratio of fat to carbohydrate oxidation as a predictor of weight gain: study of 24-h RQ. *Am J Physiol* 1990; 259: 650–7.
47. Maffeis C, Armellini F, Tatò L, Schutz Y. Fat oxidation and adiposity in children: exogenous versus endogenous fat utilisation. *J Clin Endocrinol Metab* 1999; 84: 654–8.
48. Flatt JP. Dietary fat, carbohydrate balance, and weight maintenance: effects of exercise. *Am J Clin Nutr* 1987; 45: 296–306.
49. Tremblay A, Coveney S, Despres JP, *et al.* Increased resting metabolic rate and lipid oxidation in exercise-trained individuals: evidence for a role of β-adrenergic stimulation. *Can J Physiol Pharmacol* 1992; 70: 1342–7.
50. Henriksson J. Training induced adaptation of skeletal muscle and metabolism during submaximal exercise. *J Physiol (Lond)* 1977; 270: 661–75.
51. Martin WH, Dalsky GP, Hurley BF, *et al.* Effect of endurance training on plasma free fatty acid turnover and oxidation during exercise. *Am J Physiol* 1993; 265: 708–14.
52. Martin WH. Effects of acute and chronic exercise on fat metabolism. *Exerc Sports Sci Rev* 1996; 24: 203–31.
53. Maffeis C, Zaffanello M, Schutz Y. Relationship between physical inactivity and adiposity in prepubertal boys. *J Pediatr* 1997; 131: 288–92.
54. King NA, Burley VJ, Blundell JE, *et al.* Exercise-induced suppression of appetite: effects on food intake and implications for energy balance. *Eur J Clin Nutr* 1994; 48: 715–24.
55. Deheeger M, Rolland-Cacherà MF, Fontvieille AM. Physical activity and body composition in 10-year-old French children: linkages with nutritional intake? *Int J Obes* 1997; 21: 372–9.

56. Von Kries R, Koletzko B, Sauerwald T, *et al.* Breast feeding and obesity: cross sectional study. *BMJ* 1999; 319: 147–50.
57. Neville MC, Keller RP, Seacat J, *et al.* Studies on human lactation. I. Within-feed and between-breast variation in selected components of human milk. *Am J Clin Nutr* 1984; 40: 635–46.
58. Sullivan SA, Birch LL. Infant dietary experience and acceptance of solid foods. *Pediatrics* 1994; 93: 271–7.
59. Stunkard AJ, Berkowitz RI, Stallings VA, Schoeller DA. Energy intake, not energy output, is a determinant of body size in infants. *Am J Clin Nutr* 1999; 69: 524–30.
60. Agras WS, Kraemer HC, Boekowitz RI, Korner AF, Hammer LD. Does a vigorous feeding style influence early development of adiposity? *J Pediatr* 1987; 110: 799–804.
61. Maffeis C, Micciolo R, Must A, Zaffanello M, Pinelli L. Parental and perinatal factors associated with childhood obesity in north-east Italy. *Int J Obes* 1994; 18: 301–5.
62. Kramer MS. Do breast-feeding and delayed introduction of solid foods protect against subsequent obesity? *J Pediatr* 1981; 98: 883–7.
63. Klesges RC, Stein RJ, Eck LH, *et al.* Parental influence on food selection in young children and its relationship to childhood obesity. *Am J Clin Nutr* 1991; 53: 859–64.
64. Nguyen VT, Larson DE, Johnson RK, Goran MI. Fat intake and adiposity in children of lean and obese parents. *Am J Clin Nutr* 1996; 63: 507–13.
65. Birch LL. Effects of peer models' food choices and eating behaviors on preschoolers' food preferences. *Child Dev* 1980; 51: 489–96.
66. Gortmaker SL, Must A, Sobol AM, *et al.* Television viewing as a cause of increasing obesity among children in the United States, 1986–1990. *Arch Pediatr Adolesc Med* 1996; 150: 356–62.
67. Taras HL, Sallis JF, Patterson TL, *et al.* Television's influence on children's diet and physical activity. *Dev Behav Pediatr* 1989; 10: 176–80.
68. Maffeis C, Provera S, Filippi L, *et al.* Distribution of food intake as a risk factor for childhood obesity. *Int J Obes Relat Metab Disord* 2000; 24: 75–80.

DISCUSSION

Dr. Zainudin: You showed data on the increase in fat oxidation rate among trained athletes and nontrained individuals. What duration of training program would be required to effectively increase the fat oxidation rate in children?

Dr. Maffeis: Muscle activity is associated with fat oxidation. If you chronically increase skeletal muscle activity, you have a contemporaneous increase in fat oxidation. But if you want this to be a persistent phenomenon, you need to prolong the exercise to the extent that muscle prefers to oxidize fat for energy. To stimulate fat oxidation in muscle in the long term, resistance training is best.

Dr. Dulloo: When you do experiments in the laboratory and compare high-fat versus high-carbohydrate intakes, it is an artificial situation. In real life, when we eat high-fat foods, we also drink coffee or Coca-Cola, which contain caffeine, and this increases fat oxidation, or we take polyphenols from vegetables or from green tea, which are also known to increase fat oxidation. In some countries they eat a diet high in coconut oil, which behaves like medium-chain triglycerides and increases fat oxidation. Thus in real life we take a lot of things that may balance our fat intake much better than laboratory experiments suggest.

Dr. Maffeis: I think that is a good point. However, in the Cambridge study (1), where they compared three different diets with a different fat content, they clearly showed that a high-fat diet is associated with a rapid increase in fatness and body weight, so there was definitely a positive energy balance. You are right, though, under real-life conditions we do indeed take in many different nutrients and combine them. However, on my knowledge, no data are available in children on the comparison between thermogenesis induced by mixed meals with different fat/carbohydrate ratios, supplemented or not with substances as caffeine, polyphenoles, etc.

Dr. Uauy: Do you have any comments about the quality of carbohydrate or fat relative to storage versus oxidation? For example, the effect of a high glycemic or low glycemic index for carbohydrates, and in the case of the fat the presence of omega-3 fatty acids, which may be preferentially oxidized or may even alter mitochondrial oxidation?

Dr. Maffeis: The composition of the fat or carbohydrate does affect thermogenesis, but the effect is relatively small. Moreover, no studies in children, on my knowledge, explored the meal induced thermogenesis after mixed meals with different glycemic index or fatty acid composition.

Dr. Uauy: You said the effect is not great, but 2% may make a significant contribution to body adiposity over time.

Dr. Maffeis: Yes, I agree. However, with common mixed diets is difficult to obtain a difference of 2% or total daily energy expenditure.

Dr. Buenaluz: Could you comment on the rationale of small frequent feeds? You said that this increases thermogenesis.

Dr. Maffeis: We have no experience of measuring thermogenesis in children after small meals taken often compared with larger meals taken infrequently. But Dr. F. Bellisle from France has reviewed all the published reports in children on this specific topic, concluding that there is not a significant protective effect of frequent small meals. I think this topic needs to be studied further.

REFERENCES

1. Stubbs RJ, Ritz P, Coward WA, Prentice AM. Covert manipulation of the ratio of dietary fat to carbo-hydrate and energy density: effect on food intake and energy balance in free-living men eating ad libi-tum. *Am J Clin Nutr* 1995; 62: 330–7.

Obesity in Childhood and Adolescence, edited by
Chunming Chen and William H. Dietz. Nestlé
Nutrition Workshop Series, Pediatric Program,
Vol. 49. Nestec Ltd., Vevey/Lippincott
Williams & Wilkins, Philadelphia © 2002.

Toward Understanding the Genetic Basis of Human Susceptibility to Obesity: A Systemic Approach

Abdul G. Dulloo and *Jean Jacquet

*Department of Medicine, Institute of Physiology, University of Fribourg, Fribourg,
Switzerland; *Computer Unit, Faculty of Medicine, University of Geneva,
Geneva, Switzerland*

ETIOLOGY OF HUMAN OBESITY

Epidemiologic studies of the past decades have provided overwhelming evidence that the prevalence of obesity increases rapidly, often reaching epidemic proportions, in subsistence communities emerging into affluence (1). These transitions may occur within a generation, and hence are too rapid to be explained by changes in genetic make-up of the population. It is therefore tempting to blame gluttony and sloth as virtually the sole culprits in the pandemic of obesity that has occurred in environments where highly varied and palatable energy-dense foods have become accessible all year round and where physical activity demands are low. However, interpretations of data based on prevalences and trends can often suffer from what may be referred to as the phenomenon of "meaningless means" if interindividual variations are overlooked. Within any given environment that promotes excessive energy intake and discourages physical activity, a section of the population, often large, does not become overweight or obese. One can still propose that family, social, and cultural habits—clustered under environmental factors that include learned lifestyle behaviors—play a protective role against their "obesigenic" environments (2), but equally valid are the arguments that lifestyle effects and behaviors may also be inherited, thereby propelling us into the complex area of gene–environment interactions. For example, a genetic predisposition to select high-fat foods or to be sedentary will depend on the availability of such foods or the need to perform physical activities. Moreover, the prime cause of obesity cannot be attributed to excess food intake or to low physical activity alone, as it has repeatedly been shown that not all individuals become obese when experimentally overfed (3), and there are lean habitual high-fat consumers with an overall higher energy intake and lower physical activity level than low-fat consumers (4). It is therefore evident that the efficiency of the metabolic machinery is not a constant; it varies in response to the plane of nutrition, and it varies among individuals.

Role of Genes

By far the most convincing evidence that fatness is heritable derives from adoption studies showing that identical twins have similar body weights and body fat, even when reared apart, and that adopted children tend to have body mass indices (BMI) and fat distributions that are better correlated with those of their biological than of their adopted parents (5–8). These associations have been followed by studies in twins and across families, showing a role for genotype in the interindividual variability in metabolic rate (9), and how a low energy expenditure may be a risk factor for excess weight gain both during growth (10,11) and during adult life (12). It would seem therefore that two conditions predispose to obesity: an ample supply of food and a genetic predisposition to accumulate fat. In subsistence environments, the genes that confer a high susceptibility to fatness may be expressed, but in the absence of sufficient food, obesity cannot occur. The trigger for the rise in obesity worldwide is certainly the environmental changes that favor overeating and low physical activity, but the extent to which a given individual within that population will actually develop or resist obesity resides in the interaction between his genetic makeup and the environment.

Nature-Versus-Nurture Debate

It is probably futile to try to separate the contribution of genes from that of the environment for a phenotype as complex as body weight, the regulation of which comprises a high degree of lifestyle behaviors vis-à-vis food intake and physical activity. How can we separate what is innate from what is learned when these factors are so intertwined? To quote the Swiss primatologist Hans Kummer, "It is as if we wanted to determine the relative contributions of the musician and his musical instrument in the melody! By contrast, if the melody changes, we can then legitimately raise the question about whether it is the musician or the musical instrument (*genes or environment*) which has changed."

In the analysis of genes versus environment therefore the pertinent question is, "What is the percentage change in the *variance* of the phenotype that is contributed by genes and by the environment?" In this context, the "level of heritability"—which is often estimated as the fraction of the population variation in a given obesity phenotype that can be explained by genetic transmission (13)—is highly dependent on how the study was conducted, on the kinds of relatives upon which they were based, and on what was used as the obesity phenotype (BMI, % fat). One can also expect that these values will be altered if appropriate adjustments are made for the relation between adiposity and BMI across age, sex, and ethnic groups (14). Of the three main types of study—family, twin, and adoption—that have attempted to quantify the size of the genetic contribution to the variation in BMI, those conducted with identical twins and fraternal twins reared apart have yielded the highest heritability levels, with values ranging between 60% and 85% of the variation in BMI. In contrast, adoption studies have generated the lowest heritability estimates of 20% to 35%, and family studies have generally found levels of heritability intermediate between the twin and the adoption study reports. Each design has its advantages and disadvantages and incorporates assumptions that may well be violated, with implications for the strength of the findings. Whatever the true values for heritability of fatness, however, it is undeniable that within any population in a given environment, individuals vary in the genetic makeup that renders them more prone or more resistant to obesity. Of central interest for public health and clinical medicine is how to pinpoint the genetic and metabolic basis for such susceptibility to fatness or leanness.

THE SEARCH FOR OBESITY SUSCEPTIBILITY GENES

The developments in DNA technology over the past decade, coupled with computerized bioinformation and biostatistics, have provided growing optimism that genes underlying susceptibility to obesity (commonly referred to as obesity genes) will soon be identified. Several approaches have been used, namely, variants in candidate genes, positional cloning of candidate chromosomal regions, linkage studies in families, and association studies using DNA from case and control designs or comparing genotypes in samples characterized by varying degrees of obesity.

Candidate Genes

Within a few years of the landmark cloning of the gene coding for the hormone leptin in the mid-1990s, most of the single-gene (monogenic) obesities in rodent models have been identified, and mutations with strong effects and associated with juvenile-onset morbid obesity in humans have been detected in the genes coding for leptin, leptin receptor, pro-opiomelanocortin, prohormone convertase-1, and melanocortin-4 receptor (15). Although each of these mutations is rare, they extend to 23 the list of obesity-related Mendelian disorders for which loci have previously been mapped (e.g., the Prader–Willi syndrome, the Basrdet–Biedl syndrome, and the Wilson–Turner syndrome). In the search to identify genes of importance in the much more common forms of human obesity, the relevant sequence variation in many other genes implicated in the control of food intake, thermogenesis, or substrate metabolism has been screened, including that of genes coding for the β_3 adrenoceptor, the uncoupling protein in brown adipose tissue, and its homologs (UCP2, UCP3) in other tissues, neuropeptide Y receptors 1 and 5, tumor necrosis α (TNF-α), and PPAR-γ (peroxisome-proliferator-activated receptor), to name just a few (16). In most studies, the associations were found to be absent, and in the few where associations have been reported, they were relatively weak and clouded by the high probability of false positives.

Linkage and Association Studies

Several genetic linkage studies using a genome-wide scan approach in family studies have been completed in Mexican Americans, Pima Indians, a diverse population of blacks and whites, French Canadian families, and French families. These have identified various major loci linked to obesity on chromosomes 2, 5, 10, 11, and 20, and these different quantitative trait linkages (QTLs) are believed to encode multiple genes of importance for susceptibility to obesity (17). Although the quantitatively most important locus in each of these genes is partly identified, it is not yet known exactly which genes and which mutations in the genes are associated with obesity. Those areas of the human genome will no doubt be subjected to further intense scrutiny to identify obesity susceptibility genes. However, as recently underlined by Ravussin and Bouchard (13), one must also recognize that linkages with weaker statistical significance may be important, particularly when replicated in other datasets. Genetic associations with a high level of significance ($p < 0.001$) have also been identified for variants of a number of genes, including Na/K-ATPase α_2 and β_1 with respiratory quotient, haplotypes of variants in the UCP1 gene and the β_3 adrenoceptor gene with weight loss, and the UCP2 gene with BMI or energy metabolism. However, none of these associations has proved to be the result of a mutation affecting the function or amount of a gene product. An annual update of the human obesity gene map is provided by the Quebec group (17). From association and linkage studies, it seems that putative loci affecting obesity-related phenotypes are found on all except chromosome Y of the human genome. The numbers of genes and other markers that have been associated or linked with human obesity are increasing very rapidly, and are now well over 200.

Obesity Susceptibility Genes Versus Genes for Weight Regulation

The general belief is that if genes are contributing to human susceptibility to obesity, they are doing so because of DNA sequence variation (or variations) affecting expression or function. However, the tremendous advances of the past few years— spearheaded by the identification of most of the monogenic obesities in rodent models—have been almost exclusively in the identification of molecules that play a role in the control of food intake, metabolic rate, or substrate metabolism and in adipose cell biology. While this progress is central for a better understanding of energy balance and weight regulation, there has been little or no progress with respect to the heritability of fatness. To quote Bray and Bouchard (18): "This is particularly striking when one realizes that there is not one single obese human being whose excess body mass and body fat can be explained by *a-specific mutation* in one of the genes exerting its effects in relevant energy balance pathways, with the possible exception of the mendelian syndromes, which characteristically exhibit obesity. But we knew that much before the cloning of the single-gene obesity mouse models."

   With the recent publication of the human genome, it is likely that the emphasis in research will be on a *bottom-to-top* approach (i.e., from genes to functions), with the objective of discovering the combination of genes and mutations that contributes most to the predisposition to human obesity. However, we believe that this approach, although most certainly extending the list of genes that play a role in the regulation of body weight, will not necessarily lead to the identification of the major obesity susceptibility genes. In the light of the previously mentioned disappointments, the research strategies directed at understanding the genetic basis of human susceptibility to obesity need to be reconsidered, with more emphasis on a *top-to-bottom* approach (from functions to genes). This approach, however, requires that the routes from top to bottom be better defined.

A SYSTEMIC APPROACH

Perhaps a starting point in such a reconsideration of a top-to-bottom approach is to revisit the Darwinian arguments as to why the human genome could harbor genes that predispose such a large fraction of the population to obesity. We are often reminded that the human body was designed (in evolutionary terms) to cope with recurrent food shortage periods—that is, the "famine and feast" way of life that probably prevailed during most of mammalian evolution. The general belief, as Neel has emphasized in an update of his "thrifty genotype" hypothesis (19), is that it is variations in the genes that underlie these formerly adaptive homeostatic mechanisms for survival in an environment of intermittent food availability that constitute the genetic basis of human susceptibility to fatness in our present environment. In other words, those with a genetic make-up most conducive to survival in an environment of frequent periods of food scarcity are the most susceptible to obesity in modern affluent societies. Conversely, those capable of maintaining a lean body weight without conscious effort in these same obesigenic environments are likely to be those with a genetic make-up that would put them at greatest risk of being eliminated in an environment of food scarcity. In any top-to-bottom strategy for understanding the genetic basis of human susceptibility to leanness and fatness therefore, it is of central importance to understand what these adaptive homeostatic mechanisms that optimize survival are and how they operate. From a standpoint of system physiology, the questions could be translated as follows: What are the fundamental control systems that allow a human individual to utilize the body's energy stores optimally so as to maximize survival during prolonged starvation? What are their commands and what are their specific functional roles? Furthermore, as it is also an equally high priority to reestablish these energy reserves whenever food availability increases, the questions also arise as to what the control systems are that allow the rapid rebuilding of the prestarvation capacity for survival.

Revisiting Classic Studies of Human Starvation: A Necessity

Progress in the area of human energetics and body composition regulation is, however, hampered by the need to conduct longitudinal studies of experimental starvation and refeeding. During these, food intake, metabolic rate, and body composition are documented before weight loss, and then at various points during the dynamic phases of weight loss and subsequent weight recovery. Furthermore, if a primary objective is to understand the normal physiology of weight regulation in response to starvation and refeeding, then those studies should focus on the response of healthy normal-weight (nonobese) individuals to starvation. This is a difficult, if not impossible, task in adult humans—let alone in infants, children, or adolescents—mainly because of the ethical problems that such prolonged starvation studies would entail and the practical constraints associated with long-term compliance with experimental procedures. Fortunately, the classic studies of experimental starvation and refeeding that were carried out in healthy normal-weight volunteers from 1915 to 1950 (20–22) continue to provide an invaluable source of untapped data. The desire to gain a better insight into the regulation of body weight and body composition by reanalyzing these data in the light of more modern concepts of body weight regulation has become irresistible, as similar studies can no longer be performed in humans for ethical reasons. It is primarily for these reasons that we conducted a series of reanalyses of these classic studies of starvation and refeeding, with particular emphasis on data from the 32 male volunteers who participated in the Minnesota experiment conducted at the end of World War II (22). The results of these reanalyses, which use both statistical and numerical approaches (23–25), suggest that the formerly adaptive homeostatic mechanisms for optimal survival in an environment of famine and feast are embodied in three distinct autoregulatory control systems: the control of partitioning between protein and fat (the two main energy-containing compartments in the body), and two distinct control systems for adaptive thermogenesis. In one of these (Fig. 1), the efferent limb is primarily under the control of the sympathetic nervous system, the functional state of which is dictated by overlapping or interacting signals arising from a variety of environmental stresses, including food deprivation, deficiency of essential nutrients, excess energy intake, and exposure to cold or to infections; it is thus referred to as the *nonspecific* control of thermogenesis. The other is independent of the functional state of the sympathetic nervous system and is dictated solely by signals arising from the state of depletion of the adipose tissue fat stores; it is hence referred to as the *adipose-specific* control of thermogenesis.

Compartmental Model

An overall integration of these autoregulatory control systems in the regulation of body weight and body composition during a cycle of weight loss and weight recovery is discussed with the help of a schematic diagram in Fig. 2. This diagram embodies the main finding that the control of body energy partitioning between protein and fat is an individual characteristic during weight loss and weight recovery (23), and takes into account the existence of these two distinct control systems for adaptive thermogenesis that can operate independently of each other (25,26).

During starvation, the control of partitioning determines the relative proportion of protein and fat to be mobilized from the body as fuel—the individual's partitioning characteristic (Pc) being dictated primarily by the initial body composition. The functional role of the control of partitioning is to meet the fuel needs of the individual in such a way that the energy reserve component in both the fat and protein compartments (i.e., the part that can be lost without death or irreversible damage) would reach complete depletion simultaneously—a strategy that ensures the maximum duration

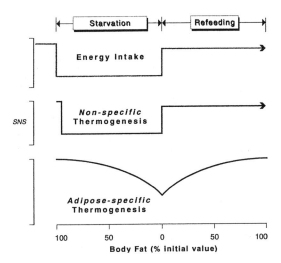

FIG. 1. Schematic representation for the two distinct control systems underlying adaptive thermogenesis during prolonged starvation and subsequent refeeding. One control system, which is a direct function of changes in the food energy supply, responds relatively rapidly to the energy deficit. Its effector mechanisms are suppressed early during the course of starvation, and upon refeeding they are restored relatively rapidly as a function of energy reavailability, and are activated further if hyperphagia occurs during refeeding. Because the efferent limb of this control system—which is primarily under sympathetic nervous system (SNS) control—is dictated not only by the dietary energy supply but also by a variety of other environmental factors such as diet composition, specific nutrient deficiencies, ambient temperature, psychological stress, and so on, it is referred to as the *nonspecific* control of thermogenesis. By contrast, the other control system has a much slower time constant by virtue of its response only to signals arising from the state of depletion/repletion of the fat stores. It is therefore referred to as the control system operating through an *adipose-specific* control of thermogenesis. From Dulloo AG (26).

of survival in a given individual during long-term food scarcity. Furthermore, the energy conserved resulting from suppressed thermogenesis is directed at reducing the energy imbalance, with the net result that there is a slowing down in the rate of protein and fat mobilization in the same proportion as defined by the partitioning characteristic of the individual. Indeed, the fact that the fraction of fuel energy derived from protein (i.e., the P_{ratio}) remains relatively constant during the course of prolonged starvation, albeit in normal-weight humans (27), implies that neither control system underlying suppressed thermogenesis is directed at sparing specifically protein or specifically fat, but at sparing both the protein and fat compartments simultaneously. During starvation therefore the functional role of both control systems underlying suppressed thermogenesis is to reduce the overall rate of fuel utilization.

During refeeding, the control of partitioning operates in such a way that protein and fat are deposited in the same relative proportion as determined by the partitioning characteristic of the individual during starvation, and this serves to reestablish the individual's prestarvation capacity for survival during long-term food scarcity. Furthermore, the increased availability of food leads to the rapid removal of suppression upon the *nonspecific* (sympathetic nervous system mediated) control of

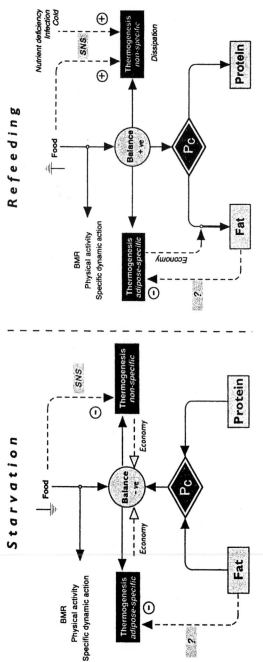

FIG. 2. Schematic representation of a compartmental model for the regulation of body weight and body composition during a cycle of weight loss (prolonged starvation) and weight recovery (refeeding). In this model, the two distinct control systems underlying adaptive thermogenesis—the *nonspecific* control and the *adipose-specific* control—are integrated with the more "basal" control of partitioning between the body fat and protein compartments, as determined by the partitioning characteristic (Pc) of the individual. (See text for details.) BMR, basal metabolic rate; SNS, sympathetic nervous system. From Dulloo AG (26).

thermogenesis. By contrast, the suppression of the thermogenesis under *adipose-specific* control is only slowly relieved as a function of fat recovery, such that the energy that continues to be spared is directed specifically at the replenishment of the fat stores. The net effect—as previously demonstrated using both statistical and numerical approaches in our reanalysis of data from the Minnesota experiment (23)—is that fat is deposited in excess of that determined by the partitioning characteristic of the individual, thereby contributing to the disproportionate rate of fat relative to lean tissue recovery. This phenomenon is often observed—both in adults after severe weight loss due to food unavailability and disease, and in infants and children recovering from protein–energy malnutrition and growth arrest (28). An adaptive process that accelerates the restitution of the fat stores rather than diverting the energy saved toward compensatory increase in body protein synthesis (an energetically costly process) would have survival value in the ancestral famine-and-feast lifestyle. This is because, by virtue of the fact that fat has a greater energy density and a lower energy cost of synthesis/maintenance than protein, it would provide the organism with a greater capacity to rebuild an efficient energy reserve rapidly, and hence to cope with recurrent food shortages. Thus the functional role of the adipose-specific control of thermogenesis during weight recovery is specifically to accelerate the replenishment of fat stores whenever food availability is increased after a long period of food deficit and severe depletion of body fat stores. This provides an alternative way of surviving without hyperphagia.

PERSPECTIVES

Genetic Basis of Human Variability in Adaptive Thermogenesis

In addition to evidence in humans from the Minnesota experiment (25,26), and more recently from the Biosphere-2 experiment (29), the existence of an adipose-specific control of thermogenesis has direct experimental support from carefully controlled energy balance and body composition studies in animals, conducted in the phase of weight recovery after starvation or growth arrest (30,31). It can also be shown to operate independently of the functional state of the sympathetic nervous system (32). It is proposed that it operates as a feedback loop between the adipose tissue fat stores and the skeletal muscle, and would hence comprise a *sensor* of the state of depletion of the fat stores, a *signal* dictating the suppression of thermogenesis as a function of the state of depletion of the fat stores, and an *effector system* mediating adaptive thermogenesis in this skeletal muscle (26). To date, however, studies of prolonged starvation and refeeding have indicated that neither free fatty acids nor leptin in blood show temporal changes that correlate with the kinetics of suppressed thermogenesis under adipose-specific control (33), nor is there evidence that the uncoupling protein homologues, UCP2 and UCP3, have a physiologic role in the mediation of skeletal muscle thermogenesis (34,35). At present, the sensors, signals, and effector system of the adipose-specific control of thermogenesis remain unknown. Their discovery will no doubt have important implications for our understanding of body composition regulation, including the identification of candidate genes underlying the susceptibility to fatness.

In the meantime, the diagram in Fig. 2 provides a structural framework to explain the apparent paradox that suppressed adipose-specific thermogenesis that results in enhanced fat deposition during refeeding—and that is postulated to occur in the skeletal muscle—persists when the nonspecific control of thermogenesis is activated in organs and tissues recruited by the sympathetic nervous system (e.g., liver, kidneys, and brown adipose tissue). Such differentially regulated control systems for thermogenesis may have arisen during the course of mammalian evolution in order to satisfy the need for energy conservation directed specifically at the rapid recovery of body fat under a variety of environmental stresses, when sympathetically mediated activation of heat production has equally important survival value. Examples of the latter include thermoregulation during weight recovery in cold environments, the generation of fever during exposure to infections, and the concomitant enhancement of thermogenesis during weight recovery on a poor diet (e.g., one that is low in protein). In this case an excess energy intake—resulting from the consumption of large quantities of the poor diet in an attempt to meet the requirements of the specific nutrients—needs to be dissipated as heat (diet-induced thermogenesis [DIT]) in order to avoid excessive weight gain.

A recent reanalysis of human overfeeding experiments by Stock (36) showed that humans seem to possess a much larger capacity for DIT than is generally recognized. Although this capacity is poorly recruited on well-balanced diets, it is much more pronounced on diets poor in essential nutrients. In this context, Stock proposed that DIT may have evolved as a mechanism for regulating the metabolic supply of essential nutrients (protein, minerals, vitamins), with only a secondary role in regulating energy balance. Our own reanalysis of the human overfeeding studies revealed the strong possibility that relatively small individual differences in DIT on balanced normal-protein diets are amplified by protein-deficient diets (37). As shown in Fig. 3, the extent to which the mechanisms underlying DIT are recruited would seem to be a function of both the individual (as judged by the interindividual variability within each diet group) and the dietary protein level, the recruitment for DIT being weak on normal-protein diets but pronounced on low-protein diets. As even small interindividual variations in the efficiency of weight gain (and hence of thermogenesis) on well-balanced diets can, over months and years, contribute to weight maintenance in some and obesity in others, the possibility arises that overfeeding low-protein diets could serve as a tool for maximizing DIT, so exaggerating individual differences in energetic efficiency. In other words, low-protein overfeeding may serve as a "magnifying glass" for unraveling the genetic and metabolic basis whereby variations in thermogenesis contribute to susceptibility to leanness and fatness during overconsumption of the typical (well-balanced) diets of our affluent societies (36,37).

Genetic Basis of Human Variability in Energy Partitioning

Apart from variability in thermogenesis, it is clear that interindividual variability in the control of partitioning between protein and fat can also contribute importantly to human susceptibility to fatness. It is indeed well established, though not often

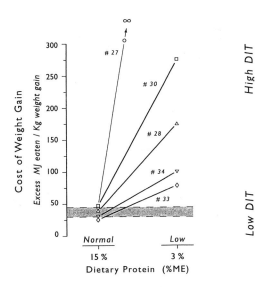

FIG. 3. Unmasking of interindividual variability in thermogenesis by low-protein overfeeding. The data represent the energy cost of weight gain (excess MJ consumed per kg weight gained) during 3 to 4 weeks of overfeeding in five volunteer subjects (Nos. 27, 28, 30, 33, and 34) who participated in both normal-protein (15%) and low-protein (3%) overfeeding in the gluttony experiments of Miller and coworkers (38,39). The two horizontal broken lines (enclosing the shaded area) correspond to predicted energy cost of weight gain on the assumption that weight gain is either 100% fat (45 MJ/kg) or 60% fat (30 MJ/kg), the latter value including cost of fat-free mass gain. The greater the deviation from the predicted values, the greater the likelihood that the excess energy was dissipated through enhanced diet induced thermogenesis (DIT). ME, metabolizable energy. From Dulloo AG (37).

appreciated, that the extra weight gain during the development of obesity reflects an increase not only in adipose mass (i.e., fat) but also in lean tissue (protein), and that the composition of the excess weight gained is a variable (40). Consequently, for the same surplus of food energy, an individual with a low partitioning characteristic will gain less protein and more fat than an individual with a high partitioning characteristic, which favors body protein deposition.

The importance of genotype in such partitioning between protein and fat has been demonstrated in the responses of 12 pairs of identical twins to experimental overfeeding, during which they all consumed an excess of 1,000 kcal/d, 6 days a week for a period of 3 months (41). Although mean weight gain was 8 kg, it ranged from 4 to 13 kg, and 37% of the variation in weight gain was associated with energy partitioning, assessed as the ratio of fat mass to fat-free mass. The mean value for this dimension of energy partitioning was 2:1, but it varied from 1:2 to 4:1 among the 24 individuals. In addition, the variance in response was at least three times greater between twin pairs than within pairs for gain in body weight and body fat. This therefore provides strong evidence that there are inherited differences not only in body weight and BMI, but also in the composition of the weight gained in response to overfeeding. A tendency to gain fat or lean tissues—that is, variability in their partitioning characteristics—seems to be a major genetically determined factor in the susceptibility to obesity. These observations underscore the need for a better characterization of interindividual variability in energy partitioning, particularly in the area of susceptibility to fatness during the growth process.

Clues to the primary determinants of such variations in energy partitioning may also be derived from our reappraisal of the physiology of human starvation, where the interindividual variability in the control of partitioning between protein and fat during weight loss and weight recovery has now been reasonably well characterized. It has been shown that this is primarily determined not only by the prestarvation ratio of fat to fat-free mass (i.e., by the initial percentage of fat [Fig. 4]), but also by the size of energy reserve fraction in the protein compartment (r_p)—the fraction of the protein compartment that could be lost without death or irreversible consequences

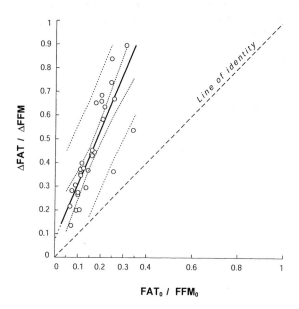

FIG. 4. Linear relation between the initial body composition (FAT_0, fat mass; FFM_0, fat-free mass) and the composition of weight loss (ΔFAT: ΔFFM) among the normal-weight men subjected to 24 weeks of semistarvation in the Minnesota experiment ($N = 31$; $r^2 = 0.7$, $p < 0.001$). The data for ΔFAT: ΔFFM are the values for change in body fat and FFM over the entire 24 weeks of semistarvation. The data for FAT_0: FFM_0 (range 0.06 to 0.34) follows a normal distribution, with a threefold variability between the 10th and the 90th centile values (range, 0.08 to 0.26). For the regression, the 95% confidence intervals are within the inner dotted lines, whereas the predictive intervals are within the outer dotted lines. The significance of the overall linear model is high (F value, 55.5; $p < 0.001$) with a significant slope (b) of 2.29 (SD 0.31) ($p < 0.001$) and a nonsignificant constant intercept (a) of 0.078 (SD 0.055). The broken diagonal line represents the line of identity between the two ratios. This relation constitutes a cardinal feature that led to the construction of a mathematical model for predicting the partitioning characteristic (Pc) of an individual during starvation (42). According to this model, the Pc has only two determinants: the FAT_0:FFM_0 ratio (which is essentially the initial percentage of fat) and r_p (which is the protein reserve fraction (r_p)—that is, the fraction of the protein compartment that could be lost without death or irreversible consequences. From Dulloo AG (42).

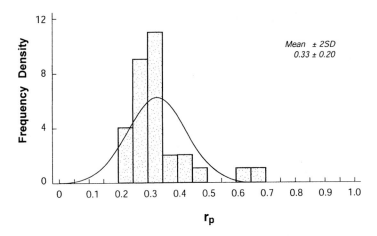

FIG. 5. Histograms showing frequency distribution for the protein reserve fraction (r_p) of the men volunteers from the Minnesota experiment (22). The values of r_p are calculated using a mathematical model for studying interindividual variability in fuel partitioning during starvation (42). A normal curve is superimposed over the histogram for comparison. Although the data r_p appear skewed, the application of the Wilk–Shapiro/Rankit normality statistical test shows that this variable could conform to a normal distribution, with Wilk–Shapiro value of 0.80. If the two possible outliers (r_p values > 0.5) are omitted, the Wilk–Shapiro value is improved from 0.80 to 0.95. From Dulloo AG (42).

(42). The application of a mathematical model for predicting the partitioning characteristic of an individual during starvation (42) to the Minnesota data on the changes in body composition during weight loss showed that there was a large—at least twofold—variability in estimates of r_p among the Minnesota men (Fig. 5). Future studies would need to explore whether interindividual variability in r_p resides in the relative proportion of organ (visceral) mass to skeletal mass, in the fiber or biochemical composition of the skeletal muscle, or in variability in skeletal muscle metabolism. Whatever the phenotypes by which this large variability in r_p expresses itself, it is likely to contribute in an important way to genetically determined variability in lean-to-fat tissue deposition, whether during weight gain in adults or during the growth process across infancy, childhood, and adolescence.

CONCLUSIONS

It is our contention that the origin of the genetic basis of human susceptibilities to fatness and leanness, most certainly polygenic, resides primarily within the three control systems that constitute the most important formerly adaptive homeostatic mechanisms in a hunter-gatherer or subsistence-farmer lifestyle of famine and feast. They probably conferred varying capacities to defend the body's protein and fat stores in an ancestral lifestyle of recurrent periods of food scarcity but now underlie our varying susceptibilities to fatness in a world where palatable foods are abundant all year round. Our understanding of the genes controlling them will depend upon the extent to which these systems can be studied in isolation from each other, let alone from all kinds of environmental or pathophysiologic disturbances. The greatest challenges nowadays are therefore to find or design the experimental conditions most likely to unravel the molecular physiologic processes underlying each of these control systems.

The components of the control system underlying the *adipose-specific* suppression of thermogenesis—namely its sensors, signals, and effectors—can certainly be studied in isolation from the other control systems regulating body composition, but within the type of constraints that can only be imposed in animal experimentation.

Subtle differences among humans in their capacity for *nonspecific* control of thermogenesis in response to diet (i.e., in diet-induced thermogenesis)—while of quantitative importance in their different susceptibilities to obesity when cumulated over months or years—are unlikely to be picked up by conventional techniques during the relatively short durations of human experimentation. It may prove necessary to simulate the appropriate unbalanced dietary conditions (i.e., low-protein overfeeding) under which diet-induced thermogenesis is recruited to unmask some of the genetic and metabolic machinery responsible for human variability in thermogenesis.

Finally, in our pursuit of a better understanding of the determinants of susceptibility to obesity in childhood and adolescence, it is necessary first to understand the determinants that underlie interindividual variability in the *partitioning between protein and fat* during growth.

To reach these objectives, there are no alternatives except robust analysis of data on changes in body composition during longitudinal studies. In this context, the application of adequate statistical or numerical approaches that allow linearization of the relation between lean and fat tissues during growth—while taking into account the synchronization between the changes in height, muscle mass, and the mass of vital organs—is certainly a vital prerequisite.

ACKNOWLEDGMENTS

This work is dedicated to the late Professor Michael J. Stock, who revolutionized the area of weight regulation and thermogenesis and traced key pathways for a better understanding of human susceptibilities to obesity and leanness. This work was supported by grant No. 3200.061687 of the Swiss National Science Foundation.

REFERENCES

1. World Health Organisation. *Obesity: preventing and managing the global epidemic.* Geneva: WHO, 1998.
2. Egger G, Swinburn B. An "ecological" approach to the obesity pandemic. *BMJ* 1997; 315: 477–80.
3. Miller DS. Factors affecting energy expenditure. *Proc Nutr Soc* 1982; 41: 193–202.
4. Blundell JE, Cooling J. Routes to obesity: phenotypes, food choices and activity. *Br J Nutr* 2000; 83: 33–8.
5. Stunkard AJ, Sorensen TIA, Hanis C, *et al.* An adoption study of human obesity. *N Engl J Med* 1986; 314: 193–8.
6. Stunkard AJ, Harris JR, Pedersen NL, McClearn GE. The body mass index of twins who have been reared apart. *N Engl J Med* 1990; 322: 1483–7.

7. Price RA, Gotterman II. Body fat in identical twins reared apart: roles for genes and environment. *Behav Genet* 1991; 21: 1–7.

8. Allison DB, Kaprio J, Korkeilla M, Koskenvuo M, Neale MC, Hayakawa K. The heritability of body mass index among an international sample of monozygotic twins reared apart. *Int J Obes* 1996; 20: 501–6.

9. Bouchard C, Tremblay A, Nadeau A, Després JP. Genetic effect in resting and exercise metabolic rates. *Metabolism* 1989; 8: 464–70.

10. Griffiths M, Payne PR, Stunkard AJ, Rivers JPW, Cox M. Metabolic rate and physical development in children at risk of obesity. *Lancet* 1990; 336: 76–8.

11. Roberts SB, Savage J, Coward WA, Chew B, Lucas A. Energy expenditure and intake of infants born to lean and overweight mothers. *N Engl J Med* 1998; 318: 461–6.

12. Ravussin E, Lillilioja E, Knowler WC, *et al.* Reduced rate of energy expenditure as a risk factor for body weight gain. *N Engl J Med* 1988; 318: 461–6.

13. Ravussin E, Bouchard C. Human genomics and obesity: finding appropriate drug targets. *Eur J Pharmacol* 2000; 410: 131–45.

14. Deurenberg P. Universal cut-off points for obesity are not appropriate. *Br J Nutr* 2001; 85: 135–6.

15. Barsh GS, Farooqi IS, O'Rahilly S. Genetics of body weight regulation. *Nature* 2000; 404: 644–51.

16. Arner P. Obesity—a genetic disease of adipose tissue? *Br J Nutr* 2000; 83 (Suppl 1): S9–16.

17. Chagnon YC, Perusse L, Weisnagel SJ, Rankinen T, Bouchard C. The human obesity gene map: the 1999 update. *Obes Res* 2000; 1: 89–117.

18. Bray G, Bouchard C. Genetics of human obesity: research directions. *Faseb J* 1997; 11: 937–45.

19. Neel JV. The "thrifty genotype" in 1998. *Nutr Rev* 1999; 57: 2–9.

20. Benedict FG. *A study of prolonged fasting.* Carnegie Institute of Washington Publication No 203. Washington, DC: Carnegie Institute, 1915.

21. Takahira H. *Metabolism during fasting and subsequent refeeding.* Tokyo: Imperial Government Institute for Nutrition, 1925: 63–82.

22. Keys A, Brozek J, Henschel A, Mickelson O, Taylor HL. *The biology of human starvation.* Minneapolis: University of Minnesota Press, 1950.

23. Dulloo AG, Jacquet J, Girardier L. Autoregulation of body composition during weight recovery in humans: the Minnesota Experiment revisited. *Int J Obes* 1996; 20: 393–405.

24. Dulloo AG, Jacquet J, Girardier L. Poststarvation hyperphagia and body fat overshooting in humans: a role for feedback signals from lean and fat tissues. *Am J Clin Nutr* 1997; 65: 717–23.

25. Dulloo AG, Jacquet J. Adaptive reduction in basal metabolic rate in response to food deprivation in humans: a role for feedback signals from fat stores. *Am J Clin Nutr* 1998; 68: 599–606.

26. Dulloo AG, Jacquet J. An adipose-specific control of thermogenesis in body weight regulation. *Int J Obesity* 2001; 25: S22–S90.

27. Henry CJK, Rivers, Payne PR. Protein and energy metabolism in starvation reconsidered. *Eur J Clin Nutr* 1998; 42: 543–9.

28. Dulloo AG. Human pattern of food intake and fuel partitioning during weight recovery after starvation: a theory of autoregulation of body composition. *Proc Nutr Soc* 1997; 56: 25–40.

29. Weyer C, Walford RL, Harper IT, *et al.* Energy metabolism after 2 y of energy restriction: the Biosphere 2 experiment. *Am J Clin Nutr* 2000; 72: 946–53.

30. Dulloo AG, Girardier L. Adaptive changes in energy expenditure during refeeding following low calorie intake: evidence for a specific metabolic component favouring fat storage. *Am J Clin Nutr* 1990; 52: 415–20.

31. Dulloo AG, Girardier L. Adaptive role of energy expenditure in modulating body fat and protein deposition during catch-up growth after early undernutrition. *Am J Clin Nutr* 1993; 58: 614–21.

32. Dulloo AG, Seydoux J, Girardier L. Dissociation of enhanced efficiency of fat deposition during weight recovery from sympathetic control of thermogenesis. *Am J Physiol* 1995; 269: 365–9.

33. Samec S, Assimacopoulos-Jeannet F, Giacobino JP, Seydoux J, Dulloo AG. Is there a role for leptin in the increased efficiency of fat recovery after starvation. *Int J Obes* 1997; 21: 99.

34. Samec S, Seydoux J, Dulloo AG. Role of UCP homologues in skeletal muscles and brown adipose tissue: mediators of thermogenesis or regulators of lipids as fuel substrate? *FASEB J* 1998; 12: 715–24.

35. Dulloo AG, Samec S. Uncoupling proteins: do they have a role in weight regulation? *New Physiol Sci* 2000; 15: 313–8.

36. Stock MJ. Gluttony and thermogenesis revisited. *Int J Obes* 1999; 23: 1105–17.

37. Dulloo AG, Jacquet J. Low-protein overfeeding: a tool to unmask susceptibility to obesity in humans. *Int J Obes* 1999; 23: 1118–21.

38. Miller DS, Mumford P. Gluttony 1. An experimental study of overeating low- or high-protein diets. *Am J Clin Nutr* 1967; 20: 1212–22.

39. Miller DS, Mumford P, Stock MJ. Gluttony 2. Thermogenesis in overeating man. *Am J Clin Nutr* 1967; 20: 1223–9.
40. Forbes GB. Lean body mass–body fat interrelationship in humans. *Nutr Rev* 1987; 45: 225–31.
41. Bouchard C, Tremblay A, Després JP, *et al.* The response to long-term overfeeding in identical twins. *N Engl J Med* 1990; 322: 1477–82.
42. Dulloo AG, Jacquet J. The control of partitioning between protein and fat during human starvation: its internal determinants and biological significance. *Br J Nutr* 1999; 82: 339–56.

DISCUSSION

Dr. Anantharaman: Based on your model, what do you feel would be the ideal micronutrient profile of a food used to refeed an infant who has been starved or malnourished?

Dr. Dulloo: At the moment, we don't really know the answer. There is a real need for experiments to study those specific components that seem to conserve energy and to accelerate fat deposition. In the study by Ancel Keys—which is the closest one that can get to the normal physiologic situation without infection—they used a diet that was very low in fat, less than 20%, and still saw an acceleration of fat deposition (1). In animals we know that if you give a high-fat diet, you exacerbate this phenomenon even more. We have tried different dietary compositions—polyunsaturated fats, fish oil, n-6, n-3, and so on—and we can reduce the exacerbation of fat deposition a little but cannot eliminate it. The next thing will be to look at zinc and other specific micronutrients, but this hasn't been done yet.

Dr. Uauy: You concentrated mainly on the genetics of food intake and fuel partitioning, but there are also the genes responsible for adipocyte differentiation and adipogenesis. Could you comment on that aspect?

Dr. Dulloo: I described the fundamental control systems where there may be strong genetic variability. We need to look at each of these. Would adipocyte differentiation, by whatever genes it may be mediated, be under the control of partitioning, be under the control of what we might call nonspecific thermogenesis, or be related to the suppression of thermogenesis that accelerates fat deposition specifically? We have to look at all these possibilities.

Dr. Shen: Could you give us your view on future genetically based treatment for obesity— for example, the use of gene therapy to intervene in obesity?

Dr. Dulloo: Everything is moving so fast that it is hard to foretell what is going to happen. We have problems just following the literature. Between the time I got the invitation to come here and now, at least six potentially very important obesity genes have been discovered. If you just look at intermediary metabolism, any of the enzymes in this enormous network has a potential candidate gene. Whether or not gene therapy could be applied, there are bound to be ethical concerns. Are we going to treat half the world where people are becoming obese?

Dr. Robinson: Are there methods available for looking at differential gene expression in response to manipulations in the environment, such as diet and activity? In other words, are researchers looking at gene expression in response to environmental manipulation as opposed to genes associated with different levels of obesity or physiologic states?

Dr. Dulloo: These are very expensive studies and require the characterization of physical activity in an enormous number of subjects. I don't know if anybody is doing this, but it's a difficult task to monitor activity in thousands of subjects, and then to look for genetic difference. I agree it would be the ideal approach, but perhaps not feasible.

Dr. Robinson: I was thinking more about experimental manipulation of activity, diet, or other environmental factors—so you would exercise and then look for variations in gene expression.

Dr. Dulloo: It is highly probable that people are doing such studies but I am not personally aware of any.

Dr. Gortmaker: My understanding of your presentation is that it was mainly focused on diet processing and the genetic influences. What about genetic influences on more fundamental physical activity levels? I tend to think of us as being programmed to want to sit still unless we're threatened with death, and then we may start running around! Do you have any sense of how one might partition the genetic influences into these two areas, energy intake versus energy expenditure?

Dr. Dulloo: It is futile to try to separate the effects of genes from environmental effects per se. Take the example of a musical performance. There are two parts to that—the person playing the music and the instrument. By just hearing the music, we cannot separate the contribution of the instrument from the contribution of the player. All we hear is the interaction of the two. In the end, we always deal with interactions.

Dr. Gortmaker: What I meant was that you spoke about dietary intake but not really about levels of physical activity in individuals, or the genetic basis of that physical activity. To what extent is that an important area for ongoing research?

Dr. Dulloo: It's likely to be a very important area. The best reason I can give for that is the study of overfeeding done by Levine in the United States (2). He overfed his subjects and there was tremendous variability in weight gain in response to the same excess energy intake. The explanation for this did not lie in differences in BMR or the thermogenic response to meals, so they concluded that the effect was caused by an increase in activity not detectable by accelerometers or pedometers—in other words, fidgeting or low-level unstructured activity. This must have a very important genetic component. What drives one person to do more of this would be an interesting area to look for gene and environmental interactions.

REFERENCES

1. Keys A, Brozek J, Henschel A, Mickelson O, Taylor HL. *The biology of human starvation.* Minneapolis: University of Minnesota Press, 1950.
2. Levine JA, Eberhardt NL, Jensen MD. Role of non-exercise activity thermogenesis in resistance to fat gain in humans. *Science* 1999; 283: 212–4.

Obesity in Childhood and Adolescence, edited by
Chunming Chen and William H. Dietz. Nestlé
Nutrition Workshop Series, Pediatric Program,
Vol. 49. Nestec Ltd., Vevey/Lippincott
Williams & Wilkins, Philadelphia © 2002.

Childhood Overweight:
Family Environmental Factors

Leann L. Birch

*Department of Human Development and Family Studies, The Pennsylvania State University,
University Park, Pennsylvania, USA*

Overweight parents are more likely to have children who become overweight. Family
resemblances in weight status are well documented (1–4), reflecting the interplay of
genes and family environmental factors. While children are growing up within the
family, parents provide both genes and environment. Behavioral genetics research illustrates the important contribution of genetics to the obese phenotype, with genes or
genetic similarity among family members explaining approximately 70% of the phenotypic variation in adiposity (5–7). Likewise, dramatic increases in the prevalence
of overweight among children and adults within the past 20 years (8,9) attest to the
critical role of the environment in the development and maintenance of overweight.
Although we have learned a great deal about the genetics of obesity, we still have relatively little information about environmental variables that promote childhood overweight (10).

A research challenge for behavioral scientists is to delineate aspects of the family
environment that mediate the development of family resemblances in adiposity and
promote childhood overweight. Behavior genetics has characterized environmental
effects as either shared or nonshared. Shared environments are those that are per-
fectly correlated across family members and influence the phenotype in the same
way. Nonshared environments are those that are not highly correlated and are experienced differently by individuals within the same family. Nonshared environments
result in different phenotypic outcomes across family members. Traditionally, family environments were assumed to be shared environments, affecting all children in
the same way. Nonshared environments were assumed to exist outside the family.
The assumption that family environments are shared environments, in combination
with results from behavioral genetics research indicating minimal effects of the
shared environment on phenotypic variation (2), have led to the erroneous conclusion
that family environments do not matter (11). In fact, however, research has revealed
that family environments and parenting practices do influence development but that
it is the *nonshared* experiences among siblings that explain variability in phenotypic
traits (12). Nonshared environments exist within families because parent–child interactions are bidirectional: parenting influences children and children influence

parenting (13). Because children influence parents, parenting practices differ across siblings, owing to sibling differences in age, sex, birth order, special abilities, temperament, and physical appearance (13,14). With respect to feeding environment, although siblings may eat from the same refrigerator and at the same table, feeding environments are nonshared because child feeding practices are a reaction to the child's phenotypic characteristics at that point in development (15).

Domain-specific parenting (16) proposes that parenting is tailored to the child on the basis not only of phenotypic differences among children but also of parental concerns and perceptions of the child's risk of developing a problem in that particular domain of development. Using obesity proneness in children to illustrate how domain-specific parenting works, Costanzo and Woody (16) reviewed research showing that parents modulate their child feeding practices according to the child's current weight status, parental investment in weight and appearance, and parents' perceptions of the child's risk of overweight. When parents were highly invested in weight-related issues (possibly because they were overweight themselves) and perceived their child to be at risk of overweight, they were more likely to attempt to control and regulate their child's food intake to alleviate proneness to obesity. However, they argue that these attempts to control the child's intake limit the opportunities for the child to develop self-control, thereby promoting rather than alleviating the risk of overweight that the parents are trying to avoid. This model has been tested and supported by research from our laboratory, and illustrates one of a number of ways in which the family environment can mediate familial patterns of adiposity.

A model depicting familial factors hypothesized to promote familial patterns of adiposity and childhood overweight appears in Fig. 1. Direct genetic links between parental weight and child weight are acknowledged in the model (as shown by the direct arrow between parent and child weight status), but the focus is on displaying and discussing a set of mediating behavioral patterns within the family that promote

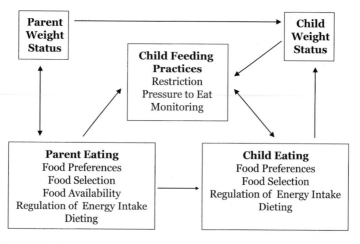

FIG. 1. Behavioral mediators of family resemblances in eating and weight status.

childhood overweight. The model illustrates how parents' weight status is linked to parents' own eating patterns and to their child feeding practices, which in turn influence children's eating behaviors and, in due course, the children's weight status. Specifically, parental eating styles, parents' food preferences, and the foods they consume and make available to their children all influence and are influenced by the parents' weight status (as shown by a double-headed arrow linking the two constructs). In turn, parent eating behaviors shape children's eating behaviors directly, as a result of social modeling and by the choice of foods available to children, and indirectly through their association with parents' child feeding practices. Child feeding practices—such as restricting children's access to food and pressuring children to eat certain foods—are largely driven by parents' own eating behaviors, children's current weight status, and parents' concern about future risk of overweight among their children (16). Finally, parent eating styles and child feeding practices shape children's eating behaviors, such as their food preferences and food selection patterns; in turn, children's eating patterns influence and are influenced by children's weight status.

Figure 1 is of limited scope, focusing exclusively on parent and child interactions and on the intake side of the energy balance equation. The focus on parenting does not imply that these are the only aspects of the family environment that may promote family resemblances in being overweight, but shows that efforts to delineate environmental variables and behavioral mediators can enhance our understanding of the modifiable factors involved in the development of childhood overweight, and point to areas where additional research is needed (10).

I will discuss aspects of this model in greater detail later. As a guide to the sections that follow, this chapter is structured around children's eating behaviors. Children's eating behaviors include food preferences, the ability to regulate energy intake on the basis of hunger and satiety cues, food selection, and meal initiation and termination. In addition, I will address the influence of parents' own eating patterns and of child feeding practices on these eating behaviors. I will also briefly discuss the larger social context in which parents feed their children (e.g., an environment that offers energy-dense, super-sized meals, places a high value on physical attractiveness and thinness in girls and women, and lacks time for food preparation). In the final section, I will review research assessing links between children's eating patterns and the risk of childhood overweight. Owing to a relative absence of research assessing behavioral mediators linking parent and child eating behaviors and weight status, most of the research relating to this model is from my own laboratory.

CHILDREN'S FOOD PREFERENCES: PARENTAL INFLUENCE

Children learn an enormous amount about food and eating during the first years of life, and this learning occurs in the family context. Through early experience with food and eating, children's genetic predispositions become patterns of food preferences and food intake, and these influence their weight status. Genetic predispositions include a preference for sweet and salty tastes, rejection of sour and bitter tastes, a tendency to reject novel foods, and the ability to learn to like and dislike foods based on the social contexts and physiologic consequences of eating (17). Young children depend on their parents to provide food, and the child's food environment is constrained and shaped by the parents' own food preferences and food selections, which in turn are determined by the larger cultural and economic context: the cost, convenience, taste, and availability of food. Although parents shape children's eating environments, determining what foods are offered and the timing and size of meals and snacks, young children's food preferences do not closely resemble their parents' food preferences (18). However, food preferences of adult children do resemble those of their parents (18,19). Perusse and Bouchard (20) reported only modest genetic effects on food preferences and found that cultural and environmental factors accounted for about 80% of the substantial within and between family variation in food preferences.

Early experience with food is especially crucial to children's developing patterns of food preference and intake because children are neophobic, initially rejecting new foods despite their need for increased dietary variety. When the child begins the transition from the exclusive milk diet during weaning, all foods are new and acceptance of these foods is critical in establishing dietary patterns that will support growth and health. Fortunately, if children have repeated opportunities to sample new foods, then some foods will be accepted. When preschool children had repeated experience with a new food, it became more familiar and their preference for the food tended to increase (21,22). Therefore children's food preferences and food intake patterns may be largely shaped by the foods the parents choose to make available to their children, and their persistence in presenting a food that is initially rejected. Our genetically determined preference for sweet and salty foods guarantees that many such foods will be readily accepted. For other foods—including meats, grains, and vegetables—relatively extensive experience is necessary for food acceptance.

Research with animal models has revealed that "learned safety" may be responsible for the reduction of neophobia through repeated consumption of new foods (23): When ingestion of a new food is not followed by illness, we learn that the food does not cause illness, and neophobia is reduced. If illness does follow, a conditioned aversion to that food may develop. Food preferences can also be learned, based on the positive postingestive effects. Rats and humans can learn to prefer flavors associated with energy-dense over energy-dilute foods or drinks (24,25). Children readily learn to prefer flavors previously associated with energy-dense over energy-dilute paired flavors (26,27). Although learned preferences for energy-dense foods may have been adaptive in times of food scarcity, in today's obesity-promoting food environment, where energy-dense foods are inexpensive and readily available in large portions, such preferences can promote overconsumption and overweight (28).

CHILDREN'S EATING: A SOCIAL ACTIVITY

Children's early eating experiences typically occur in a social context, first involving the mother–infant dyad, then, increasingly, other eaters who can serve as models, and also adults who use child feeding practices to control children's eating. Much of our research has focused on the impact of these early social contexts of feeding. For example, to examine the effects of common child feeding practices on children's food preferences, we simulated them in the laboratory (29–31). Parents often use sweet foods to reward children for finishing their vegetables. We found that when palatable foods were used as rewards for a desired behavior, those foods become even more preferred by children (29). Although parents believe that pressuring children to eat a "healthy" food is an effective way to increase the child's liking for that food (32), we have repeatedly found that, rather than fostering food acceptance, pressuring and coercing children to eat particular foods promotes dislike of those foods (no wonder American children tend not to eat their vegetables) (30,31). Thus the effects of child feeding practices on children's food preferences and food intake are often not those that their parents intend. In fact, the evidence indicates that many of these practices may promote a liking for foods high in energy, sugar, and fat, while also fostering a dislike of vegetables and other healthy foods.

CHILDREN'S RESPONSIVENESS TO HUNGER AND SATIETY CUES: EFFECTS OF EXPERIENCE AND LEARNING

Infants are able to regulate their energy intake on the basis of their physiologic needs, reflecting a responsiveness to internal hunger and satiety cues. Infants older than about 6 weeks adjusted their formula intake in response to differences in the energy density of the formula, consuming greater volumes of a formula with a low energy density than of one with a high energy density, so that the total energy intake remained similar (33). Preschool children can also adjust the amount of food they consume in response to changes in the energy density of their food, maintaining a relatively constant energy intake across changes in energy density (34,35). In addition, over 24-hour periods children maintained relatively consistent total daily energy intakes, and this was attributable to meal-to-meal adjustments in energy intake (36). When olestra was substituted for dietary fat for about 10% of the total daily energy intake, thus diluting the energy density of the diet, children increased their self-selected intake to maintain total 24-hour energy intake at levels similar to the control condition (37). The ability to regulate energy intake closely, based on physiologic need, is an adaptive behavior preventing overweight. With increasing age, we see increasing individual differences in children's responsiveness to energy density as a factor controlling food intake.

The substantial individual differences among children in their ability to regulate their energy intake led us to investigate whether feeding practices could foster differences in regulatory behavior. Parents' feeding practices provide guidance for their children about which cues they should be responsive to in controlling their food intake. A child who reports she is full but is told to clean her plate may learn to ignore her internal feedback signaling feelings of fullness, and focus instead on finishing the portion served to her. When a child says, "I'm hungry" and is told, "Not now, wait until mealtime," the child may learn that it is the presence of food, not hunger, that should initiate eating. Finally, if parents chronically restrict children's access to palatable snacks, children may learn to eat in the presence of food, whether or not they are hungry. Research from our laboratory supports these ideas. In one particular study, adults encouraged children to focus on feelings of hunger and fullness ("internal" condition), or in the contrasting "external" condition children were pressured to "clean up the plate" (38). Over a series of subsequent meals, children who were focused on hunger and satiety cues adjusted their intake to compensate for manipulations in the energy density of the meal so that they maintained a consistent total energy intake. However, children in the external context did adjust their intake in response to changes in energy density, showing that their responsiveness to energy density was easily overridden by feeding practices that emphasized external cues, such as pressure to finish the portion. We have also found that heavier girls were subjected to greater parental control, thus illustrating nonshared environmental influences, and they showed less capacity to adjust their intake in response to differences in energy density (39); no consistent relation was noted for boys. Thus, although parents need to set limits, there appears to be an inherent tension between socializing children into eating at mealtimes while supporting their capacity for self-regulation.

FAMILY RESEMBLANCES IN FOOD INTAKE PATTERNS

Children's food intake patterns are influenced by their food preferences and sensitivity to hunger and satiety cues. The foods that parents make available to children, the extent to which parents restrict their children's access to food, and their own eating behaviors all contribute to the context in which children learn about food and eating. Many years ago, Davis demonstrated that when young children were offered a variety of healthful foods in the absence of adult attempts to control or coerce their eating, the children selected diets that supported adequate growth and health (40,41). She pointed out that the secret to the children's success was in the array of healthy, unseasoned, unprocessed foods offered to them. This context is radically different from that provided today for a child in the United States or other Westernized cultures, and the effects of the contemporary food environment on children's dietary intake and weight status must be systematically examined. Current data reveal that today's children—living in an obesity-promoting food environment that provides readily available, cheap, energy-dense, palatable foods in large portions (42)—are consuming diets that are too high in sugar and fat and that contain too few servings of fruits, vegetables, grains, and dairy products (43). Given this larger cultural and economic context, what are parents to do to foster healthy eating patterns in their children?

One straightforward approach to teaching children moderation in their intake of snack foods high in sugar, fat, and energy density involves restricting children's access to palatable snacks or "junk" food. However, research suggests that potentially problematic eating styles in children may be fostered by parents' well-intended attempts to help children control their food intake. Using both experimental and naturalistic research designs, we have found that restricting preschool children's access to certain foods promoted children's attention to, and intake of, the restricted foods when they became available, even if they were not hungry (44,45). There is also limited evidence that these practices shape individual differences in styles of intake control, including dietary restraint and eating in the absence of hunger, and aspects of dietary disinhibition. Five-year-old girls' perceptions of parental use of pressure and restriction in child feeding predicted the development of dietary restraint and disinhibition among girls (46). Pressure to eat can be interpreted as "coaching" children to eat in response to the presence of food, even in the absence of hunger. This may, in turn, lead girls toward disinhibited eating styles, and finally toward attempting to control their intake cognitively rather than relying on hunger and satiety cues. As in other domains of children's development, parental imposition of high levels of external control may promote problems in self-regulation (47). These parenting practices can promote problems of self-regulation in the feeding domain, fostering children's intake of "forbidden" foods, avoidance of "healthy" foods, and development of styles of intake control that can place children at risk of chronic dieting, dietary restraint and disinhibition, binge eating, problems of energy balance, and overweight.

PARENTS AS MODELS FOR CHILDREN'S EATING

There is some evidence that parents are also models for children's eating. One change in children's diets during the last 30 years is a dramatic increase in soft drink consumption, and increased soft drink consumption is linked to greater increases in weight status (48). Harnack *et al.* (49) reported that children who were high consumers of soft drinks also consumed significantly more total energy, more sugars, and less milk. We have asked whether parental patterns of soda intake may influence children's soda intake. Mothers' and daughters' milk and soft drink intake are negatively correlated, and mothers' patterns of beverage intake influence their daughters' intakes; mothers' milk and soft drink consumption predicted daughters' intake of these beverages (50). Mother–daughter similarities in intake have also been reported for fruits and vegetables (51) and for diet composition. When Lee *et al.* (52) compared the diets of girls meeting the American Academy of Pediatrics guidelines for dietary fat (more than 20% but less than 30% of energy from fat) with diets of children consuming diets containing more than 30% of energy from fat, results showed that girls' diets reflected their mothers' diets. Mothers of girls consuming diets with more than 30% of energy from fat also had diets higher in fat, lower in fiber, and lower in vitamin A and C, riboflavin, folate, and calcium than mothers of girls consuming diets with less than 30% of energy from fat. These findings collectively highlight the importance of parents' food selection and intake patterns in shaping children's dietary intake and suggest that parents need to lead by example when encouraging children to select healthy diets. As depicted in Fig. 1, parents' eating habits and their use of child feeding practices such as restriction and pressure are intricately linked to each other and to the parents' weight status, thereby illustrating that each of these factors is likely to be an intermediary linking parent and child weight status. Using structural equation modeling, we tested the influence of maternal characteristics and practices on daughters' eating and weight (53) and found that the mother's own dietary restraint (or the cognitive and behavioral restriction of food intake) predicted her use of restrictive feeding practices with her daughter, and restrictive feeding predicted daughters' weight status independently of maternal weight. Similarly, we found that mothers' disinhibited eating, or overeating in the presence of palatable foods, mediated resemblances in weight status in mothers and their preschool-aged daughters (54). When girls were given unrestricted access to palatable snack foods, including chocolate chip cookies and potato chips, following a meal eaten to satiety, girls' intake of these foods was associated with their mothers' reports of disinhibited eating and with their mothers' weight status—mothers who were more overweight were more likely to report disinhibited eating, which in turn was associated with greater free access intake among girls, independent of girls' weight status. Daughters' free access intake of palatable snack foods and mothers' disinhibition accounted for 49% of the variance in daughters' weight status. Family resemblances between mothers' and daughters' eating and weight status reflect genetic factors, modeling effects, food availability, and child feeding strategies. Research is needed to delineate the relative contributions of genetics, modeling, and feeding practices to the emergence of family resemblances in eating behaviors that may mediate family resemblances in adiposity.

CHILD FEEDING IN AN OBESITY-PROMOTING ENVIRONMENT

Child-feeding practices, including restriction and pressure, that promote children's overeating in response to the availability of palatable foods may be especially problematic in today's "obesigenic" food environment (42). For example, American portion sizes have become very large (42), especially relative to children's energy needs, and food is inexpensive, energy-dense, and readily available. Fast food stores, convenience marts, and vending machines have expanded the availability of energy-dense, inexpensive, palatable foods. Lifestyle changes include the expansion of eating beyond mealtimes to a wide variety of work and leisure settings, and there is evidence that snacking is increasingly frequent. Popkin and colleagues (55) have reported that during the period when the prevalence of childhood overweight has doubled for children and adolescents (56), the frequency of snacking by children and adolescents also increased significantly. In addition, snacks tended to be more energy-dense and to be higher in fat than meals during that period, contributing to the increased energy and fat intakes.

Portion sizes have increased in recent years, and are often very large, especially relative to children's energy needs. Large portions are the norm, particularly for meals purchased away from home, and inexpensive "super-sized" or "value-sized" foods are common. When adults are served larger portions, they eat more (57,58). What impact do these large portions have on children's intake? Recently, we investigated the effects of portion size on young children's intake: The younger group's mean age was 3.5 years, whereas the older group's was 5. Children consumed a series of lunches differing in the portion size of the entrée (macaroni and cheese). Although the 3-year-olds' intakes were not related to the portion sizes they were served, the 5-year-olds increased their intake significantly as portion size increased—a pattern similar to that noted for adults. This pattern of findings reflects the child's increasing awareness and emphasis on external cues as controls of food intake from 3 to 5 years. Additional research is needed to determine how children learn about appropriate portion sizes, and whether child-feeding practices can shape individual differences in children's responsiveness to portion size.

CHILDREN'S EATING: LINKS TO OVERWEIGHT?

In this chapter, I have focused on familial factors, outlined in Fig. 1, that shape children's eating patterns, and on how these factors are linked to parents' weight status. A discussion of behavioral mediators of familial similarity in weight status is not complete, however, without considering links between the children's eating patterns—including food preferences, energy regulation, and food intake—and their body weight. Heavier children report a greater preference for fat (59), and such children also tend to regulate their energy intakes less precisely (39). Links between children's dietary intake and childhood overweight have been investigated, with a focus on whether diet composition, differences in the percentage of energy from fat, or patterns of food group intake can predict differences in body weight. Although most research has revealed higher energy intakes among obese than among normal-weight children, these findings do not shed light on the etiology of overweight, bearing in mind that higher energy intakes are needed to maintain energy balance in overweight children, given their greater lean body mass and fat mass (60). Relations between children's weight status and macronutrient composition of the diet have also been reported, with overweight children consuming diets that provide a greater proportion of energy from fat (59,61,62). Among adults, there is extensive evidence that the percentage of energy from fat is linked to overweight (63,64). (Ref. 64 is a rebuttal of this point.) As a result of the cross-sectional nature of these studies, it is difficult to determine whether children are overweight because they have a preference for fat, have difficulties regulating intake, and consume diets high in fat, or whether the reverse is true. It is likely that both are true; that is, children's eating styles contribute to their becoming overweight and their overweight status is maintained or exacerbated as a result of their eating styles.

Longitudinal data are the key to determining how dietary intake patterns may contribute to the development of childhood overweight. Several recent longitudinal studies (52,65–68) show that higher levels of dietary fat intake are associated with greater increases in weight among children. Eck *et al.* (65) followed children who differed in risk for overweight based on their parents' weight status and noted that the high risk group gained more weight over a 1 year period and consumed a greater proportion of their energy from fat. Klesges *et al.* (66) examined weight change among 146 children over a 3-year period, and noted that the percentage of energy from fat predicted weight change over that period. Lee *et al.* (52) categorized children on the basis of whether they met or exceeded the American Academy of Pediatrics guidelines for dietary fat intake (more than 20% but less than 30% of energy from fat, or more than

30% of energy from fat), and found that children consuming diets with more than 30% of energy from fat showed significantly greater gains in both body mass index and in skinfold thickness from ages 5 to 7 years. As reported previously, mothers of girls consuming higher-fat diets also consumed diets that were higher in fat (52). Taken together, these findings implicate the percentage of energy from fat in the development of childhood overweight and provide additional evidence for environmental mediation of familial patterns of overweight through parent–child similarities in dietary fat intake.

CONCLUSIONS

Although research has assessed genetic links between parent and child weight status, relatively little research has assessed the extent to which parents (particularly parents who are overweight) select and provide environments that promote overweight among their children. Parents provide food environments for their children's early experiences with food and eating. These family eating environments include the foods parents make available to children, parents' own eating behaviors, and child-feeding practices. There is evidence that all these facets of the family eating environment shape the development of eating behaviors in children: Behavioral mediators of familial patterns of overweight include parents' own eating behaviors and their parenting practices, which influence the development of children's eating behaviors and mediate familial patterns of overweight. In particular, parents who are overweight, have problems controlling their own food intake, or are concerned about their child's risk for overweight may adopt controlling child-feeding practices in attempts to prevent overweight in their children. Unfortunately, evidence suggests that these parental control attempts may interact with genetic predispositions to promote the development of problematic eating styles and childhood overweight. Although we have argued that behavioral mediators of family resemblances in weight status— such as disinhibited or binge eating and parenting practices—are shaped largely by environmental factors, individual differences in these behaviors also have genetic bases (69–72).

A primary public health goal involves the development of family-based prevention programs for childhood overweight. Taken together, the findings I have reviewed here suggest that effective prevention programs must focus first on providing anticipatory guidance to help parents foster patterns of preference and food selection in their children that are more consistent with healthy diets; and second, on promoting their children's ability to self-regulate their intakes. Guidance for parents should include information on how children develop patterns of food intake in the family context, and practical advice on how to foster children's preferences for healthy foods and promote their acceptance of new foods. Parents need to understand the costs of coercive feeding practices and be given alternates to the use of restriction and pressuring children to eat. Providing parents with easy-to-use information regarding appropriate portion sizes for children is also essential, as are suggestions on the appropriate timing and frequency of meals and snacks. Especially during early and middle childhood, the family environment is the key to the development of food preferences, patterns of food intake, and eating styles, as well as activity preferences and patterns that shape children's developing weight status.

To design effective prevention programs, more complete knowledge is needed on behavioral intermediaries that foster overweight, including the family factors that shape activity patterns, meals taken away from home, the impact of stress on family members' eating styles, food intake, activity patterns, and weight gain. The research I have presented in this chapter illustrates how ideas regarding the effects of environmental factors and behavioral mediators on childhood overweight can be investigated. Such research requires the development of reliable and valid measures of environmental variables and behaviors. Because childhood overweight is a multifactorial problem, additional research is needed to develop and test theoretical models describing how a wide range of environmental factors and behavioral intermediaries can work in concert with genetic predisposition to promote the development of childhood overweight. The critical test of these theoretical models will be the success of preventive interventions based on such models.

REFERENCES

1. Garn SM, Sullivan TV, Hawthorne VM. Fatness and obesity of the parents of obese individuals. *Am J Clin Nutr* 1989; 50: 1308–13.
2. Grilo CM, Pogue-Geile MF. The nature of environmental influences on weight and obesity: a behavior genetic analysis. *Psychol Bull* 1991; 110: 520–37.
3. Whitaker RC, Wright JA, Pepe MS, Seidel KD, Dietz WH. Predicting obesity in young adulthood from childhood and parental obesity. *N Engl J Med* 1997; 337: 869–73.
4. Morrison JA, Payne G, Barton BA, Khoury PR, Crawford P. Mother–daughter correlations of obesity and cardiovascular disease risk factors in black and white households: the NHLBI growth and health. *Am J Public Health* 1994; 84: 1761–7.
5. Maes HH, Neale MC, Eaves LJ. Genetic and environmental factors in relative body weight and human adiposity. *Behav Genet* 1997; 27: 325–51.
6. Jacobson KC, Rowe DC. Genetic and shared environmental influences on adolescent BMI: interactions with race and sex. *Behav Genet* 1998; 28: 265–78.
7. Faith MS, Pietrobelli A, Nunez C, Heo M, Heymsfield SB, Allison DB. Evidence for independent genetic influences on fat mass and body mass index in a pediatric twin sample. *Pediatrics* 1999;104: 61–7.
8. Troiano RP, Flegal KM, Kuczmarski RJ, Campbell SM, Johnson CL. Overweight prevalence and trends for children and adolescents: the National Health and Nutrition Examination Surveys, 1963 to 1991. *Arch Pediatr Adolesc Med* 1995; 149: 1085–91.
9. Ogden CL, Troiano RP, Briefel RR, *et al.* Prevalence of overweight among preschool children in the United States, 1971 through 1994. *Pediatrics* 1997; 99: 1.
10. Faith MS, Johnson SL, Allison DB. Putting the *behavior* into the behavior genetics of obesity. *Behav Genet* 1997; 27: 423–39.
11. Harris J. Where is the child's environment? A group socialization theory of development. *Psychol Rev* 1995; 102: 458–89.
12. Plomin R, Daniels D. Why are children in the same family so different from one another? *Behav Brain Sci* 1987; 10: 1–60.
13. Holden GW, Miller PC. Enduring and different: a meta-analysis of the similarity in parents' child rearing. *Psychol Bull* 1999; 125: 223–54.
14. Magnusson D, Stattin H. Person–context interaction theories. In: Lerner R, ed. *The handbook of child psychology,* vol 1. *Theoretical models of human development,* 5th ed. New York: John Wiley & Sons, 1997: 685–740.
15. Turkheimer E, Waldron M. Nonshared environment: a theoretical, methodological, and quantitative review. *Psychol Bull* 2000; 126: 78–108.

16. Costanzo PR, Woody EZ. Domain specific parenting styles and their impact on the child's development of particular deviance: the example of obesity proneness. *J Soc Clin Psychol* 1985; 3: 425–45.
17. Birch LL. Development of food preferences. *Annu Rev Nutr* 1999; 19: 41–62.
18. Birch LL. The relationship between children's food preferences and those of their parents. *J Nutr Educ* 1980; 12: 14–8.
19. Rozin P, Fallon A, Mandell R. Family resemblance in attitudes to foods. *Dev Psychol* 1984; 20: 309–14.
20. Perusse L, Bouchard C. Genetics of energy intake and food preferences. In: Bouchard C, ed. *The genetics of obesity*. Boca Raton, Florida: CRC Press, 1994: 125–34.
21. Birch LL. Dimensions of preschool children's food preferences. *J Nutr Educ* 1979; 11: 91–5.
22. Birch LL, Marlin DW. I don't like it; I never tried it: effects of exposure on two-year-old children's food preferences. *Appetite* 1982; 3: 353–60.
23. Kalat JW, Rozin P. "Learned safety" as a mechanism in long-delay taste aversion learning in rats. *J Comp Physiol Psychol* 1973; 83: 198–207.
24. Booth D. Food-conditioned eating preferences and aversions with interoceptive elements: conditioned appetites and satieties. *Ann NY Acad Sci* 1985; 443: 22–41.
25. Sclafani A. Nutritionally based learned flavor preferences in rats. In: Capaldi E, Powley T, eds. *Taste, experience, and feeding*. Washington, DC: American Psychological Association, 1990: 139–56.
26. Kern DL, McPhee L, Fisher J, et al. The postingestive consequences of fat condition preferences for flavors associated with high dietary fat. *Physiol Behav* 1993; 54: 71–6.
27. Johnson SL, McPhee L, Birch LL. Conditioned preferences: young children prefer flavors associated with high dietary fat. *Physiol Behav* 1991; 50: 1245–51.
28. Birch LL. Children's preferences for high-fat foods. *Nutr Rev* 1992; 50: 249–55.
29. Birch LL, Zimmerman S, Hind H. The influence of social affective context on preschool children's food preferences. *Child Dev* 1980; 51: 856–61.
30. Birch LL, Birch D, Marlin D, Kramer L. Effects of instrumental eating on children's food preferences. *Appetite* 1982; 3: 125–34.
31. Birch LL, Marlin D, Rotter J. Eating as the "means" activity in a contingency: effects on young children's food preference. *Child Dev* 1984; 55: 532–9.
32. Casey R, Rozin P. Changing children's food preferences: parent opinions. *Appetite* 1989; 12: 171–82.
33. Fomon S. *Nutrition of normal infants*. St Louis: Mosby Year-Book, 1993.
34. Birch LL, Deysher M. Caloric compensation and sensory specific satiety: evidence for self regulation of food intake by young children. *Appetite* 1986; 7: 323–31.
35. Birch LL, McPhee L, Sullivan S. Children's food intake following drinks sweetened with sucrose or aspartame: time course effects. *Physiol Behav* 1989; 45: 387–95.
36. Birch LL, Johnson SL, Andresen G, et al. The variability of young children's energy intake. *N Engl J Med* 1991; 324: 232–5.
37. Birch LL, Johnson SL, Jones MB, Peters JC. Effects of a non-energy fat substitute on children's energy and macronutrient intake. *Am J Clin Nutr* 1993; 58: 326–33.
38. Birch L, McPhee L, Shoba B, Steinberg L, Krehbiel R. "Clean up your plate": effects of child feeding practices on the development of intake regulation. *Learning Motiv* 1987; 18: 301–17.
39. Johnson SL, Birch LL. Parent's and children's adiposity and eating style. *Pediatrics* 1994; 94: 653–61.
40. Davis C. Self selection of diet by newly weaned infants. *Am J Dis Child* 1928; 36: 651–79.
41. Davis C. Results of the self selection of diets by young children. *Can Med Assoc J* 1939; 41: 257–61.
42. Hill JO, Peters JC. Environmental contributions to the obesity epidemic. *Science* 1998; 280: 1371–4.
43. Munoz KA, Krebs-Smith SM, Ballard-Barbash R, Cleveland LE. Food intakes of US children and adolescents compared with recommendation. *Pediatrics* 1997; 100: 323–9.
44. Fisher JO, Birch LL. Restricting access to a palatable food affects children's behavioral response, food selection and intake. *Am J Clin Nutr* 1999; 69: 1264–72.
45. Fisher JO, Birch LL. Restricting access to foods and children's eating. *Appetite* 1999; 32: 405–19.
46. Carper J, Fisher J, Birch L. Young girls' emerging dietary restraint and disinhibition are related to parental control in child feeding. *Appetite* 2000; 35: 121–9.
47. Baumrind D. Current patterns of parental authority. *Dev Psychol* 1971; 4: 1–103.
48. Ludwig D, Peterson K, Gortmaker S. Relation between consumption of sugar-sweetened drinks and childhood obesity: a prospective, observational analysis. *Lancet* 2001; 357: 505–8.
49. Harnack L, Stang J, Story M. Soft drink consumption among US children and adolescents: nutritional consequences. *J Am Diet Assoc* 1999; 99: 436–41.

50. Fisher JO, Mitchell DC, Smiciklas-Wright H, Birch LL. Maternal milk consumption predicts the trade-off between milk and soft drinks in young girls' diets. *J Nutr* 2001; 131: 246–50.
51. Fisher JO, Birch LL. Parents' restrictive feeding practices are associated with young girls' negative self-evaluation about eating. *J Am Diet Assoc* 2000; 100: 1341–6.
52. Lee Y, Mitchell D, Smiciklas-Wright H, Birch L. Diet quality, nutrient intake, weight status, and feeding environments of girls meeting or exceeding the AAP recommendations for total dietary fat. *Pediatrics* 2001; 107: 95.
53. Birch LL, Fisher JO. Mothers' child-feeding practices influence daughters' eating and weight. *Am J Clin Nutr* 2000; 71: 1054–61.
54. Cutting TM, Fisher JO, Grimm-Thomas K, Birch LL. Like mother, like daughter: familial patterns of overweight are mediated by mothers' dietary disinhibition. *Am J Clin Nutr* 1999; 69: 608–13.
55. Jahns L, Siega-Riz A, Popkin B. The increasing prevalence of snacking among US children from 1977–1996. *J Pediatr* 2001; 138: 493–8.
56. Troiano RP, Flegal KM. Overweight children and adolescents: description, epidemiology, and demographics. *Pediatrics* 1998; 101: 497–504.
57. Engell D, Kramer M, Zaring D, Birch L, Rolls B. Effects of serving size on food intake in children and adults. *Obesity Res* 1995; 3: 381.
58. Booth D, Fuller J, Lewis V. Human control of body weight: cognitive or physiological? Some energy-related perceptions and misperceptions. In: Coiffi L, James W, Van Itallie T, eds. *The body weight regulatory system: normal and disturbed mechanisms.* New York: Raven Press, 1981.
59. Fisher JA, Birch LL. Fat preferences and fat consumption of 3- to 5 year-old children are related to parental adiposity. *J Am Diet Assoc* 1995; 95: 759–64.
60. Goran M. Measurement issues related to studies of childhood obesity: assessment of body composition, body fat distribution, physical activity, and food intake. *Pediatrics* 1998; 101: 505–18.
61. Gazzaniga JM, Burns TL. Relationship between diet composition and body fatness, with adjustment for resting expenditure and physical activity, in preadolescent children. *Am J Clin Nutr* 1993; 58: 21–8.
62. Nguyen VT, Larson DE, Johnson RK, Goran MI. Fat intake and adiposity in children of lean and obese parents. *Am J Clin Nutr* 1996; 63: 507–13.
63. Bray G, Popkin B. Dietary fat intake does affect obesity. *Am J Clin Nutr* 1998; 68: 1157–73.
64. Willett WC. Dietary fat and obesity: an unconvincing relation. *Am J Clin Nutr* 1998; 68: 1149–50.
65. Eck LH, Klesges RC, Hanson CL, Slawson D. Children at familial risk for obesity: an examination of dietary intake, physical activity and weight status. *Int J Obes* 1992; 16: 71–8.
66. Klesges RC, Klesges LM, Eck LH, Shelton ML. A longitudinal analysis of accelerated weight gain in preschool children. *Pediatrics* 1995; 95: 126–32.
67. Robertson S, Cullen K, Baranowski J, *et al.* Factors related to adiposity among children aged 3 to 7 years. *J Am Diet Assoc* 1999; 99: 938–43.
68. Davison KK, Birch LL. Child and parent characteristics as predictors of change in girls' body mass index. *Int J Obes* 2001; 25: 1834–42.
69. Deater-Deckard K, Fulker D, Plomin R. A genetic study of the family environment in the transition to early adolescence. *J Child Psychol Psychiatry* 1999; 40: 769–75.
70. Plomin R. Genetics and children's experiences in the family. *J Child Psychol Psychiatry* 1995; 36: 33–68.
71. Sullivan P, Bulik C, Kendler K. Genetic epidemiology of binging and vomiting. *Br J Psychiatry* 1998; 173: 75–9.
72. Bulik C, Sullivan P, Kendler K. Heritability of binge-eating and broadly defined bulimia nervosa. *Biol Psychiatry* 1998; 44: 1210–8.

DISCUSSION

Dr. Uauy: I'm surprised you did not put more emphasis on advertising to children. How can we counteract the effects of advertising?

Dr. Birch: It's obviously extremely important, though it's difficult to measure. Our focus has been more on whether we can help parents with parenting skills than on taking on the advertising industry or the food industry. But clearly it's enormously important and we are not going to make progress without that as well. I appreciate your comment.

Dr. Endres: In relation to TV advertising and the blackmailing of mothers by their children at the supermarket, an investigation in Germany (Diehl JM, Giessen, Germany, personal communication, 1998) has shown that 5- to 8-year-old children already put pressure on their mother to buy certain things they have seen advertised in the media. What is your experience in the United States?

Dr. Birch: Various published studies have confirmed that this is happening in the United States (1). This is a huge issue, and one we have to find a way to address. Just teaching mothers to deal with it in the supermarket is probably not enough.

Dr. Bellizzi: One of your later slides referred to the importance of experiences with food and eating. From my personal experience, food, eating, and cooking are all important in helping a child to understand about food in a way that is fun. What is the influence of nurseries on children's eating habits? Nowadays, young children spend a great deal of time at nurseries and may take most of their meals there. How does that affect the exposure they are getting at home?

Dr. Birch: We know very little about that. In the United States a large proportion of young children are in day care centers for 30 or more hours a week and that's got to be very important in this context, especially as their caregivers often come from very different socioeconomic and ethnic groups. We find the parents' influence remains strong even in cases where their children are in childcare for 30 to 40 hours a week, but it is inevitable that the caregivers will also exert powerful effects. Parents whose children are in childcare all day long may only see them eating at breakfast and in the evening, and this can be a source of anxiety, especially when their children may not be particularly interested in eating because they have been eating during the day.

Dr. Bellizzi: I also have a question about your chips experiment, where you showed that children who were 3.5 years old regulated their intake regardless of the portion size, whereas older children ate according to the portion size. Is that because we lose the ability to distinguish how much food we eat, or is it because of an environmental impact?

Dr. Birch: What happens with most people is that there is an overlay of all kinds of cultural factors, and the eating becomes increasingly culturally determined as you get older, so that things like the time of day, the presence of foods, whether or not other people are eating, and expectations of various kinds come into play. What we are seeing with these very young children is the transition period from a food depletion drive to a drive that is increasingly controlled by a variety of external factors. This is really a most important time for preventing the development of overweight.

Dr. Endres: I have a question about salt foods for young children. There is an ongoing discussion of how much sodium young children may eat. In processed foods, at least in Europe, the upper limit is normally 200 mg/100 g. It is known that in homemade foods the sodium content is often much higher, say 500 to 700 mg/100 g. What is your experience in this respect?

Dr. Birch: I think immediately of Beauchamp's work, where he showed that very young toddlers and preschool children have preferences for high levels of salt in, for example, soup—much higher than they probably ever experienced in daily eating (2). This parallels work showing that people on low-salt diets increase their salt intakes quite dramatically as soon as they have the opportunity to consume higher-sodium diets. I don't think that is a good thing—I'm just saying that this is what tends to happen given our predispositions.

Dr. Endres: I think that if the upper level is set too low there is a high risk that mothers will add extra salt. I believe that the level should be somewhat higher than at present, say, 300 mg/100 g.

Dr. Anantharaman: I have a question concerning variety. Is there anything to suggest that a breast-fed child is more willing to accept variety in the weaning diet because of exposure to different flavors in breast milk?

Dr. Birch: There is not much in the literature yet, although there will soon be more. For example, Mennella has done a whole series of elegant studies looking at the effects of including different substances in the maternal diet—garlic, vanilla, alcohol, and so on—and studying their presence in breast milk and the acceptance of those foods by infants and toddlers (3). We ourselves did some work years ago which was published in *Pediatrics* (4), looking at breast-fed versus formula-fed infants and their acceptance of initial solids. We found that breast-fed infants were more ready to accept solids, and this is consistent with the animal work showing that the flavors from the maternal milk lead to preferences for the maternal diet, and that early variety tends to lead to the later, more ready acceptance of new diets (5).

Dr. Anantharaman: So in that context, would you expect that in the preparation of weaning foods, something that might facilitate weaning could be the addition of flavors that a breast-fed child might have been exposed to, a weaning food with a garlicky flavor or whatever?

Dr. Birch: This is a really interesting area, and it's amazing to me that there hasn't been more work done on it. There has been some discussion in the industry about adding flavors to formula or to puréed transition foods, but to my knowledge that hasn't got very far yet. We know a lot more about rat pups than we do about humans, and in the rat the transition to solids is clearly facilitated by the cues the mothers' diets give to the pups (6).

Dr. Jiang: I was very interested in your presentation. Can you suggest a good way to prevent a child from overeating?

Dr. Birch: If I could answer that I'd be rich and famous! One thing is to assist children to prefer food that are not so energy-dense. This requires giving them lots of opportunities to eat complex carbohydrates, fruits, vegetables, and so on. Another thing that is very important is parental education about appropriate portion sizes. This may be different in China, but in the United States, parents often have very inflated ideas of how much young children need to eat to sustain growth. For example, they may expect 2-year-olds to eat portions that are two or three times as big as the child needs. We need to help children to have opportunities to self-regulate and self-select rather than thinking we can impose all the controls from without, because that doesn't work!

Dr. Bar-Or: It seems to me that your data relate mostly to children from the general population who are not necessarily obese. Are there any data on learning patterns in toddlers or preschool children who do become obese, and if so do they differ from children who are not yet obese?

Dr. Birch: There is some indirect evidence that relates to your point. For example, Agras and his colleagues (7) have shown that differences occurring very early on in terms of suckling performance are related to the development of obesity—that is, the infants who are the most lively feeders at the breast or the bottle tend to be the ones who become obese later on. We found in our own work that there is a relation between children's responsiveness to energy density, both in the short term and over 24-hour periods, and their weight status. As to whether or not there are differences in the learning process that might be related to weight status, I don't know whether anybody has done that work. It needs to be done.

Dr. Chen: In China, we are increasingly providing education in nutrition—dietary guidelines, what foods are nutritious, and so on. But we don't teach the children much about food and eating, or about how to make good choices about food, and about which are energy-dense foods. These things are not well taught to children in China.

Dr. Birch: For years, we have been telling our children "eat this; it is good for you," or "don't eat that; it's not good for you," but we know that this is just not effective. For both adults and children, preferences tend to drive intake within the constraints of what is available. So we need to learn to help children to *like* what it is that we think they should eat.

REFERENCES

1. Robinson TN, Saphir MN, Kraemer HC, *et al.* Effects of reducing television viewing on children's re-quests for toys: a randomised controlled trial. *J Dev Behav Pediatr* 2001; 22: 179–84.
2. Cowart BJ, Beauchamp GK. The importance of sensory context in young children's acceptance of salty tastes. *Child Dev* 1986; 57: 1034–9.
3. Mennella JA, Jagnow CP, Beauchamp GK. Prenatal and postnatal flavor learning by human infants. *Pediatrics* 2001; 107: 88.
4. Sullivan SA, Birch LL. Infant dietary experience and acceptance of solid foods. *Pediatrics* 1994; 93: 271–7.
5. Capretta PJ, Rawls LH. Establishment of a flavor preference in rats: Importance of nursing and wean-ing experience. *J Comp Physiol* 1974; 86: 670–3.
6. Galef BG, Jr. A historical perspective on recent studies of social learning about foods by Norway rats. *Can J Psychol* 1990; 44: 311–29.
7. Agras WS, Kraemer HC, Berkowitz RI, *et al.* Influence of early feeding style on adiposity at 6 years of age. *J Pediatr* 1990; 116: 805–9.

Obesity in Childhood and Adolescence, edited by
Chunming Chen and William H. Dietz. Nestlé
Nutrition Workshop Series, Pediatric Program,
Vol. 49. Nestec Ltd., Vevey/Lippincott
Williams & Wilkins, Philadelphia © 2002.

The Role of the Physical Activity Environment in Obesity Among Children and Adolescents in the Industrialized World

Steven L. Gortmaker

*Department of Health and Social Behavior, Harvard School of Public Health,
Boston, Massachusetts, USA*

The prevalence of obesity among children and adolescents has been increasing rapidly in the in the United States and other industrialized countries (1). While the etiology of obesity is complex and is related to both genetic and environmental determinants, obesity ultimately results from an imbalance of energy intake over energy expenditure (2). Because both energy intake and energy expended through physical activity have substantial discretionary components, they can be influenced by the social and physical environment, and hence are the foci of intervention and policy.

This chapter is focused on describing patterns of physical activity among children and adolescents in industrialized societies, reviewing evidence for how these patterns influence energy imbalance and obesity prevalence, and documenting how these physical activity patterns are in turn influenced by social, economic, and physical environments.

In discussing these issues, I will first examine the entire distribution of physical activity levels among children and adolescents, ranging from very inactive to very physically active. Using computerized electronic monitoring data among adolescents aged 13 to 15 in the United States, I will document the very low levels of activity found in this free ranging youth population, and note the potentially significant contribution to physical activity of habitual patterns such as school attendance.

I will next examine in detail evidence for the potential impact of both low levels of activity—including sitting in school and television viewing—and moderate and vigorous physical activity levels on obesity. These analyses point to the strong evidence for the unique influence of broadcast television in the industrialized world on childhood obesity, the effect reflecting a mixture of time spent in an inactive state and the influence on dietary intake. I review research concerning impact of the social,

---

Assumptions: We use the same equations predicting resting metabolic rate for boys and girls as noted earlier. This leads to an estimate of kcal expended per minute, which is then multiplied by the MET to obtain the total kcal per minute expended under different physical activity regimens.

economic, and physical environment on physical activity levels of children and adolescents, and find little solid evidence but much speculation. I discuss the implications of this science base and gaps in knowledge for programs and policies aimed at reducing obesity in the industrialized societies.

METHODS

Subjects

Data for results reported in this study were collected as part of the Planet Health intervention and evaluation program that took place in schools located in four communities in the Boston (Massachusetts) metropolitan area between autumn 1995 and spring 1997. For the present analyses, subjects were from the five randomly assigned control schools that did not take part in the intervention program designed to reduce obesity prevalence (3). The median household income of zip code areas where the five schools were located averaged $34,200. This median is lower than that for all households in Massachusetts in the 1990 census ($41,000), but similar to the US figure ($33,952) (3). Sixty-five percent of those eligible completed the baseline evaluation in autumn 1995, after exclusion of individuals who transferred schools at baseline, were in special education classes, were in grades other than sixth or seventh, or did not complete the English language version of the questionnaire. Follow-up data were collected in spring 1997 (19 months later) for 84% of the baseline sample.

From all subjects with baseline and follow-up data, we subsequently selected a random sample (stratified by school, sex, and grade) of students in these five schools in the winter of 1997. These 139 students wore Tritrac monitors on their hip using an elasticized belt; with activity data stored electronically every minute in three (triaxial) dimensions. Staff recorded time of initiation and instructed the participants to return the monitors in either 3 days (if they received the monitor on a Tuesday), or 4 days (if they received the monitor on a Friday). Students were paid $5 for their assistance upon return of the monitor. All students who agreed to wear the monitors in one participating school also wore the monitors a second time a few weeks later, and also completed repeat 24-hour activity recalls. These participants were paid $10 for their assistance. The activity monitor data were collected during the period February through April 1997. Upon return of the monitor, staff noted the time and date of return, and interviewed the participant concerning times they may have removed the monitor during the days they had it. The study was approved by the Committee on Human Subjects at the Harvard School of Public Health.

Design and Measures

Television and Video

Time spent in television and video viewing was measured with the 11-item television and video measure (TVM) (3). Questions were asked about hours of television typically viewed during each day of the week, as well as use of video recorders and video and computer games. Items were appropriately weighted and summed to obtain a total viewing hour-per-day estimate. In a validation sample ($N = 53$), we found a deattenuated correlation of television viewing assessed by the TVM versus repeat 24-hour recalls of $r = 0.54$, with equivalent means.

Demographic, Social, and Behavioral Variables

Age was calculated based on birth date and date of anthropometric examinations; in a few cases of missing birth date, self-reported age from the Food and Activity (FAS) survey was used. Sex was classified at the time of examination by measurers, except for a few missing cases where sex data from school list data were used. Ethnic categories were based on responses of students who were asked to mark all the responses that applied to the question, "How do you describe yourself?" The response categories were as follows: "white," "black," "Hispanic," "Asian or Pacific Islander," "American Indian or Alaskan Native," "other." Participants indicating "black" were classified "African-American."

Tritrac Accelerometer Data

Tritrac data included activity vector magnitude readings for each minute over the time period sampled. Recent studies in children and adolescents (4–6) indicate excellent validity of triaxial accelerometers, with reported prediction of objective measures of oxygen consumption ranging from $R^2 = 0.93$ to $R^2 = 0.90$. Previous study with another computerized accelerometer indicates that a reasonable approximation of individual activity levels requires 3 days of data collection, owing to the significant intraindividual variability from day to day (7). Studies of data from each of the three planes indicate that the vector magnitude measure (the geometric mean of the measures of activity in each of the three planes) is the best overall indicator of energy expenditure (4).

An individual with 3 days of Tritrac data would provide 4,320 data points. For assessment of activity levels, we used data on weekdays collected between 07:00 and 21:59, and on weekends from 09:00 to 21:59. We derived these intervals by examining the extent to which participants had removed their monitors (we used an indicator whereby if there was virtually no movement recorded on the Tritrac for 30 consecutive minutes—indicated by a vector magnitude of less than 10—we considered the monitor removed). These analyses indicated that the time periods chosen corresponded to the times at which most of the participants had started using the monitor for the day. At both the chosen time points, the uptake of use and decrease in use changed rapidly over the previous and succeeding half-hour intervals. In estimating activity levels, we coded as missing those time intervals where there was virtually no indicated movement (a vector magnitude less than 10 for 30 consecutive minutes). We also conducted parallel analyses where we used different limits—a minimum of 3 days of data, a minimum of 9 hours a day, as well as no movement (indicated by 30 consecutive minutes of vector magnitude zero)—and the results were quite similar.

In estimating physical activity levels, we used two cutoff points: vector magnitudes of 250 and 1,000. The derivation of these cutoff points was based on the translation of accelerometer vector magnitude estimates into estimated MET (metabolic equivalent) values. For this calculation, a few equations describing assumptions are needed. One approach is to simply use the equations that come with the Tritrac monitors (8). However, these use adult equations for calculation of basal metabolic rate (BMR). Instead, we estimated BMR for participants using the WHO equations for boys and girls of this age range (9). We then calculated the equation the Tritrac software uses to estimate energy expenditure from activity (EEA), for each minute interval: EEA = 0.00037 × [weight of subject in kg] × [vector magnitude]. We calculated regressions using Tritrac estimated energy expenditure from physical activity versus the Tritrac vector magnitude readings. These regressions were calculated using thousands of data points, for a series of individuals with known weights. The R^2 for these equations was always greater than 0.99, indicating an excellent fit. We defined a MET value for each minute interval as [EEA + BMR]/BMR. The estimated MET values using these equations for EEA and BMR are highly correlated with the values calculated by the Tritrac software. There is little difference between the two approaches.

Given these equations, we then solved for the vector magnitude as a function of MET level and the weight of the subject (kg):

For girls 10 years of age or more: vector magnitude = [MET − 1][229 + 14,002/weight];

For boys 10 years of age or more: vector magnitude = [MET − 1][328 + 12,218/weight].

Using these equations and assuming an average weight for boys of 59 kg and for girls of 56 kg (the means of these variables in our sample), we see that a MET of 1.5 corresponds to a vector magnitude of about 250 for girls and 269 for boys, and a MET of 3 corresponds to a vector magnitude of about 958 for girls and 1,072 for boys.

Studies of the Tritrac (and other computerized accelerometers) indicate that on average they underestimate total energy expenditure during a given time period by anywhere from 30% to 70% among free-ranging populations (10,11). This underestimation makes theoretical sense, as the accelerometers, worn typically on the hip, will provide underestimates of upper-body movement, will underestimate expenditure during certain activities (e.g., bike riding, walking up stairs), and do not typically take into account other aspects of energy expenditure, such as carrying heavy loads (like a backpack) or weight training.

We report activity in terms of estimated minutes per day. The basic analyses of the Tritrac data estimated the proportion of the time period that corresponds to various MET levels. Thus if in the sample there were 30,000 data points gathered on weekdays between 09:00 and 09:29, and 7% of these points were spent at activity ≥ 3.0 MET, we report 7% for this period, and this can be translated into 7% of a 30-minute interval, or 2.1 minutes. Note that in other analyses (not shown) we examine individual level variability, including duration of bouts of activity.

RESULTS

Physical Activity Levels Among Youngsters Throughout the Day

These Tritrac data indicate a relatively sedentary population of youngsters 11 to 14 years of age (Fig. 1). Data were collected from 139 subjects who contributed a total of 1,017,421 person-minutes of data—an average of 7,320 observations per subject. A typical weekday for this sample (07:00 to 22:00) consists of 73% of the day—or about 11 hours—spent at sedentary activities (1.0 to 1.5 MET). These results are consistent with our sense of the sedentary nature of industrialized society. There is some evidence for slightly greater levels of inactivity among girls than among boys. In Fig. 1 the charted line for female inactivity is generally higher throughout the day than the line for male inactivity (an average of 74% of the day versus 72%).

An examination of these data taken half-hour by half-hour clearly indicates two low points of inactivity on these weekdays: These occur at about 07:30 and at about 14:00. These low points of inactivity coincide with the times that youngsters are going to school in the morning and leaving school in the afternoon.

These results are mirrored in our analysis of time spent in moderate and vigorous activity (time spent at ≥ 3.0 MET) (Fig. 2). The time of day with the highest level of ≥ 3.0 MET activity in the population appears to occur after school, at around 14:00, with substantial activity also occurring early before school begins at 07:30. In general, boys showed higher rates of physical activity of ≥ 3.0 MET during much of the day, but particularly during the period 14:00 to 19:00. Overall, boys spend on average about 1.2 hours a day at activities involving ≥ 3.0 MET, and girls spend an average of 0.8 hours a day at this level. Note that this time at 3.0 MET or greater for a particular individual can consist of many short intervals or a few larger intervals.

An important fact about the inactivity time spent by youngsters is that only part of this time is spent viewing television and other video activities such as video games. Our estimates of total video use per day in the sample in 1997 was about 3.2 hours (based both on self-report survey and on 24-hour diary estimates) (3), or less than 30% of the average day's level of inactivity time.

We found a minimal empirical relation between time spent in moderate and vigorous physical activity and time spent in a specific inactivity such as television viewing (12). Although it is obvious that increased time spent in inactivity automatically constrains the time spent in more vigorous activity, because there is a relatively small amount of moderate and vigorous activity in the lives of youngsters (on average) in industrialized societies—and television viewing comprises just a fraction of inactive time—this means there are many ways to fit in small amounts of active time with patterns of television viewing. Hence average daily hours viewing television and time spent at ≥ 3.0 MET are generally minimally correlated variables.

Analytic Estimates of Changes in Physical Activity Levels on Obesity

It is helpful to distinguish the potentially different roles of moderate and vigorous physical activity versus the impact of inactivity, including television viewing, on

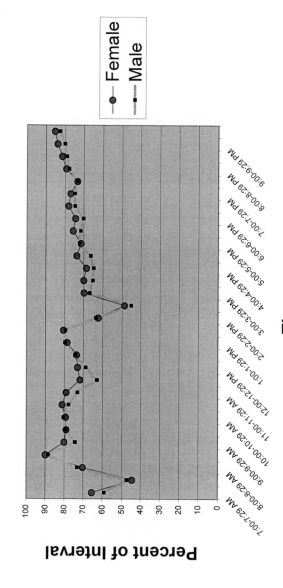

FIG. 1. Percentage of half-hour weekday time periods with Tritrac vector magnitude of <250 ($\leq$1.5 MET); $N = 139$; 1,017,421 person-minutes.

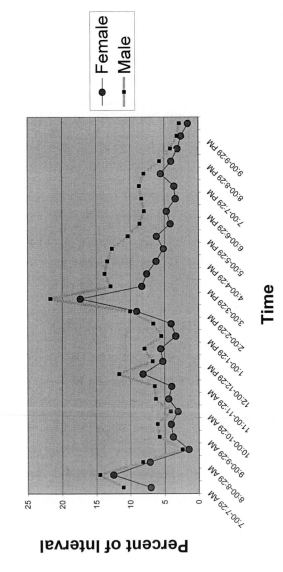

FIG. 2. Percentage of half-hour weekday time periods with Tritrac vector magnitude of >1,000 (≥3.0 MET); *N* = 139; 1,017,421 person-minutes.

obesity. One perspective would be simply to note the energy expended on these activities. Analysis of physical activity from this perspective indicates that both inactivity and moderate and vigorous activity can alter risk of excess weight gain significantly. For example, here are two scenarios where altering physical activity levels could affect the risk of obesity:

Reduce inactivity: If we assume that youngsters watch about 3 hours of television a day, imagine replacing this 3 hours with less viewing time: 2.5 hours of television (assuming 1.1 MET) and 0.5 hours of walking (assuming 3.0 MET). For a girl aged 12 (weight 46 kg), this translates into a difference in energy expenditure of an additional 52 kcal/day.[1] Based on the assumption that a 1-lb (454 g) weight gain is equivalent to 3,500 kcal, an imbalance of 52 kcal/day could account for a difference in weight of 5.4 lb (2.45 kg) in a year (13).

Increase vigorous activity: In contrast, let us assume another change, this time in vigorous activity. Let us assume that this same individual moves from virtually no activity of 5 MET or higher to 20 minutes of physical activity at 5.0 MET or higher three times a week, consistent with one of our national goals. This shift would produce (20 × 3)/7, or about 8.6 minutes a day of new activity greater than 5.0 MET. If we assume the replaced activity was at 1.1 MET, the extra expended energy for a female subject of 46 kg would total about 32 kcal/day, an imbalance that has the potential to produce a difference in weight of 3.3 pounds (1.5 kg) in a year.

A wide range of such scenarios is possible. However, simply from the perspective of energy expenditure, these scenarios illustrate that the potential long-term consequences of relatively minor changes in levels of both inactivity and vigorous physical activity can be significant. The key issue is that relatively small daily differences aggregated over the course of a year or more can produce substantial shifts in relative weight.

Empirical Evidence for the Impact of Physical Activity on Obesity

A review of epidemiologic and experimental studies indicates that the strongest relation between obesity and physical activity is found with a specific form of inactivity—television viewing. Television viewing has been cited as one cause of the increasing prevalence of obesity, based on both longitudinal (14,18) and cross-sectional observational studies (15,16,17). These observational studies have recently been corroborated by randomized controlled trials of reduced levels of television viewing designed to reduce obesity (3,19,20). The impact of television viewing on obesity most probably reflects both the displacement of more vigorous activities by television, as illustrated above, and also effects on diet. Foods are heavily advertised on children's television (21), and television viewing is associated with between-meal snacking by children (22). Similar findings of an independent effect of television viewing on obesity have been reported from adult prospective studies (23,24).

There are substantial numbers of observational studies that indicate an inverse relation between moderate and vigorous physical activity levels and obesity in children and adolescents (25–29). In contrast, there is more limited evidence that programs of increased physical activity can reduce obesity, although increased physical activity can clearly assist in maintaining energy balance. Long-term effectiveness in reducing obesity has been demonstrated in intensive clinical programs for obese children (30) that require parental participation and which focus on modifications in both diet and physical activity. There is also evidence for short-term effects following forced increases in physical activity (31). All this evidence points to the potentially important role that increased physical activity levels can play in the prevention of obesity (32,33).

A useful intervention strategy may be to encourage replacing television time with physical activities of the youngster's choice (34,35). This approach has been found effective in school-based (3,36) and clinical interventions (37).

Social, Economic, and Physical Environmental Effects on Physical Activity Levels

How the environment influences physical activity levels of children and adolescents has not been well studied as a science, but some areas of influence are apparent. As noted in the recent report to the president of the United States:

> Behavior is shaped, in large measure, by one's environment. Our young people live in a social and physical environment that makes it easy to be sedentary and inconvenient to be active. Developments in our culture and society over the past few decades that have discouraged youth physical activity include the following:
>
> • Community design centered around the automobile has discouraged walking and bicycling and made it more difficult for children to get together to play.
> • Increased concerns about safety have limited the time and area in which children are allowed to play outside.
> • New technology has conditioned our young people to be less active, while new electronic media (for example, videos and computer games, cable and satellite television) have made sedentary activities more appealing.
> • States and school districts have reduced the amount of time students are required to spend in physical education classes, and many of those classes have so many students that teachers cannot give students the individual attention they need.
> • Communities have failed to invest adequately in close-to-home physical activity facilities (e.g., parks, recreation centers). [38]

Although these assertions appear reasonable, in fact very few potential policy and environmental changes have been documented to affect either physical activity levels or obesity (39,40). Although data are very limited, the potential impact of "environmental limitations" seems obvious: If there are no neighborhood parks or traffic-free places to play, few youngsters will engage in such activities. While most published reports have focused on individual level risk factors and behaviors, some environmental factors have been identified (41–43). Studies among adolescents and young adults indicate that a range of environmental barriers, including neighborhood safety, influence physical activity (44,45). We have examined data from the National Longitudinal Survey of Youth, and the corresponding surveys of their children aged

10 to 15 years in 1992, a nationally representative sample of 1,513. Fifty-one percent of the children of parents who rate their child's schools unsafe are reported to watch 5 or more hours of television a day, compared with 31% among those rating their schools safest ($p < 0.001$). A study of a multiethnic sample of youth indicated that racial/ethnic disparities in exercise levels were mediated by disparities in access to exercise facilities and programs (46). Another study of a multiethnic sample of high school students (47) indicated that the "primary SES difference appeared to be related to participation in activity lessons or classes and higher quality physical education in the school serving more affluent students." Some European studies have shown an association of areas of cities with physical activity levels among adults (48), disparities in physical activity resources (49), and variations in physical activity levels of adolescents (50).

Walking and cycling are common pastimes with children and adults (51). Research indicates that fear of walking or cycling in traffic is a frequently cited reason for not choosing these ways of travel (52). In a recent study of police districts, Macpherson *et al.* (53) found correlations between traffic patterns and injury rates at the neighborhood level, as well as an inverse association between street crossings and the area socioeconomic status. Other reports have shown that pedestrian and bicycle injuries in low-income areas are significantly more common than in affluent areas (54–56) and for certain racial and ethnic groups. Evaluations of traffic-calming interventions showed increases in bicycle traffic following environmental changes (57). These environmental strategies point to the importance of looking at the physical characteristics of a neighborhood as important influences on the physical activity patterns of its residents.

There is some evidence that school- and community-based programs may increase physical activity in young people. However, data from the Centers for Disease Control Youth Risk Behavior Surveillance System (YRBSS) suggest that opportunities for formal physical activity are limited in school settings, where youngsters spend the most time. An estimated 42% of high school students surveyed in 1991 were enrolled in daily physical education classes, well below the *Year 2000* objective of 50%. A more recent report indicates that by 1997 this rate had fallen to 27% (58). The School Health Policies and Programs Study in 1994 (59) also found that school-based physical education in the United States was limited, that classes rarely focus on lifetime physical activity as recommended by the CDC (1), and that only a fraction (15%) of physical education teachers required students to develop individualized fitness programs (60).

Some data on transportation reinforce the assertion about community design: "National transportation surveys found that walking and bicycling by children aged 5 to 15 dropped 40% between 1977 and 1995" (38). However, we do not know if these changes can be attributed to community design, or perhaps to a search for efficiency among busy households (many with two wage earners), attempting to minimize transit time. Our Tritrac data, however, provide one reassuring note: Although youngsters may be generally inactive, the data clearly indicate that the one active thing they do on weekdays is to go to and from school. This transit journey may provide a good opportunity to add activity to the lives of all youngsters. It has been reported in the United States that "more than one third (37%) of all trips to school are made from one mile away or less, but only 31% of these trips are made by walking" (38). The journey to and from school may offer a fine opportunity for community interventions at relatively low cost that could significantly boost activity levels among young people in the United States. Comparative data from other industrialized countries would be informative. Right now we have no experimental data indicating the impact of new "walk-and-bike-to-school" programs, but clearly the potential is substantial.

Environmental and policy change offers the opportunity to create environments for children and adolescents that increase physical activity, reduce inactivity, and prevent obesity. Unfortunately, our science base is very limited for making informed policy and environmental choices. However, programs and policies that reduce television viewing by providing alternatives and increasing opportunities for physically active play and sport will be unlikely to do harm, and in fact were the norm in many communities in the past. A return to less television and more play seems essential (61).

DISCUSSION

Modern industrialized society is generally characterized by low levels of physical activity, where individuals typically use motorized transport rather than walking or running, most work (including schooling for children) involves sedentary days, and vigorous physical activity consists of rare leisure-time pursuits. The quantitative work from our research group, using both 24-hour physical activity recalls and computerized electronic monitoring of physical activity levels, has confirmed these views in a study of children and adolescents (62). A larger sample of data in the present study has clearly indicated these same patterns of pervasive inactivity and moderate and vigorous activity. Because of the general underestimation of energy expenditure by the Tritrac monitors in free-living populations, these are probably underestimates of time spent daily at 3.0 MET or more. Our estimates of an average of 1 hour a day spent at 3.0 MET activity or more is consistent with two other studies using computerized accelerometers (63,64).

If accurate and generalizable, these objective data could have important implications for surveillance and monitoring of physical activity levels among young people in the United States. Yet there is a serious gap between what these Tritrac estimates indicate and the national goals for physical activity of children and adolescents. Various national panels have recommended that youngsters engage in physical activity levels that vary widely, as follows:

1. "Some of the child's activity each day should be in periods lasting 10 to 15 minutes or more and include moderate to vigorous activity" (65).
2. "[There should be] three or more sessions per week of activity that last 20 or more minutes at a time and that require moderate to vigorous levels of exertion" (66,67).

Children and teenagers are advised by the 2000 version of the Dietary Guidelines for Americans to "aim for at least 60 minutes of moderate physical activity most days of the week, preferably daily" (67).

Clearly, these three goals represent different levels of activity among youngsters, with daily averages ranging from 9 to 60 minutes of moderate (≥ 3.0 MET) activity. Our studies using Tritrac computerized accelerometers indicate that the vast majority of youngsters are on average meeting a goal of 30 minutes a day of moderate and vigorous activity (≥ 3.0 MET), with a conservative estimate of a mean of 60 minutes a day.

These results are in contrast to other estimated levels of physical activity among young people in the United States. The Surgeon General's *Report on Physical Activity and Health* cites inadequate levels of physical activity among only a small percentage of youngsters, but also notes the limited evidence for these self-reported data (51). We know very little about the validity of the self-report measures used to assess national goals.

The *Healthy People 2010* goal for television viewing is that youngsters watch no more than 1 or 2 hours a day (69). National estimates of television viewing indicate levels of about 3 hours a day (70–72). These goals are clearly lower than the averages found in our study and others.

When we recently designed a school-based intervention trial, we encouraged students to meet a goal of 30 minutes of moderate to vigorous physical activity every day (3). Our intervention was not successful in increasing moderate and vigorous physical activity, although it reduced television viewing, reduced obesity, and improved diet among girls. One hypothesis is that students at baseline considered they were already engaging in more than 1 hour of physical activity a day—including walking to and from school, sports, walking at school, and so on. This is what they reported in their surveys, and, as noted earlier, this is what the Tritrac data indicated. Our failure may have been in setting the wrong goals.

What are the right physical activity goals? The present findings may lead us to question how these various physical activity and inactivity goals were derived, and whether the goals, when objectively measured and targeted, represent our best science. Are these goals set too low because previous research could not measure precisely all the small bursts of activity that occur throughout a typical day? Are these goals optimal to both improve cardiovascular health and reduce obesity risk? Do we need sustained bursts of activity for 10 or 20 minutes or more a day, or are smaller bursts adequate? Are our goals for television viewing realistic? Do we need to revise them in the light of the internet revolution? What are youngsters thinking?

We need objective data on physical activity among children and adolescents to both create surveillance systems and examine their impact on outcome. We need to validate our surveillance measures, and we need to understand these data in relation to the perceptions of children and adolescents. Finally, we need to document effective policy and environmental changes that can affect physical activity and obesity. We have much work to occupy us in the future.

ACKNOWLEDGMENTS

We thank Arthur Sobol for crucial assistance with statistical programming. This work was supported by the National Institutes of Child Health and Human Development (HD-30780), and the Centers for Disease Control and Prevention (Prevention Research Centers grant U48/CCU115807). This work is solely the responsibility of the author and does not represent official views of the Centers for Disease Control and Prevention.

REFERENCES

1. US Department of Health and Human Services. *Healthy People 2000: National health promotion and disease prevention objectives.* Atlanta: US Department of Health and Human Services, Public Health Service, 1990.
2. Koplan JP, Dietz WH. Caloric imbalance and public health policy. *JAMA* 1999; 282: 1579–81.
3. Gortmaker SL, Peterson K, Wiecha J, *et al.* Reducing obesity via a school-based interdisciplinary intervention among youth: Planet Health. *Arch Pediatr Adolesc Med* 1999; 153: 409–18.
4. Bouten CV, Westerterp KR, Verduin M, Janssen JD. Assessment of energy expenditure for physical activity using a triaxial accelerometer. *Med Sci Sports Exerc* 1994; 26: 1516–23.
5. Melanson EL, Freedson PS. Physical activity assessment: a review of methods. *Crit Rev Food Sci Nutr* 1996; 36: 385–96.
6. Eston RG, Rowlands AV, Ingledew DK. Validity of heart rate, pedometry, and accelerometry for predicting the energy cost of children's activities. *J Appl Physiol* 1998; 84: 362–71.
7. Janz KF, Witt J, Mahoney LT. The stability of children's physical activity as measured by accelerometry and self-report. *Med Sci Sports Exerc* 1995; 27: 1326–32.
8. Hemokinetics Inc. *TriTrac-R3D activity monitor instruction manual.* Madison, Wisconsin: Hemokinetics Inc, 1995.
9. *Recommended dietary allowances,* 10th ed. Washington, DC: National Academy Press, 2000.
10. Hendelman D, Miller K, Baggett C, Debold E, Freedson P. Validity of accelerometry for the assessment of moderate intensity physical activity in the field. *Med Sci Sports Exerc* 2000; 32: 442–9.
11. Welk GJ, Blair SN, Wood K, Jones S, Thompson RW. A comparative evaluation of three accelerometry-based physical activity monitors. *Med Sci Sports Exerc* 2000; 32: 489–97.
12. Gortmaker SL, Dietz WH, Cheung L. Inactivity, diet and the fattening of America. *J Am Diet Assoc* 1990; 90: 1247–55.
13. Bennett WI. Dieting: ideology versus physiology. *Psychiatr Clin North Am* 1984; 7: 321.
14. Dietz WH, Gortmaker SL. Do we fatten our children at the TV set? Obesity and television viewing in children and adolescents. *Pediatrics* 1985; 75: 807–12.
15. Gortmaker SL, Must A, Sobol AM, Peterson K, Colditz GA, Dietz WH. Television viewing as a cause of increasing obesity among children in the United States, 1986–1990. *Arch Pediatr Adolesc Med* 1996; 150: 356–62.
16. Shannon B, Peacock J, Brown MJ. Body fatness, television viewing and calorie-intake of a sample of Pennsylvania sixth grade school children. *J Nutr Educ* 1991; 23: 262–8.
17. Obarzanek E, Schreiber GB, Crawford PB, *et al.* Energy intake and physical activity in relation to indexes of body fat: the National Heart, Lung, and Blood Institute Growth and Health Study. *Am J Clin Nutr* 1994; 60: 15–22.
18. Berkey CS, Rockett HR, Field AE, *et al.* Activity, dietary intake, and weight changes in a longitudinal study of preadolescent and adolescent boys and girls. *Pediatrics* 2000; 105: 56.
19. Robinson TN. Reducing children's television viewing to prevent obesity: a randomized controlled trial. *JAMA* 1999; 282: 1561–7.
20. Epstein LH, Valoski AM, Smith JA, *et al.* Effects of decreasing sedentary behavior and increasing activity on weight change in obese children. *Health Psychol* 1995; 14: 1–7.
21. Taras HL, Gage M. Advertised foods on children's television. *Arch Pediatr Adolesc Med* 1995; 149: 649–52.
22. Clancy-Hepburn K, Hickey AA, Nevill G. Children's behavior responses to TV food advertisements. *J Nutr Educ* 1974; 6: 93–6.
23. Ching PLYH, Willett WC, Rimm EB, Colditz GA, Gortmaker SL, Stampfer MJ. Activity level and risk of overweight in male health professionals. *Am J Public Health* 1996; 86: 25–30.

24. Fung TT, Hu FB, Yu J, *et al.* Leisure-time physical activity, television watching, and plasma bio-markers of obesity and cardiovascular disease risk. *Am J Epidemiol* 2000; 152: 1171–8.
25. Wolf AM, Gortmaker SL, Cheung L, Gray HM, Herzog DB, Colditz GA. Activity, inactivity, and obesity: racial, ethnic, and age differences among schoolgirls. *Am J Public Health* 1993; 83: 1625–7.
26. Raitakari OT, Porkka KV, Taimela S, Telama R, Rasanen L, Viikari JS. Effects of persistent physical activity and inactivity on coronary risk factors in children and young adults. The Cardiovascular Risk in Young Finns Study. *Am J Epidemiol* 1994; 140: 195–205.
27. Hernandez B, Gortmaker SL, Colditz GA, Peterson KE, Laird NM, Parra-Cabrera S. Association of obesity with physical activity, television programs and other forms of video viewing among children in Mexico City. *Int J Obes Relat Metab Disord* 1999; 23: 845–54.
28. Berkey CS, Rockett HR, Field AE, *et al.* Activity, dietary intake, and weight changes in a longitudinal study of preadolescent and adolescent boys and girls. *Pediatrics* 2000; 105: 56.
29. O'Loughlin J, Gray-Donald K, Paradis G, Meshefedjian G. One- and two-year predictors of excess weight gain among elementary schoolchildren in multiethnic, low-income, inner-city neighborhoods. *Am J Epidemiol* 2000; 152: 739–46.
30. Epstein LH, Valoski MS, Wing RR, McCurley J. Ten-year follow-up of behavioral, family-based treatment for obese children. *JAMA* 1990; 264: 2519–23.
31. Lee L, Kumar S, Leong LC. The impact of five-month basic military training on the body weight and body fat of 197 moderately to severely obese Singaporean males aged 17 to 19 years. *Int J Obes Relat Metab Disord* 1994; 18: 105–9.
32. Gutin B, Manos TM. Physical activity in the prevention of childhood obesity. *Ann NY Acad Sci* 1993; 699: 115–26.
33. Goran MI, Reynolds KD, Lindquist CH. Role of physical activity in the prevention of obesity in children. *Int J Obes Relat Metab Disord* 1999; 23: 18–33.
34. Carter J, Wiecha J, Peterson KE, Gortmaker SL. *Planet Health.* Champaign, IL: Human Kinetics Press, 2001.
35. Cheung LWY, Gortmaker SL, Dent H. Eat Well and Keep Moving. Champaign, IL: Human Kinetics Press, 2001.
36. Gortmaker SL, Cheung LWY, Peterson KE, *et al.* Impact of a school-based interdisciplinary intervention on diet and physical activity among urban primary school children: Eat Well and Keep Moving. *Arch Pediatr Adolesc Med* 1999; 153: 975–83.
37. Epstein LH, Valoski MS, Wing RR, McCurley J. Ten-year follow-up of behavioral, family-based treatment for obese children. *JAMA* 1990; 264: 2519–23.
38. Secretary of Health and Human Services and the Secretary of Education. *Promoting better health for young people through physical activity and sports.* A Report to the President. Washington, DC: Government Printing Office, 2000.
39. Sallis JF, Bauman A, Pratt M. Environmental and policy interventions to promote physical activity. *Am J Prev Med* 1998; 15: 379–97.
40. Blair SN, Booth M, Gyarfas I, *et al.* Development of public policy and physical activity initiatives internationally. *Sports Med* 1996; 21: 157–63.
41. Dishman RK, Dunn AL. Exercise adherence in children and youth: implications for adulthood. In: Dishman RK, ed. *Exercise adherence: its impact on public health.* Champaign, IL. Human Kinetics Press, 1988: 155–200.
42. Sallis JF, Simons-Morton BG, Stone EG, *et al.* Determinants of physical activity and interventions in youth. *Med Sci Sports Exerc* 1992; 24: 248–57.
43. Sallis JF, Prochaska, Taylor WC. A review of correlates of physical activity of children and adolescents. *Med Sci Sports Exerc* 2000; 32: 963–75.
44. Sallis JF, Johnson MF, Calfas KJ, Caparosa S, Nichols JF. Assessing perceived physical environmental variables that may influence physical activity. *Res Q Exerc Sport* 1997; 58: 345–51.
45. Myers RS, Roth DL. Perceived benefits of and barriers to exercise and stage of exercise adoption in young adults. *Health Psychol* 1997; 16: 277–83.
46. Garcia AW, Broda MA, Frenn M, Coviak C, Pender NJ, Ronis DL. Gender and developmental differences in exercise beliefs among youth and prediction of their exercise behavior. *J School Health* 1995; 65: 213–9.
47. Sallis JF, Zakarian JF, Hovell MF, Hofstetter CR. Ethnic, socioeconomic and sex differences in physical activity among adolescents. *J Clin Epidemiol* 1996; 2: 125–34.
48. Ellaway A, Macintyre S. Does where you live predict health related behaviors? A case study in Glasgow. *Health Bull (Edinb)* 1996; 54: 443–6.

49. Macintyre S, Maciver S, Sooman A. Area, class and health: should we be focusing on places or people? *Int Soc Pol* 113; 22: 213–34.
50. Karvonen S, Rimpela AH. Urban small area variation in adolescents health behavior. *Soc Sci Med* 1997; 45: 1089–98.
51. US Department of Health and Human Services. *Physical activity and health: a report of the Surgeon General.* Centers for Disease Control and Prevention, National Center for Chronic Disease Prevention and Health Promotion. Atlanta: US Department of Health and Human Services, 1996.
52. Federal Highway Administration. *The National bicycling and walking study: transportation choices for a changing America* (publication No. FHWA-PD-94-023). Washington, DC; US Department of Transportation, 1994.
53. Macpherson A, Roberts I, Pless IB. Children's exposure to traffic and pedestrian injuries. *Am J Public Health* 1998; 88: 1840–3.
54. Pless IB, Verreault R, Arsenault L, Frappier J, Stulginskas J. The epidemiology of road accidents. *Am J Public Health* 1987; 77: 358–60.
55. Roberts I, Norton R, Jackson R, Dunn R, Hassall I. Effect of environmental factors on risk of injury of child pedestrians by motor vehicles: a case–control study. *BMJ* 1995; 310: 91–4.
56. Stevenson M, Jamrozik K, Spittle J. A case–control study of traffic risk factors and child pedestrian injury. *Int J Epidemiol* 1995; 24: 957–64.
57. Clarke A, Dornfeld M. *Traffic calming, auto restricted zones, and other traffic management techniques: their effect on bicyclists and pedestrians.* Federal Highway Administration publication No FHWA-PD-93-028. Washington, DC; US Department of Transportation, 1994.
58. Americans are closer to US health goal, but Satcher sees huge disparities between races. *New York Times* June 11, 1999.
59. Kann L, Collins JL, Pateman BC, Small ML, Ross JC, Kolbe LJ. The School Health Policies and Programs Study (SHPPS). *J School Health* 1995; 65: 291–4.
60. Pate RR, Small ML, Ross JG, Young JC, Flint KH, Warren CW. School physical education. *J School Health* 1995; 65: 312–18.
61. Dietz WH. The obesity epidemic in young children. Reduce television viewing and promote playing. *BMJ* 2001; 322: 313–14.
62. Cradock A, Gortmaker SL, Peterson K, Sobol A, Wiecha J. Are youth less active than they say? Youth recall and TriTrac accelerometer estimates of physical activity levels. Proceedings of a meeting of the Ambulatory Pediatric Association, Boston, MA, May 15, 2000.
63. McMurray RG, Harrell JS, Bradley CB, Webb JP, Goodman EM. Comparison of a computerized physical activity recall with a triaxial motion sensor in middle-school youth. *Am J Prev Med* 1998; 15: 379–97.
64. Janz KF, Witt J, Mahoney LT. The stability of children's physical activity as measured by accelerometry and self-report. *Med Sci Sports Exerc* 1995; 27: 1326–32.
65. Corbin CB, Pangrazi RP. Physical activity for children: a statement of guidelines. Reston, VA: National Association for Sport and Physical Education, 1998.
66. Sallis JF, Patrick K. Physical activity guidelines for adolescents: consensus statement. *Pediatric Exerc Sci* 1994; 6: 302–14.
67. US Department of Agriculture and Department of Health and Human Services. *Nutrition and your health: dietary guidelines for Americans,* 5th ed. Washington, DC: Government Printing Office, 2000.
68. Roberts DF, Foehr UG, Rideout VJ, Brodie M. *Kids & Media @ the New Millennium: a comprehensive national analysis of children's media use.* Menlo Park, CA: Kaiser Family Foundation, 1999.
69. US Department of Health and Human Services. *Healthy people 2010: understanding and improving health.* Washington, DC: Government Printing Office, 2000.
70. Stanger JD, Gridina N. Media in the home 1999: the fourth annual survey of parents and children. Philadelphia: Annenberg Public Policy Center of the University of Pennsylvania, 1998.
71. Andersen RE, Crespo CJ, Bartlett SH, Cheskin LJ, Pratt M. Relationship of physical activity and television watching with body weight and level of fatness among children: results from the Third National Health and Nutrition Examination Survey. *JAMA* 1998; 279: 938–42.
72. Nielsen Media Research. 1998 Report on Television. New York, 1998 [online]. Available from: URL: *http://www.nielsenmedia.com.*

DISCUSSION

Dr. Strauss: I think there is an important type of activity that is very much ignored, involving between 1.5 and 3 METs, and this corresponds to play and pre-play activity. People either focus on complete sedentary inactivity or on vigorous activity. We just did a study sponsored by Nestlé where we put activity monitors on 100 children aged 10 to 16 years. We found that the children were vigorously active for only about 12 minutes a day. The majority of the time spent being active involved low level activity in the 1.5 to 3 METs range, and this was negatively correlated with television viewing. Do you have any comments on that?

Dr. Gortmaker: These results are consistent with our findings and make an interesting point. So you think that most of the energy that pre-teen and teenage children expend during the day is in the 1.5 to 3 METs range?

Dr. Strauss: Yes. About 80% of their time is spent inactive, 5% to 6% of their time—that is, around 12 minutes a day—is spent being vigorously active, but the majority of the time spent in physical activity involves low level activity that tends to be ignored.

Dr. Gortmaker: I think this is a very important perspective. What do you think are the intervention implications of your findings?

Dr. Strauss: I think the implication is that if you decrease television viewing, though the children would not necessarily then go out and play soccer and engage in sports, they would nonetheless be more active.

Dr. Gortmaker: I would definitely agree with that, but at the same time I would not want to emphasize only the trade-off between television viewing and low level activity. I agree that this is an important part of the mechanism, but the advertising for food on TV found is the other very important link to obesity. I don't know if you studied the patterns of activity levels over the day, but I would guess they correspond to what we have seen—that children tend to increase the level of 1.5 to 3 METs activity as they go to school and during different parts of the school day. We have found the lowest levels of overall activity on weekends, when there are fewer structured activities. The point you make suggests that if we are interested in obesity prevention, we need to think about what factors contribute to overall energy expenditure among young people. My guess is that our data are consistent with this view that energy expenditure in the 1.5 to 3 METs range explains much of the expenditure above basal that is related to physical activity.

Dr. Koletzko: I was impressed by the Tritrac data, particularly where they show that our traditional concept of children being more inactive at school—and therefore more active out of school—appears to be wrong, now that video games and computer time are becoming more popular as free time occupations. I have a couple of questions. Do the Tritrac data allow you to differentiate between active movement and passive movement, such as might occur when being driven in a car or a bus to school? Also, heart rate has been used as an index of energy expenditure in adults. Are there any data showing whether it is a useful measure of energy expenditure in children?

Dr. Gortmaker: With regard to the first question, we have investigated this a bit. Generally, when persons wearing Tritracs are in buses or cars you don't see very much movement. When you hit bumps you may get a small increase in the activity recorded, but the amount depends on the stiffness of the springs of the bus. I have worn one of these devices for many days myself, and have become embarrassed at my low level of activity! I have found that when I drive my car, which has very stiff springs, I get virtually no movement registered, so these monitors are quite accurate in that way. They don't tell you if the subjects are lifting weights or engaging in similar types of activity, so they do tend to underestimate overall energy expenditure, but I think in general they do a very good job in recording minute-to-minute activity.

With regard to your second question, there are a couple of very nice studies relating Tritrac and other computerized accelerometers to measures of energy expenditure, and they do quite well, with r^2 values around 0.8 in children engaged in a range of activities (1). So those data look quite good. Some studies using heart rate monitors show similar patterns of activity, but I have not seen direct comparisons with accelerometers and energy expenditure measures.

Dr. Jiang: Have you found that your measurements of activity level correlate with the presence or absence of obesity?

Dr. Gortmaker: We actually found very little difference in the activity levels in this age group among children who were obese or not obese. There was a slightly *higher* rate of vigorous activity among children who were obese, but the curves were remarkably similar.

Dr. Yanovski: I am interested in the role of TV in obesity. Are there any studies comparing individuals who primarily watch videos or use the computer, where they would not be getting commercial messages stimulating intake, versus those who primarily watch commercial TV, with the many child-centered food commercials? This might help to separate the reduced activity versus increased intake roles of TV viewing.

Dr. Gortmaker: A former student of ours, Dr. Bernardo Hernandez, did a nice study like that among adolescents in Mexico City. He found a strong relation between hours of broadcast TV viewing and levels of obesity in children, but no relation between the use of video games and obesity (2). These data suggest that the advertising component is more important than the inactivity component, though this is only one study and the results need to be confirmed. It is also important to note that we have found that 80% of video time of youth is still broadcast TV.

Dr. Yanovski: My other comment is that in most adult studies, until you get to extraordinary levels of activity, additional intake will balance out additional activity to a large degree and so there will not be a net weight change. Thus it seems quite plausible to me that the effects of TV might be mediated through a non-activity-related change.

Dr. Steinbeck: In the Planet Health study, why was there no observed weight loss in the boys compared with the girls?

Dr. Gortmaker: There was actually weight gain in both boys and girls, because they were all growing, but it is true we did not see effects of the intervention on obesity in boys. In this age range, girls are growing more rapidly than boys, and it could be that this is a more opportune time to see intervention effects emerging among girls. Another explanation might be that our intervention resonated less with the boys than with the girls on issues of diet. I should say that in the Planet Health intervention we never focus on obesity or talk about it; lessons discuss healthy eating, reducing saturated fats, eating more fruit and vegetables, and reducing TV time and replacing it with more active time—those are the four messages. These messages may appeal less to the boys, who at this age may want to be big and muscular. Also in the United States, though obesity is also increasing rapidly among boys, there has been very much of a focus on girls and women. We have a series of national programs now focusing on obesity in girls, but nothing focusing on obesity in boys. I do think this is an important area for research. In addition, one school in particular did not implement the program well. If we drop this school (and its control) we find effects for boys (p = 0.05). Do you have any ideas?

Dr. Steinbeck: I think you can appeal to boys much more on the grounds of physical activity and sporting prowess than you can on health. That extends into the adult age group as well.

Dr. Ruslisjarif: I have a question about physical activity for obese preschool children. In Indonesia about 40% of obese children are in the preschool age. What kind of activity can you suggest for them?

Dr. Gortmaker: That is an interesting question. In the United States, preschool children typically engage in lots of play, and most neighborhoods provide environmental and cultural support for engagement in play activities. The problems are more likely to start around later primary school, middle school, and adolescence, when cultural issues and lack of opportunities tend to limit activity. My question to you would be, "What support is available in Indonesia for children's play activities, and are there supportive environments where they can play?"

Dr. Ruslisjarif: In Indonesia, usually both parents are working, and the child is left at home with a carer. So these children are usually with their parents only at weekends and during holidays.

Dr. Gortmaker: Does anyone else have any thoughts on this problem?

Dr. Bar-Or: Maybe just to send them outdoors! Obviously, there are safety issues, but if you can satisfy those issues, then the children will find active things to do. You don't need to give them aerobic activity or structured activity. Indoors, they are much more limited, but going outdoors can be a simple and effective solution.

Dr. Cole: You have told us that television watching is strongly associated with obesity, and of course that it is also associated with very low levels of activity. This isn't meant to be as tongue-in-cheek as it may sound, but I've always thought that what is required is something like a clockwork radio—a clockwork TV that you have to cycle to allow it to be viewed. I can think of a lot of strategies you could build in so that the parent can control the child's activity level as they watch TV.

Dr. Gortmaker: Thank you. Dr. Tom Robinson has an intervention involving an electronic devise called "the TV allowance." This is not inexpensive, but it does allow you to achieve some of the things we have been talking about and to set limits in a way that puts the control more in the hands of the children. I also believe there is a study by Dr. Len Epstein's group where children did have to cycle on a bike to "power" the TV. I don't think they liked it very much, however. Dr. Robinson, do you want to comment?

Dr. Robinson: Yes, the idea is that if children have the ability to control their TV viewing time, as opposed to restrictions being imposed by parents or others, they are more motivated to try to comply with those restrictions. I've heard from many parents about how, by letting their children control their own TV time or even setting their own goals, the children find it much more rewarding, and the parents don't have to be policemen to make sure that the children are complying with the goals. In relation to pedal power, I don't believe the technology is available to generate enough energy to power a TV from a bicycle, but it is possible to devise switches that allow the power to flow to the TV when a certain level of output is achieved on a bicycle or treadmill. But this is a fairly expensive solution.

Dr. Buenaluz: In school, teachers should resort to role playing more, and involve the children in active demonstrations instead of making them sit passively at their desks. Children usually enjoy learning activities more if they are physically involved.

REFERENCES

1. Bouten CV, Westerterp KR, Verduin M, *et al.* Assessment of energy expenditure for physical activity using a triaxial accelerometer. *Med Sci Sports Exerc* 1994; 26: 1516–23.
2. Hernandez B, Gortmaker SL, Colditz GA, *et al.* Association of obesity with physical activity, television programs and other forms of video viewing among children in Mexico City. *Int J Obes Relat Metab Disord* 1999; 23: 845–54.

Obesity in Childhood and Adolescence, edited by
Chunming Chen and William H. Dietz. Nestlé
Nutrition Workshop Series, Pediatric Program,
Vol. 49. Nestec Ltd., Vevey/Lippincott
Williams & Wilkins, Philadelphia © 2002.

Environmental Factors Leading to Pediatric Obesity in the Developing World

Guansheng Ma

*Institute of Nutrition and Food Hygiene, Chinese Academy of Preventive Medicine,
Beijing, China*

A recent report of World Health Organization indicated that there is a global epidemic of obesity, affecting both developed and developing countries (1). Though there is much published information from developed countries about obesity and about its causes and its consequences for health, information from developing countries is limited, especially for childhood obesity. Onis and Blossner (2) and Martorell *et al.* (3) analyzed the prevalence of overweight and obesity in children in developing countries and concluded that—although undernutrition remained a major public health problem—obesity among children did not seem to be of great importance in such countries. However, further surveys from developing countries (1,4–6) have indicated that the prevalence of overweight and obesity in childhood and adolescence has been increasing rapidly in the past two decades and has now reached epidemic proportions. It appears that obesity has, in fact, become a public health problem in some developing countries, and intervention strategies should be put in place to try to limit its incidence.

As there is a lack of effective measures for treating obesity, the most effective and economical strategy is to prevent obesity at an early stage of life. Contributing factors to the onset and development of obesity should be identified so that an effective preventive strategy can be developed. Although genetic factors play an important role in determining individual susceptibility to obesity (7), genetics cannot explain the current obesity epidemic, as our genes have not changed substantially during the past two decades. This suggests that the primary cause of the rapid increase in obesity lies in environmental and social factors (8).

The study described in this chapter was designed to explore the environmental factors concerned with childhood obesity in China and to provide scientific information that will help in developing effective intervention strategies. These data may also serve as reference data for other developing countries.

SUBJECTS AND METHODS

Subjects

The investigation was carried out in 1999 and involved 9,356 children (4,570 boys and 4,786 girls) aged 4 to 17 years. They were selected from four eastern cities of China (Guangzhou, Shanghai, Jinan, and Haerbin) using a stratified multistage cluster random sampling method. Three kinds of questionnaire were designed to obtain information from preschool children, elementary students, junior students, and their respective parents. The questionnaires were interview administered for children aged 4 to 8 years, and self-administered for students older than 8 years and for all the parents.

The weight and height of the children were measured by trained interviewers following a standardized procedure. Overweight and obesity were defined as weight-for-height exceeded 110% and 120%, respectively, of the WHO reference for children aged 4 to 6.9 years, and of Chinese standards for children aged 7 to 17 years.

In the analysis of the prevalence of overweight and obesity, the following variables were considered: sex, age, age group (preschool, elementary, and junior school students), domicile region (northeast, east, mid-south), domicile situation (urban or suburban), domiciliary monthly per capita income in renminbi yuan (RMB) (distributed in three categories: low income, less than RMB 293.20; middle income, RMB 293.20 to 722.90; high income, over RMB 722.90) (9), educational level of the parents, breakfast frequency (0 to 1 per week, 2 to 4 per week, 5 to 7 per week), television viewing time (less than 1 hour per day, 1 to 2 hours per day, 2 to 3 hours per day, more than 3 hours per day), fast food consumption (never, 1 to 2 times per month, 3 to 4 times per month), and desired body size.

The hypothesis of no association between groups of children and the demographic characteristics of the groups was tested using the chi distribution. Logistic regression models were developed using the SAS 6.12 program to identify factors characterizing obesity, after adjustment for possible confounding and interactive effects. Factors examined were sex, age group, domicile region, domicile situation, income, educational level of parents, breakfast frequency, fast food consumption, television viewing hours, and desired body size. Odds ratios (OR) and their 95% confidence intervals (CI) were calculated. All p values were two-sided. A p value of < 0.05 was accepted as statistically significant.

RESULTS

The prevalence of overweight and obesity among children and adolescents according to age and sex are presented in Table 1. The overall prevalences of overweight and obesity were 12.1% and 11.9%, respectively. Overweight and obesity were more prevalent in boys than in girls (13.2% versus 11.0%; 14.8% versus 9.3%). The peak prevalence of obesity was 19.3% in boys 12 years of age and 13.1% in girls 13 years of age.

The prevalence of obesity in relation to the demographic characteristics of the subjects is given in Table 2. Boys were about 1.6 times more liable to obesity than girls (OR, 1.567; 95% CI, 1.345 to 1.827). The prevalence of obesity was 13.6% in the

TABLE 1. *Prevalence (%) of overweight and obesity (weight-for-height) according to age and sex*

Age	N			Obesity (%)			Overweight (%)			OW + O (%)		
	M	F	T	M	F	T	M	F	T	M	F	T
4–	334	337	671	11.1	9.2	10.1	20.1	19.0	19.5	31.2	28.2	29.6
5–	362	370	732	10.5	11.1	10.8	18.0	18.9	18.4	28.5	30.0	29.2
6–	365	344	709	11.5	9.6	10.6	16.2	12.8	14.5	27.7	22.4	25.1
7–	323	300	623	16.1	7.7	12.0	12.7	10.7	11.7	28.8	18.4	23.7
8–	332	325	657	14.8	5.2	10.1	13.9	8.9	11.4	28.7	14.1	21.5
9–	381	367	748	17.9	10.6	14.3	11.3	10.1	10.7	29.2	20.7	25.0
10–	369	407	776	14.4	11.8	13.0	15.2	10.6	12.8	29.6	22.4	25.8
11–	396	400	796	17.4	13.0	15.2	12.9	10.3	11.6	30.3	23.3	26.8
12–	400	466	866	19.3	10.1	14.3	12.3	10.3	11.2	31.6	20.4	25.5
13–	391	374	765	17.1	13.1	15.2	11.3	10.2	10.7	28.4	23.3	25.9
14–	392	484	876	11.2	7.2	9.0	6.4	6.4	6.4	17.6	13.6	15.4
15–	376	424	800	13.6	5.0	9.0	11.2	9.2	10.1	24.8	14.2	19.1
16–	149	188	337	18.1	3.7	10.1	11.4	5.3	8.0	29.5	9.0	18.1
Total	4570	4786	9356	14.8	9.3	11.9	13.2	11.0	12.1	28.0	20.3	24.0

Abbreviations: F, female; M, male; N, number of subjects; OW + O, overweight and obesity; T, total.
Note: Obesity is defined as weight-for-height exceeding 120% of the WHO reference for children aged 4–6.9 years and exceeding 120% of Chinese standard for children aged 7–17 years.

elementary school students, which was significantly higher than that in preschool children or junior students. The prevalence of obesity was greatest in northeast China, least in mid-south China, and intermediate in east China. Obesity was more prevalent in urban than in suburban areas, with odds ratios ranging between 0.982 and 1.282. There were significantly more obese children in high-income families than in low-income families. In relation to food consumption, the risk of obesity was related to the frequency of breakfast eating, in that children who often skipped breakfast were more likely to be obese than their counterparts who ate breakfast daily; and children who often consumed fast food were more likely to be obese than those who consumed fast food less often. With regard to television viewing, obese children watched more television daily than their nonobese counterparts: the prevalence of obesity increased by about 1.5% for each additional hour of television viewed.

By chi testing with no adjustment for other variables, obesity in children tended to be greater in those with better educated parents. The prevalence of obesity was 13.8% in children claiming to prefer a larger body size; this was significantly higher than in those who preferred a normal or small body size. Children with parents preferring a larger body size were also more likely to be obese.

DISCUSSION

Prevalence and Trends of Obesity in Developing Countries

Onis and Blossner (2) analyzed 160 nationally representative cross-sectional surveys from 94 countries and found that the global prevalence of overweight in preschool children was 3.3% (defined as a weight-for-height > 2 SD above the NCHS/WHO reference median). The percentage of overweight children was highest in Latin America and the Caribbean (4.4%), followed by Africa (3.9%), and Asia (2.9%). The

TABLE 2. *Prevalence of obesity with odds ratios (OR) and 95% confidence intervals (CI)*

Variable	N	Obesity (%)	OR (CI) crude	OR (CI) adjusted
Sex[a]				
Female	4,786	9.3	1.000	1.000
Male	4,570	14.8	1.696 (1.495–1.925)	1.567 (1.345–1.827)
Age group[a]				
Preschool	2,329	10.7	1.000	1.000
Elementary	4,474	13.6	1.322 (1.131–1.546)	1.358 (1.138–1.620)
Junior	2,553	10.2	0.951 (0.792–1.143)	0.988 (0.803–1.215)
Domicile region[a]				
Mid-south	2,390	10.2	1.000	1.000
East China	4,638	12.2	1.228 (1.048–1.440)	1.347 (1.143–1.588)
Northeast	2,328	13.2	1.347 (1.127–1.610)	1.415 (1.172–1.708)
Domicile situation[b]				
Suburb	4,115	11.0	1.000	1.000
Urban	5,241	12.7	1.178 (1.037–1.337)	1.122 (0.982–1.282)
Income[b]				
Low	2,883	11.6	1.000	1.000
Middle	5,180	11.9	1.032 (0.896–1.189)	1.069 (0.919–1.243)
High	1,293	12.8	1.124 (0.921–1.371)	1.207 (0.967–1.507)
Educational level of parents				
Low	207	9.2	1.000	1.000
Mediate	6,266	11.7	1.305 (0.810–2.102)	1.365 (0.839–2.221)
High	2,883	12.8	1.448 (0.894–2.344)	1.502 (0.908–2.482)
Breakfast frequency[a]				
5–7/week	8,726	11.8	1.000	1.000
2–4/week	490	13.5	1.170 (0.895–1.528)	1.230 (0.936–1.615)
0–1/week	140	18.6	1.714 (1.119–2.623)	1.742 (1.123–2.702)
Fast food frequency[b]				
No	1,900	10.5	1.000	1.000
1–2/month	7139	12.2	1.184 (1.007–1.393)	1.180 (0.996–1.400)
3–4/month	311	13.9	1.370 (0.966–1.943)	1.277 (0.891–1.832)
TV viewing time[a]				
<1 h/d	3,012	10.9	1.000	1.000
1–2 h/d	4,255	11.8	1.089 (0.941–1.260)	1.102 (0.949–1.279)
2–3 h/d	1,427	13.2	1.233 (1.019–1.490)	1.253 (1.031–1.523)
>3 h/d	56	15.1	1.444 (1.119–1.865)	1.398 (1.075–1.819)
Desired body size by children				
Small	1,381	10.6		1.000
Normal	4,029	10.6	0.988 (0.818–1.217)	1.078 (0.869–1.337)
Large	3,946	13.8	1.358 (1.120–1.648)	1.083 (0.870–1.349)
Desired body size by parents				
Small	575	9.9	1.000	1.000
Normal	4,880	10.4	1.054 (0.790–1.406)	1.051 (0.782–1.410)
Large	3,901	14.2	1.501 (1.127–1.999)	1.198 (0.880–1.632)

Note: Obesity defined as weight-for-height exceeding 120% of the WHO reference for children aged 4–6.9 years and exceeding 120% of Chinese standard for children aged 7–17 years.
[a] $p < 0.1$ (logistic regression analysis).
[b] $p < 0.05$.

percentage of overweight children in different countries ranged from 0.1% in Sri Lanka to 14.4% in Uzbekistan. It was concluded that obesity did not appear to be a public health problem among preschool children in Asia. However, although undernutrition remains a major problem in developing countries, it is now apparent that obesity is becoming prevalent in some of these countries, especially in urban areas that are undergoing a rapid transition in their economies and lifestyles. The prevalence of obesity in preschool children and schoolchildren has increased at an alarming rate in those countries in the past two decades. For example, the prevalence of obesity among Singaporean preschool children increased from 2.6% in 1988 to 6.8% in 1991, and among schoolchildren from 5.4% in 1980 to 8.8% in 1985 and to 13.2% in 1990 (5). A similar trend is present in other developing countries (2), including China (4,10). The prevalence of obesity among children aged 0 to 7 years increased from 0.91% in 1986 to 2.0% in 1996 (4), whereas among schoolchildren it increased by two- to threefold between 1985 and 1995 (10). This increasing trend is observed in both urban and rural areas of China (11). Our results show that the prevalence of obesity among children in urban China has reached the level found in developed countries (12). The total number of children aged 0 to 17 years in China is 361.7 million, accounting for 29.0% of the total population. If the increasing trend to obesity persists, very large numbers of children will be affected. The economic cost of controlling this problem will be tremendous, considering that obese children are much more likely than normal-weight children to become obese adults, and thus may be at increased risk of obesity-related morbidity and mortality. Action should be taken immediately to control this emerging public health problem.

Domicile Region

Dietz and Gortmaker (13) found regional variations in childhood obesity in American children. They showed that the prevalence of obesity was greatest in the northeast of the country, followed in descending order by the midwest, the south, and the west. Ding *et al.* (14) also showed regional variation in the prevalence of obesity in Chinese children. Neutzling *et al.* (6) also found such variation in Brazilian adolescents. In our study we found that the prevalence of obesity was greater in northeast China than in south China, whereas in east China the prevalence was intermediate. These findings are in agreement with those of Ding. It is of interest that the increasing prevalence of obesity between 1986 and 1996 was greatest in south China (17.5%), followed by central China (12.2%), and north China (1.4%) (4). Differences in economic development may play a role in this trend.

Socioeconomic Status

The relation between the prevalence of obesity and socioeconomic status has been reviewed by Sobal and Stunkard (15). They concluded that obesity was negatively correlated with socioeconomic status in developed countries but positively correlated in developing countries.

Neutzling *et al.* (6) found that Brazilian adolescents in a high-income group were two to three times more liable to overweight and obesity than their lower-income counterparts. This confirmed previous findings in Brazil (16) and in China (17). In our study we found a similar relation between the prevalence of obesity and income levels.

Martorell *et al.* (3) showed that in developing countries overweight was more common in children of mothers with higher educational achievement. We also found that children of well-educated parents tended to be more obese than their counterparts with poorly educated parents.

There is an urban–rural divide, with urban children showing significantly higher rates of obesity than their rural counterparts (3). The results of our study showed that children living in urban areas were more likely to be obese than their counterparts in suburban areas. A possible explanation is that parents with a higher income and better education, living in urban areas, are more likely to be "westernized," thus increasing the risk of obesity.

Eating Practices

Breakfast

The relation between obesity and breakfast eating has been identified in studies conducted in both developed and developing countries. A positive association between skipping breakfast and being overweight was found in American children (18). The same correlation has been shown in Chinese children (19,20). Our results in the present study indicated that breakfast skippers were more likely to be obese than their counterparts who had breakfast daily, with an odds ratio of 1.7. The underlying mechanism is unclear. Children who skip breakfast may eat more in the day, or be less active, or make poor food choices over the rest of the day and thus increase the risk of obesity in the long term (21). On the other hand, children who are already overweight may tend to skip breakfast in an attempt to lose weight (18).

Fast Food Consumption

A positive association between fast food consumption and obesity has been identified in American adults (22), but there is limited information on children. "Western" fast food is very popular in big cities in China, and there has been a dramatic increase in the numbers of restaurants selling these types of food in the past decade. More than 20% of preschool children and schoolchildren in cities consume fast foods at least once a month (23). Fast foods are high in fat and energy and low in fiber. Frequent consumption of fast foods will increase the intake of fat and total energy, which increases the risk of developing obesity.

Television Viewing

Significant associations between the time spent watching television and the prevalence of obesity have been observed among American children and adolescents.

Youngsters who watch more television daily are significantly more obese than their counterparts who watch less television (24). There is a dose–response relation between the obesity, superobesity, and time spent watching television, with an increase in obesity prevalence of 2% for each additional hour of television viewed (25). A similar relation between the prevalence of obesity and television watching has been observed in Chinese children (19) and was reconfirmed in our present study.

The number of television sets owned per 100 households increased from 17.2 in 1985 to 89.8 in 1995, and to 111.6 in 1999 in China (9). More than half of the urban children in China watch television for more than 1 hour daily. Urban children spend increasing amounts of time playing with computers and video games, and there has been a rapid expansion in retail sales of computer electronics in China.

Possible explanations for the relation between television viewing and obesity are that TV viewing is inversely associated with time spent in physical activity and that commercials on TV influence children's food choices and eating practices.

Dietary Factors and Physical Activity Pattern

Obesity is a result of an energy imbalance, where energy intake exceeds energy expenditure over a long period of time. Many studies have focused on dietary factors or physical activity alone, but the results have been inconsistent (26–29). It is now clear that obesity is not simply a result of overeating or of a lack of physical activity; nevertheless, high-fat and energy-dense diets and a sedentary lifestyle are the two characteristics most strongly associated with the increased prevalence of obesity worldwide (1).

Dietary patterns have changed rapidly in China over the past two decades. Fat intake in both rural and urban children increased dramatically between 1989 and 1993 (14). Although the physical activity pattern of Chinese children has not been investigated, adults in urban China were more likely to be sedentary 1991 than in 1989 (30).

The interaction of dietary factors and physical activity on the development of childhood obesity has not been documented in developing countries because of the lack of sophisticated population-based instruments for measuring physical activity patterns. Research in this area should be strengthened in the future.

Social Factors

In addition to the genetic and environmental factors, the influence of social factors on the development of obesity should not be neglected. In parallel with the transformations that are occurring in economic development and lifestyle, changes in social structure, social norms and perceptions, and attitudes to health and body image will unavoidably take place. This may have a profound influence on the trend to obesity.

Throughout most of human history, an increase in weight and girth has been viewed as a sign of health and prosperity. In Chinese culture this is still the case for young children in urban areas and for both children and adults in rural areas. Our study found that children and their parents preferred a large body size for boys and a small body size for girls. The prevalence of obesity in children who preferred a large body size was significantly increased. Children of parents who preferred a large body size were also more likely to be obese. Perceptions of body size may affect eating behavior and the management of body weight, which in turn will influence the development of obesity. The underlying mechanism of these phenomena needs to be explored in the future.

SUGGESTIONS

The following are some suggestions for reducing obesity in children:

1. **Identify factors influencing the trend to obesity in developing countries.** There is limited information from developing countries on factors contributing to the development of childhood obesity. The influence of current changes in dietary patterns, lifestyle, social structure, and culture on the increasing trend to obesity should be analyzed. Recommendations can then be made for developing public health policies and programs for preventing and managing obesity nationwide.
2. **Develop a national prevention strategy.** As undernutrition is still the major public health problem in developing countries, obesity has not received enough attention in most of these countries, although its prevalence has increased dramatically in the past two decades. It is clear that obesity is difficult to cure once it is established; the most effective and economical strategy is to prevent it. National public policy should be developed to face this new challenge in public health. The strategy should be targeted at reducing the prevalence of obesity in the population as a whole. A framework of health promotion in schools should be adopted to foster a healthy lifestyle in children.

REFERENCES

1. World Health Organization. *Obesity: preventing and managing the global epidemic.* Report on a WHO consultation on obesity (WHO/NUT/NCD/98.1). Geneva: WHO, 1997.
2. Onis M, Blossner M. Prevalence and trends of overweight among preschool children in developing countries. *Am J Clin Nutr* 2000; 72: 1032–9.
3. Martorell R, Khan K, Hughes ML, Grummer-Strawn LM. Overweight and obesity in preschool children from developing countries. *Int J Obes* 2000; 24: 959–67.
4. Ding ZY, He Q, Fan ZH, *et al.* National epidemiological study on obesity of children aged 0–7 years in China 1996. *Natl Med J China* 1998; 78: 121–3.
5. Kei LK. National strategies to reduce the incidence of obesity (Singapore). Symposium proceedings of 12th International Symposium on Maternal and Infant Nutrition. Heinz Institute of Nutritional Science, Guangzhou, 1998: 158–64.
6. Neutzling MB, Taddei JAAC, Rodrigues EM, Sigulem DM. Overweight and obesity in Brazilian adolescents. *Int J Obes* 2000; 24: 869–74.
7. Comuzzie AG, Allison DB. The search for human obesity genes. *Science* 1998; 280: 1374–7.
8. Hill JO, Peters JC. Environmental contributions to the obesity epidemic. *Science* 1998; 29: 1371–4.
9. National Bureau of Statistics. *China statistical yearbook 2000.* Beijing: China Statistics Press, 2000.
10. Research Group on Physical Fitness and Health Surveillance in Chinese School Children. *Report of the 1995 national survey on physical fitness and health status in Chinese students.* Jilin: Jilin Scientific Technology Publishing House, 1996.
11. Chen CHM. Fat intake and nutritional status of children in China. *Am J Clin Nutr* 2000; 72: 1368–72.
12. Centers for Disease Control. Update: prevalence of overweight among children, adolescents, and adults in the United States, 1988–1994. *MMWR* 1997; 46: 199–202.

13. Dietz WH, Gortmaker ST. Factors within the physical environment associated with childhood obesity. *Am J Clin Nutr* 1984; 39: 619–24.

14. Ding ZY, Zhang X, Huang Z. The epidemiological study on obesity of children 0–7 years old in urban area in China. *Acta Nutr Sinica* 1989; 11: 266–75.

15. Sobal J, Stunkard AJ. Socioeconomic status and obesity: a review of literature. *Psychol Bull* 1989; 105: 260–75.

16. Arteaga H, Dos Santos JE, Dutra de Oliveira JE. Obesity among schoolchildren of different socioeconomic levels in a developing country. *Int J Obes* 1982; 6: 291–7.

17. Ge KY, Zhai FY. *The dietary and nutritional status of the Chinese population – children and adolescents.* Beijing: People's Medical Publishing House, 1999.

18. Wolfe WS, Campbell CC, Frongillo EA, Haas JD, Melnik TA, Overweight schoolchildren in New York State: prevalence and characteristics. *Am J Public Health* 1994; 84: 807–13.

19. Yang NH, Zhou YZH, Mao LM. Survey on the prevalence and factors affecting obesity in schoolchildren in Wuhan. Proceedings of Danone Institute China, 3rd Annual Symposium, Beijing, 2000: 62–5.

20. Guldan GS, Cheung ILT, Chui KKH, Childhood obesity in Hong Kong: embracing an unhealthy lifestyle before puberty. Proceedings of the 12th International Symposium on Maternal and Infant Nutrition, Heinz Institute of Nutritional Sciences, Guangzhou, 1998: 35–57.

21. Ortega RM, Requejo AM, Lopez-Sobaler AM, *et al.* Difference in the breakfast habits of overweight/obese and normal weight schoolchildren. *Int J Vitam Nutr Res* 1998; 68: 125–32.

22. Jeffery RW, French SA. Epidemic obesity in the United States: are fast foods and television viewing contributing? *Am J Public Health* 1998; 88: 277–80.

23. Wu J, Ma GS, Hu XQ, *et al.* Eating fast food practices of Chinese children and adolescents in four cities. *Chinese J School Health* 2000; 21: 244–6.

24. Dietz WH, Gortmaker SL. Do we fatten our children at the television set? Obesity and television viewing in children and adolescents. *Pediatrics* 1985; 75: 807–12.

25. Gortmaker SL, Must A, Sobol AM, *et al.* Television viewing as a cause of increasing obesity among children in the United States, 1986–1990. *Arch Pediatr Adolesc Med* 1996; 150: 356–62.

26. Lissner L, Heitmann BL. Dietary fat and obesity: evidence from epidemiology. *Eur J Clin Nutr* 1995; 49: 79–90.

27. Shapiro LR, Crawford PB, Clark, MJ, Pearson DL, Raz J, Huenemann RL. Obesity prognosis: a longitudinal study of children from children age of 6 months to 9 years. *Am J Public Health* 1984; 74: 968–72.

28. Maffeis C, Talamini G, Tato L. Influence of diet, physical activity, and parent's obesity on children's adiposity: a four year longitudinal study. *Int J Obes* 1998; 22: 758–64.

29. Moore LL, Nguyen USD, Rothman KJ, Cupples LA, Ellison RC. Preschool physical activity level and change in body fatness in young children. The Framingham children's study. *Am J Epidemiol* 1995; 142: 982–8.

30. Popkin BM. The nutrition transition in low-income countries: an emerging crisis. *Nutr Rev* 1994; 52: 285–98.

DISCUSSION

Dr. Ismail: In your summary, you said that television viewing was related to obesity in China, but from the bar graph you showed, this did not seem to have much influence on boys, though it had a rather big effect on girls. Could you comment on that?

Dr. Ma: You are right, there were sex differences in obesity prevalence for girls and boys, and their TV viewing times were different. I don't have any explanation for this phenomenon at present—these are just the preliminary results of my study and I don't know the underlying mechanism.

Dr. Dietz: It's fascinating to see the parallels with obesity in the United States and elsewhere. Does your recognition, and Dr. Chen's, of obesity as a public health problem make this a priority public health concern for China? If not, what institutional changes would have to occur to make it a public health problem?

Dr. Ma: In the scientific arena we believe that obesity in urban China has now definitely become a health concern. We know that obese children are more likely to become obese adults, and that the prevalence of obesity in children has reached epidemic levels, so if we don't take action now the problem will get out of hand. We also know that obesity is related to certain chronic diseases, and that the direct and indirect costs of obesity amount to a substantial proportion of national health care. For these reasons, we believe that in urban China obesity should be regarded as a public health priority.

Dr. Dietz: I agree, but what I was asking was how do you *know* when you have made it a priority? For example, in the United States, the CDC recognizes obesity as a priority public health problem, the surgeon general of the United States has recognized obesity as a priority problem, but Congress has not. So what I am asking is whether it is sufficient for the Chinese Academy of Preventive Medicine to recognize this as a problem, or how will you know that you have succeeded in making it a priority?

Dr. Ma: I think that question should be answered by Madam Chen, as she represents the Chinese Obesity Task Force.

Dr. Chen: Your question is of critical importance, because obesity has not yet been established in China as a public health concern. Even among the medical fraternity it is not taken very seriously. We therefore organized a working group on obesity in China to collect scientific evidence that would convince the policy makers about the cost and future danger of obesity in children and adults. Obesity is a big problem in China, the prevalence of overweight being about 30% in adults. The policy makers need to be informed about the economic costs this will entail in the future. The current priority is to collect evidence. At present, we don't have good data on physical activity and the factors associated with obesity in children. We are considering the possibility of international collaboration to investigate the current situation and make informed predictions of future economic and health implications of obesity in China.

Dr. Shen: I also have a comment about this issue. I absolutely agree with Dr. Chen's view that we need evidence to convince the government. Everybody in this room believes that obesity has become a serious problem. However, it is another matter to convince government officials, who need the evidence to be presented in understandable form. In the next 5 or 10 years, epidemiologic studies will be of critical importance. Furthermore they should not be limited to the east coast of China but should be done nationwide. If all the Chinese delegates in this room, who come from different parts of China, can work together to undertake a nationwide epidemiologic study, that would be of the greatest value.

Dr. Bar-Or: Following up this question, let's suppose we are now 10 years older and you have the evidence. How do you think the Chinese authorities will implement the recommendations? As a Canadian, the scene I'm familiar with is that it's very hard to convince the Canadian government that something should be done, and even if we do manage to convince them, they often do not have a very clear idea of what to do about it. So what would you think would happen in the Chinese scenario when the evidence is provided?

Dr. Ma: We can only provide the evidence and hope we can persuade the government to develop an obesity intervention policy. The Scientific Committee can continue to press for obesity intervention as well. The involvement of the mass media is also very important. Many people are aware that obesity is a public health concern, and sometimes if the push comes at grass roots level this may be an effective way of persuading the government to take action.

Dr. Shen: I can give you an example of the government's response to another problem. My research area is mainly related to the prevention of lead poisoning in Chinese children. I started working on this problem 12 years ago. Before that time, although lead poisoning was considered a problem in the United States and Western Europe, this was not the case in China. However, about 12 years ago I discovered that the blood lead level of children in Shanghai was extremely high—much higher than in children in the United States. I therefore decided to do a nationwide epidemiologic study and found the prevalence of lead poisoning to be very high by the standards provided by the US CDC. I also found that the high lead level was extremely harmful to children's development, reducing the IQ and causing behavior problems. And after 3 to 5 years of work on this problem, I found that the principal source of lead in China is leaded gasoline. In a pilot study I proved that removal of lead from gasoline resulted in a reduction in the blood lead level. I presented these data to the Ministry of Public Health and the Mayor of Shanghai, and they were very supportive, providing me with a very large grant for a large-scale study. About 5 years later, that is 3 years ago, the government decided on the basis of my data that leaded gasoline should be phased out in the whole of China. This is a success story about how the government responds to scientific research. I believe that if we can provide sufficient evidence about obesity, the government will respond appropriately.

Dr. Sung: I'm interested in the different prevalences of obesity in the four cities you investigated. Obesity appears to be most common in the northeast of China, which is less well off economically than the other regions you studied. What is the reason for that? Do you use one growth chart for the whole country? I have the impression that people in the north are of a larger build than in the south. If you use the same growth chart for both regions, this may give the impression of more obesity in the north.

Dr. Ma: Well, as you know, the dietary pattern in China varies according to region. For example, in the south of China rice is the staple, whereas in the north it is wheat. I carried out analyses between 1982 and 1992 but found no difference in average energy intakes in the different regions. Maybe genetic factors play a role. People in the northern part of China are usually taller than in the south. Regarding growth charts, we use a Chinese standard for weight for height, based on the Chinese Physical Fitness and Health Survey conducted in 1985. We use the same weight-for-height standard in the whole country. There are some arguments about the validity of this standard, but if we were to use different standards in different regions it would be very hard to make comparisons.

Dr. Buenaluz: You had a chart showing increased energy consumption from fat in Chinese children. How were these data obtained? Did you do a dietary survey?

Dr. Ma: Yes, this result was based on a dietary survey. We obtained data on food intakes of all the individuals in the household and then calculated the individual dietary intakes.

Dr. Buenaluz: My concern is that when we have conducted dietary surveys in this way we find that sometimes the family does not want to reveal their actual consumption.

Dr. Chen: Consumption was assessed by weighing and by diary records, so we feel the assessments were quite accurate. The observations were summed for each household member, and the housewife also made an assessment of the proportions consumed by individual family members. We think that the fat measurements were probably more accurate than the other nutrients, because all the oils were weighed by the interviewers.

Dr. Huang: I'm interested in your finding that obesity is more common in boys than in girls in China. How do you explain that phenomenon?

Dr. Ma: That is an interesting question. One possible explanation may be a genetic effect. There could also be sociocultural influences. For example, most parents and indeed children think that a desirable body size for boys is large and for girls is small. People think that if you are a boy you should eat more food and look stronger. Also, boys like movie action stars, and there are many role models on TV commercials.

Dr. Dulloo: When dietary fat increases, one needs to consider the type of fat. In Malaysia it's palm oil; in Thailand it's coconut oil. What kind of oil do you use in China? That would be relevant to the effect on plasma fatty acids.

Dr. Ma: We use mainly vegetable oils such as soy oil and corn oil.

Dr. Dulloo: Is it polyunsaturated? φ-6? Is it like palm oil, which is very different in its fatty acid composition? These aspects can affect energy balance.

Dr. Ma: The soy oil and corn oil are similar to what is used in other countries such as the United States. In some parts of China animal fats are popular, particularly pig fat.

Dr. Dulloo: This would need to be quantified in the future.

Dr. Ma: Yes, a lot needs to be done, especially in relation to the correlations between physical activity patterns, diet, and the development of obesity. This was just a preliminary study. There have been very few studies focusing on the factors contributing to obesity. We need to do more in the future.

Obesity in Childhood and Adolescence, edited by
Chunming Chen and William H. Dietz. Nestlé
Nutrition Workshop Series, Pediatric Program,
Vol. 49. Nestec Ltd., Vevey/Lippincott
Williams & Wilkins, Philadelphia © 2002.

Conventional Treatment for Childhood and Adolescent Obesity

Kate S. Steinbeck

Departments of Endocrinology and Adolescent Medicine, Royal Prince Alfred Hospital and University of Sydney, Sydney, Australia

The WHO International Obesity Task Force (IOTF) concluded that the growing worldwide prevalence of obesity in children (and adults) is today's neglected public health problem (1). The IOTF argues that obesity management to achieve weight loss in the overweight and obese and obesity prevention to prevent weight gain in those of normal weight should not be considered separate clinical and public health issues. This approach runs counter to the manner in which conventional treatment of obesity is generally provided.

There has been an increase over the past decades in the number of publications on the treatment of childhood and adolescent obesity (Fig. 1). Most of these publications do not provide a strong evidence base for obesity management, being short term and uncontrolled.

CONVENTIONAL TREATMENT

The accepted components of obesity management in children and adolescents, as indeed for adults, are shown in Table 1 (1). Evidence supporting the efficacy of these strategies, particularly in the medium term (≥ 12 months), is quite limited. The 1997 systematic review of the treatment and prevention of obesity by Glenny *et al.* (3) identified 13 randomized controlled trials in children and adolescents with a minimum of 12 months of follow-up, including intervention time. The studies were small, usually less than 20 subjects per group, and although all were randomized, attrition rates ranged up to 56% and only one study provided an "intention-to-treat" analysis. Outcome data were almost exclusively concerned with changes in the degree of overweight, and none reported broader health outcomes.

Overall, the studies to guide evidence-based practice in the management of childhood and adolescent obesity are limited in number, scope, quality, and size. However, the work of Epstein and colleagues, spanning more than 20 years (4–7), demands attention. The children in Epstein's studies were between 8 and 12 years of age, were at least 20% heavier than ideal body weight (IBW), and had one parent willing to attend the sessions. Main exclusions were psychiatric disturbance,

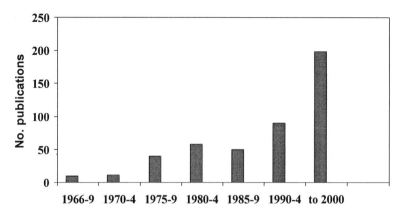

FIG. 1. The number of publications on childhood and adolescent obesity management over the last four decades.

learning disability, and significant medical illness. The families recruited were predominantly white, intact families from higher socioeconomic groups. There was a cash deposit, which was returned according to the number of sessions attended.

Subjects were seen in groups, generally with children and parents separately. The intervention was between 2 and 6 months with decreasing frequency of contact, followed by a maintenance period of 12 months. The intervention was structured behavioral modification and diet, either with or without prescribed physical activity. Prescribed physical activity included programmed group aerobic exercise, lifestyle exercise, home walking programs, and reduction in sedentary activity. Attrition rates were about 20%. Follow-up weight data on children and parents exist for up to 120 months.

The main findings of Epstein's studies are as follows:

- Better weight outcomes were achieved if parents and children were seen separately.
- The addition of physical activity improved 12-month weight outcomes.
- Children were better at maintaining weight loss in the long term than their parents.

Adolescents are generally viewed as a more difficult therapeutic group. The normal issues and tasks of adolescence, which include independence from family and conformity with peer group, detract from conventional management regimens. In

TABLE 1. *Conventional treatments for childhood and adolescent obesity*

1. Reduction of energy intake by dietary modification, and using conventional foods
2. Increase in energy expenditure by an increase in physical activity
   2.1 Planned
   2.2 Lifestyle or incidental
3. Increase in energy expenditure by a decrease in sedentary activity
4. Modification of behaviors and habits associated with eating and activity
5. Involvement of the family in the process of change

addition, older adolescents have lost height growth as a means of weight reduction. Puberty may already have exacerbated the degree of overweight, and medical morbidity is more prevalent. Earlier studies have identified parental participation and frequency of contact as improving weight loss (8,9).

Brownell *et al.* (8) treated 12- to 16-year-olds using three different therapeutic strategies—child alone, mother and child together, and mother and child separately (MCS). Although numbers were small, MCS showed both the greatest loss and the greatest maintenance of loss. MCS had a -17.1% relative overweight change at the end of the 4-month intervention, which was maintained at the 6- and 12-month follow-up, compared with the other two groups, which achieved a -5% change at these time points. Blood pressure as an index of morbidity fell with successful weight management. Weight change in children was not associated with significant weight change in mothers.

Coates *et al.* (9) required study subjects to attend a 1-hour group session five times a week for 10 weeks, with emphasis on reduced energy intake and behavioral modification. Subjects were followed for another 5 weeks of problem-solving sessions and then at weekly weigh-ins to week 20. The group, which had daily contact and had a monetary reward contingent on weight loss, achieved the most weight reduction: $+37.5\%$ overweight to $+25\%$ overweight at week 15, although a trend to slow regain was already apparent by week 20.

In 1987 Mellin *et al.* (10) published an evaluation of a practical intervention for adolescents—the *Shapedown Program.* The program can be used as self-instruction, individual counseling, or group program and is in a self-directed change format that encourages sustainable, successive modifications in diet, exercise, relationships, lifestyle, communications, and attitudes. There is separate parental material, which considers strategies for support, modification of the environment, and improved parenting style. There were 14 90-minute weekly adolescent sessions and two parent sessions. Subjects were between 14 and 18 years of age and most were female. The mean change for the intervention group was -5.9%, -6.2%, -9.9% reduction in relative overweight at 3, 6, and 15 months, respectively, compared with control figures of -0.3%, -5.2%, and -0.1%, respectively.

MEDIUM- TO LONG-TERM FOLLOW-UP DATA FOR WEIGHT MANAGEMENT OUTCOMES

Though it appears that various weight management programs in children and adolescents can achieve short-term results, there is a need for evidence about interventions that achieve success in the long term. Only Epstein's group has very long-term data over 10 years (4). The mean percentage change in overweight was -18%, -5%, and -5% at 6, 60, and 160 months, respectively, with children stabilizing their degree of overweight at 5 years. Thirty percent of children achieved a 20% reduction in overweight at 10 years (compared with 3% of parents). The longer the loss sustained in the early postintervention period, the better the long-term outcome. No negative effects on long-term growth and development were found.

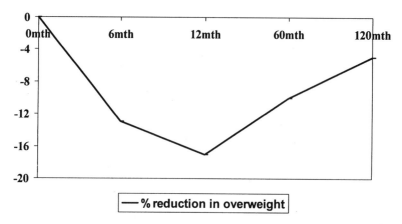

FIG. 2. The pattern of percent reduction in overweight children and adolescents subjected to conventional weight management strategies of up to 6 months' duration. This figure is a composite of five studies of varying duration of follow-up (maximum 10 years).

Gately *et al.* (11) reported a study in nearly 200 overweight children (mean age, 12.6 years) who attended an 8-week summer camp specifically for weight loss. Conventional strategies included increased physical activity, moderate dietary restriction, and behavior modification. Fifty percent of the original group reenrolled in 12 months, having had no formal follow-up. The mean standardized body mass index (BMI) scores for those reenrolling were +3.6, +2.4, and +2.7 at 0, 8, and 52 weeks, indicating weight loss and maintenance of that loss.

Nuutinen and Knip (12) treated 48 children between 6 and 16 years of age. Individual, group-, and school-based interventions were used, which concentrated on diet and behavioral change. The intervention was 12 months, followed by 12 months of observation and another review at 60 months. There was no difference in the success rate between the three treatment groups, with success defined as a 10% or more reduction in relative overweight. At the end of 12 months the mean change in overweight in the successful group was -24.7%, and -17.8% at 5 years. At 5 years, one-third of those measured had a normal weight for height. There were no recorded predictors of success at weight loss, but those who had success in weight management achieved a more favorable lipid profile and a 30% reduction in fasting insulin.

Figure 2, taken from combined datasets, represents pictorially the expected pattern of long-term weight loss outcomes using conventional management strategies.

HOW CHILDREN REACH CONVENTIONAL TREATMENT

Not every child and adolescent who needs treatment is referred. The choice of referral is made for them. Such referral figures are not generally accessible, but the gatekeeper is often the primary care physician. Knowledge and beliefs about childhood obesity may dictate the frequency of referral.

THE PROVIDERS OF CONVENTIONAL TREATMENT

If only published data are considered, then the conventional treatment of childhood and adolescent obesity generally uses a multidisciplinary team. Physicians, dietitians, physiotherapists, nurse practitioners, and counselors may be involved. In view of the high prevalence of overweight and obesity in the community, it should be possible for weight management to be provided by a number of different types of health professionals and by those whose time does not come at high monetary cost. Given the strong genetic component of obesity, the management of childhood and adolescent obesity could also be addressed in adult weight management programs.

SETTINGS FOR CONVENTIONAL TREATMENT

Overall management strategies need to be transferable and not dependent on a particular setting for success. Many settings have been utilized (Table 2). Inpatient treatment is not strictly conventional, is high cost and short-term, but can demonstrate that weight loss is possible. A hospital clinic allows contact with multiple health professionals but may have limited access. The doctor's office provides local access and a medical assessment, but expertise, time constraints, and cost may influence the quality of the service.

Community health centers provide local access, a multidisciplinary approach, and competence in group programs. Camps provide day-long intervention, with a high physical activity component, structure, and supervision, but are short term and somewhat artificial. School-based management acknowledges that children and adolescents spend a significant portion of time in school, and a weight management program can be combined with an established health syllabus. There are, however, disadvantages, which include targeting of children who may already be experiencing teasing and bullying.

Braet *et al.* (13) have recently reviewed their group's experience of different settings for their basic program: group, individual, summer camp, or "advice in one session." The basic program incorporated healthy eating combined with cognitive behavior therapy. The group and individual settings were seven 90-minute, twice-monthly sessions, followed by seven monthly family follow-up sessions. The 10-day camp included daily lifestyle exercises for 5 hours a day and then monthly follow-up. The mean weight losses for group, individual, camp, and "advice-in-one-session" settings at the end of 12 months were 13.1%, 9.8%, 14.7%, and 6.8%, respectively, with controls showing a 2.5% gain. Those children who were less than 55% overweight and less than 14 years of age showed the greatest relative weight loss. The more time-efficient options (one-session advice, group, and camp) did as well as individual management. Additionally, group-based approaches match established

TABLE 2. *Settings for conventional treatment of obese children and adolescents*

1. Hospital	3. Community health service	5. School
2. Doctor's office	4. Camps	

health care delivery patterns in community settings, are accessible to large numbers of overweight children and their families, foster social support, share problem solving, and provide access to successful models.

THE EVIDENCE FOR THE COMPONENTS OF CONVENTIONAL TREATMENT

Dietary Modification

Dietary intervention in children tends to reflect adult management trends. Thus older studies were rather prescriptive. More recently, low fat and healthy eating utilizing general guidelines have been employed. A low-glycemic-index diet has been suggested as useful in childhood obesity management, but the study was short term and retrospective (14).

Epidemiologic evidence suggests a positive association between dietary fat intake and obesity (15). A recent metaanalysis (16) concluded that a reduction in dietary fat without restriction of total energy intake is effective in producing weight loss in overweight *adult* subjects. There is some cross-sectional evidence that children who are overweight have higher fat intakes (17), but no prospective data. Thus there are no studies in obese children or adolescents that evaluate the role of low-fat diets for weight loss. There are numerous metabolic reasons why a high-fat diet may compromise the regulation of energy balance, particularly in those with a genetic predisposition to obesity and low levels of activity. Focusing on fat—and hence on eating habits, food shopping, and the type of food, rather than on quantity and dietary restriction—may also be an important strategy to support the development of the child's capacity to self-regulate intake. The Dietary Intervention Study in Children (DISC) used a low-fat *ad libitum* diet in children for the primary purpose of reducing low-density lipoprotein (LDL) cholesterol (18). DISC has provided long-term evidence in a population of children between 8 and 10 years of age and not selected for obesity showing that such a diet does not compromise nutritional status or growth and development. There was also no sustained weight change over time with the intervention group.

A low-fat *ad libitum* diet will generally provide a daily fat intake of 55 g, which approximates to 25% of the energy intake. This level of fat intake was achieved by 10% of Australian children 6 to 10 years of age in the 1995 National Nutrition Survey, whereas an additional 20% of children had fat intakes of around 25% to 30% of dietary energy. This level of fat intake is recommended by the IOTF as necessary to minimize energy imbalance in sedentary individuals, can be readily achieved while maintaining palatability and acceptability, will principally reduce saturated fat, and will not compromise micronutrient intake (19).

Dietary intervention should follow the national nutrition guidelines, use low-fat food preparation, and choose low-fat protein foods. The quantity of animal protein often needs to be reduced and meat alternatives considered. More fruit and vegetables should be consumed and healthier snack food choices need to be available. Such an intervention thus aims for an overall reduction in energy intake by reducing both energy-dense (high-fat) foods and portion size. Low-fat *ad libitum* diets in the clinical situation must be prescribed as "until you no longer feel hungry," and do not mean "as much as you want." Additionally, special-occasion or "treat" foods need to be limited. Healthier take-out food choices need to be encouraged, and parties and social occasions should be actively managed. Breakfast must always be eaten. Obese children tend to avoid eating in public (because of teasing) and therefore tend to overeat in the evening. As a result, they do not feel hungry at breakfast. The amount of nutrients taken as liquid should be limited, with water used for quenching thirst.

It is advisable to refrain from calorie counting or food weighing. These practices are difficult, time-consuming, and inaccurate, and they have a low compliance. One or two dietary changes at a time should be made, and when these are well in place, the next ones should be made. The therapist must be sensitive to sociocultural issues and preferences, and should continue to emphasize that the changes are *forever*. It is best to avoid the word *diet,* which for most persons has very temporary connotations. All family members, whatever their body mass, should consume similar types of food.

Increasing Physical Activity

Energy expenditure as a result of movement is of great importance when addressing the treatment of overweight and obesity (20). Physical activity in children can be planned or incidental, and incidental activity includes spontaneous physical activity (wriggling and fidgeting), a behavior that is often actively discouraged in children.

Although the enhancement of physical activity is a component of weight management programs, studies tend not to define the relative contribution of physical activities or to quantify compliance. Only recently has this been done in adults (21), in a study that showed that if the energy deficit induced by exercise was identical to that induced by dietary intervention, then the weight loss was identical. The enhanced activity prescriptions in childhood obesity management are unlikely to induce such a large degree of energy deficit. Epstein and co-workers provide some evidence for an additional advantage of physical activity, and this group has shown that decreasing sedentary behavior is as effective in short-term weight management in children as increasing active behavior (5).

Prompting children to be active increases activity, and parental physical activity has an influence on children's activity. It appears that the parent–child relation for inactivity is stronger than the relation for more vigorous activity, for both obese and control children (22). Thus interventions to raise energy expenditure should involve strategic targeting at both individual and family levels to increase physical activity and modify sedentary behavior (23). An emphasis on choice and a reduction in sedentary behavior are likely to be more successful in producing long-term weight control. Programs that encourage skill development can affect longer-term activity patterns and choices in children through to adulthood (24), and may be beneficial for longer-term weight maintenance.

Parental involvement is essential in a range of practical ways: encouragement, accompanying children to recreation areas, increasing their own physical involvement in the chosen activities, monitoring TV use, and providing alternatives to sedentary behavior. There are no pediatric data to support a specific time or intensity-based activity prescription in obesity management. A range of daily after-school activities and weekly family-based initiatives, with an emphasis on outside activities, should be prescribed, as these characteristics of activity reflect total activity patterns (25).

In summary, any activity where energy has to be used can be included, with the aim of doing more than previously. In the beginning, not too much emphasis should be placed on intensity. The duration and intensity of any chosen activity should be gradually increased. Children and adolescents should choose activities that they like and that are fun. Families need to be reminded that physical activity is not just sport or similar planned activity. There needs to be a strong emphasis on increased lifestyle or incidental activity, and a constant goal of decreasing sedentary time.

Behavioral Modification Interventions and Habit Change

These interventions are based on the use of cognitive strategies, behavioral strategies, education, and motivation. As most obesity studies use some type of behavioral intervention, it is difficult to isolate the individual effect of this component, and such strategies should be considered integral to any management program that seeks long-term changes in human behavior.

Parenting skills training may well facilitate behavioral change in children. Family interactions and the parents' role in determining and responding to their children's food choice and mealtime behavior play an important role in problem eating behavior in children, which may contribute to the development of obesity (25). There is a paucity of controlled outcome research examining the role of parenting interventions in the management of childhood obesity. The work of Golan *et al.* (26,27) provides some interesting evidence for parents as the sole agents of change in weight management in children. Their hypothesis is that the "focus on manipulating the environment using parents as the main agent of change and strengthening their leadership skills would help the children overcome resistance to change and take the focus off them being identified as the (obese) patient." Children between 6 and 11 years of age, more than 20% above expected weight, with both parents living at home and agreeable to meeting all study requirements formed the study group. In the experimental intervention only the parents attended group sessions, whereas in the conventional intervention only the children attended the group sessions. Dietary instruction (centered on reduced saturated fat), alteration in sedentary behavior, and behavioral modification were the management strategies. In the parent group there was an emphasis on general parenting skills.

The main outcomes were:

- Children in the experimental group decreased overweight by 14.6% (compared with 8.4% in the conventional intervention).
- Neither intervention resulted in an increase in physical activity time for children.
- There was a positive relation between reduction in overweight and changes in eating styles, particularly a decrease in eating between meals and in eating with accompanied activity.

Golan's work accords with clinical experience and the recognition that a developmentally appropriate approach to management of obesity in childhood is important.

Behavioral interventions focus on dietary and activity change. Such behavioral modification has to be addressed in an age-appropriate manner. In the preschool years a wide range of foods should be encouraged and children must ask for and not just take food. Continuous grazing should be avoided, as should manipulative battles over food. Play must be taught and encouraged and television limited. Walking should be encouraged so that endurance is increased, even though the obese child may initially complain of discomfort. Habits start at this age, so parents need to work on those habits that they do not wish continued.

For primary school–age children, parents should still be in control of foods coming into the house, but they are not totally in control of what their children eat outside the house. Parents should ensure that breakfast is eaten and still encourage children to ask for rather than take food. Encouraging play and playmates, and limiting computer and video games as well as television are still important strategies. Involving the child in physical household tasks is an effective means of increasing physical activity and spending time with the child. Children of this age will respond well to self-monitoring of behavior change, using star or sticker charts.

During adolescence eating is often independent of family and home, but families can still set healthy eating examples. Adolescents need involvement in both meal choice and food preparation. Healthy food choices should be praised, but families should avoid making a big issue of less healthy choices. Weight maintenance may have to be accepted if progress to weight loss is too difficult. Parents and therapists should recognize the adolescent's emerging maturity, but continue to set limits and define boundaries. The overweight adolescent is likely to have already experienced personal failure at weight loss and observed similar failures in other family members. Adolescents need to gain confidence in managing other aspects of their life before they have enough confidence to manage their weight.

Active parenting is a specific aspect of family behavioral change, where behavior modeling is as important as instruction. An assertive parenting style is necessary, rather than being too aggressive or too passive. Discipline is a way of setting controls or boundaries and is required by all children and adolescents. Discipline can be achieved by modeling, using various and positive rewards and having realistic expectations.

BARRIERS TO CONVENTIONAL TREATMENT

In any conventional management of obesity in children and adolescents it is important to address beliefs that are likely to interfere with effective management.

Obesity will reduce or disappear during puberty. Tracking data clearly do not support this belief.

Restrictive food practices in childhood will induce an eating disorder. This concern emphasizes the importance of physical activity as a weight management strategy, because attention is deflected from food and eating. Data show that obese children and adolescents are at risk of, or already have, disordered eating (28).

Dietary restriction will impair normal growth and development. Approximately 2% to 4% of daily energy requirements are used for growth. Obese children are overnourished, and a slowing of excessive growth velocity (in response to overnourishment) is a normal phenomenon in successful management.

Obesity equates with health. This belief is more prevalent in cultures where deprivation and poor childhood health are within parental memory. Obese children have well-documented morbidity.

OUTCOME INDICATORS IN THE CONVENTIONAL MANAGEMENT OF CHILDHOOD AND ADOLESCENT OBESITY

Outcome indicators are shown in Table 3. Weight change remains the primary outcome, but there are no data to indicate how much is enough or optimal. Children and adolescents are generally still growing. It may be necessary only to halt weight gain and to allow the child or adolescent to grow into their current body weight. This observation does not apply to the older adolescent or the extremely obese child.

In children and adolescents there must be standardization of fatness measures. BMI must be age adjusted. The BMI SD score is excellent for statistical manipulation but is clinically impractical. Monitoring of height and weight on a growth centile chart has practical clinical value. This is particularly so if weight maintenance is the agreed goal. As children continue to attain height, their weight centiles come closer to matching their height centiles. Waist circumference can be used as an indirect measure of reducing truncal adiposity (29). Skinfold measurements are not clinically useful owing to measurement difficulties, including subject acceptability and intra- and intertester reliability.

A reduction in BMI has been associated with improved metabolic indicators in adults. There is no Level One (high quality) evidence from trials in children. The study by Sasaki *et al.* (30) focused on cardiovascular risk reduction in 41 children. This was a school-based program, and the obese children had an extra 300-kcal daily deficit of aerobic activity, but with no dietary intervention. There was a 50% reduction in the degree of overweight at 12 months, with a slight further change at 24 months. There was a significant increase in high-density lipoprotein cholesterol and a less marked change in triglycerides over the same period.

The Nuutinen and Knip study (12) discussed earlier also shows the value of improvements in metabolic profile in a conventional treatment program. Even in the

TABLE 3. *Outcome indicators in the conventional treatment of obesity in children and adolescents*

Primary	Secondary
Body fatness (weight)	Medical morbidity: sleep apnea
	Metabolic status: hypertension, lipids, insulin
	Exercise capacity and endurance
	Eating behaviors
	Psychosocial function
	Family function

absence of significant weight change, such results would be regarded as clinically important, but their effects on long-term macrovascular morbidity associated with childhood obesity are unknown.

Habit change in weight management is important but does not always translate into weight change. Measuring dietary intake or physical activity is difficult, subject to reporting bias, and of uncertain reliability and validity. Self-monitoring of simple behavior change is, however, often incorporated, as children are familiar with this type of monitoring in other behavioral change settings.

As concerns have been raised about the effect on psychosocial well-being of weight management in obese children, it may be a fruitful area of research to use selected validated measures to assess the impact of interventions on child well-being and body image, parenting capacity, confidence, and satisfaction.

RESEARCH QUESTIONS AND POLICY DIRECTION

Suggestions for research questions and policy direction are outlined in Table 4. The prevalence of childhood and adolescent obesity demands that management occurs at a community level. Community intervention embodies principles of equity of access, knowledge of local needs, and reduced costs. Research is not a tradition at this point of care and needs to be fostered and supported by tertiary institutions. Research needs to be directed at the replication of studies such as Epstein's in primary care settings.

There is sound evidence over two decades that parental involvement is important in weight management. The relevant studies have primarily been in intact families, and the challenge is to adjust delivery to all family situations.

The messages for management should be consistent and congruent with the messages for prevention of overweight and obesity. Such messages include low-fat eating, portion size according to age, physical activity, and behavioral change. Management of established obesity could also be integrated with prevention initiatives. Evidence suggests that management has better results if the child is not excessively overweight and is younger, whereas the practice is often to adopt a "wait-and-see" approach. Increasing activity as a management focus still lags behind diet prescription and behavioral change. It is difficult both to increase physical activity consistently and to prescribe physical activity in an effective and suitably directive manner. Input from professionals, such as exercise physiologists, who traditionally have not focused on childhood and adolescent obesity, would be valuable.

TABLE 4. *Future directions in the conventional management of childhood and adolescent obesity*

1. Replication of weight management studies in children and adolescents in community settings.
2. Development of national guidelines for obesity management in children and adolescents.
3. Health professional education around obesity management in children and adolescents.
4. Long-term follow-up and evaluation of obesity management programs in children and adolescents.
5. Integration of obesity treatment with obesity prevention in children and adolescents.
6. Clinically useful measures of physical activity in children and adolescents.

There should be the development of national guidelines for the management of overweight and obesity in children and adolescents, in order to address specific local requirements. The evidence base will not at present be great, but further evidence cannot be awaited before guidelines are developed. Rather, the production of evidence should occur in parallel with well-designed demonstration studies.

Guidelines will allow for the education of health and other professionals. Obesity and overweight are not yet seen as the business of many sectors other than health. Obesity is a socially engineered problem with medical ramifications, and the responsibility for its management cannot remain exclusively in the health sector.

Therapists who treat obesity in children and adolescents need to evaluate their programs and to allow for outcome indicators other than weight change. There is little knowledge of what happens to those children and adolescents who drop out of treatment early. It is assumed that their outcomes are poor, but there is no proof of this. Evidence has been provided for short to medium-length interventions that induce a sustainable weight change. The optimum times for program delivery, review, and reinforcement to avoid significant relapse are unknown.

CONCLUSIONS

The conventional management of childhood and adolescent obesity has been addressed in the medical literature for decades. There is good evidence that children do better than adults in conventional weight management programs. There is strong evidence for the important role of parents in conventional management of childhood and adolescent obesity. Appropriate accessible management settings and long-term evaluation of the outcomes in these settings should be part of management in the twenty-first century.

REFERENCES

1. World Health Organisation. *Obesity. Preventing and managing the global epidemic.* Report of a WHO consultation on obesity (WHO/NUT/NCD/98.1). Geneva: WHO, 1998.
2. Steinbeck K, Aitken M, Droulers AM. *Growing up, not out; a weight management guide for families.* Sydney, Australia: Simon & Schuster, 1998.
3. Glenny A-M, O'Meara S, Melville A, Sheldon TA, Wilson C. The treatment and prevention of obesity: a systematic review of the literature. *Int J Obes* 1997; 21: 715–37.
4. Epstein LH, Valoski A, Wing RR, McCurley J. Ten-year follow up of behavioral family based treatment of obese children. *JAMA* 1990; 264: 2519–23.
5. Epstein LH, Paluch RA, Gordy CC, Darn J. Decreasing sedentary behaviors in treating pediatric obesity. *Arch Pediatr Adolesc Med* 2000; 154: 220–6.
6. Epstein LH, Wing RR, Koeske R, Ossip D, Beck S. A comparison of lifestyle change and programmed aerobic fitness on weight and fitness changes in obese children. *Behav Ther* 1982; 13: 651–65.
7. Epstein LH, Valoski AM, Kalarchian MA, McCurley J. Do children lose and maintain weight easier than adults: a comparison of child and parent weight changes from six months to ten years. *Obes Res* 1995; 3: 411–7.
8. Brownell KD, Kelman JH, Stunkard AJ. Treatment of obese children with and without their mothers: changes in weight and blood pressure. *Pediatrics* 1993; 71: 12–6.
9. Coates YJ, Jeffery RW, Slinkard LA, Killen JD, Danaher BG. Frequency of contact and monetary reward in weight loss, lipid change and blood pressure reduction with adolescents. *Behav Ther* 1982; 13: 175–85.
10. Mellin LM, Slinkard LA, Irwin CE. Adolescent obesity intervention: validation of the SHAPEDOWN program. *J Am Diet Assoc* 1987; 87: 333–8.

11. Gately PJ, Cooke CB, Butterly RJ, Mackreth P, Carroll S. The effects of a children's summer camp program on weight loss, with a 10 month follow-up. *Int J Obesity* 2000; 24: 1445–52.
12. Nuutinen O, Knip M. Long term weight control in obese children: persistence of treatment outcomes and metabolic change. *Int J Obes* 1992; 16: 279–87.
13. Braet C, Van Winckel M, Van Leeuwen K. Follow-up results of different treatment programs for obese children. *Acta Paediatr* 1997; 86: 397–402.
14. Speith LE, Harnish JD, Lenders CM, *et al.* A low-glycemic index diet in the treatment of pediatric obesity. *Arch Pediatr Adolesc Med* 2000; 154: 947–51.
15. Lissner L, Heitmann BL. Dietary fat and obesity:evidence from epidemiology. *Eur J Clin Nutr* 1995; 49: 79–90.
16. Astrup A, Ryan L, Grunwald GK, *et al.* The role of dietary fat in body fatness: evidence from a preliminary meta-analysis of ad-libitum low-fat dietary intervention studies. *Br J Nutr* 2000; 83: 25–32.
17. Gazzaniga JM, Burns TL. Relationship between diet composition and body fatness, with adjustment for resting energy expenditure and physical activity, in preadolescent children. *Am J Clin Nutr* 1993; 58: 21–8.
18. Writing Group for the DISC Collaborative Research Group. Efficacy and safety of lowering dietary fat and cholesterol in children with elevated low-density lipoprotein cholesterol. The Dietary Intervention Study in Children (DISC). *JAMA* 1995; 273: 1429–35.
19. Magarey AM, Daniels L, Boulton TJC. Reducing the fat content of children's diet: nutritional implications and practical considerations. *Aust J Nutr Diet* 1993; 50: 69–74.
20. Fox K. *Aetiology of obesity. III. Physical inactivity.* British Nutrition Foundation Task Force on Obesity. Oxford: Blackwell, 1999.
21. Ross R, Dagnone D, Jones PJ, *et al.* Reduction in obesity and related comorbid conditions after diet induced weight loss or exercise induced weight loss in men. A randomised controlled trial. *Ann Intern Med* 2000; 133: 92–103.
22. Fogelholm M, Nuutinen O, Pasanen M, Myohanen E, Saatela T. Parent–child relationship of physical activity patterns and obesity. *Int J Obes Relat Metab Disord* 1999; 23: 1262–8.
23. Gutin B, Riggs S, Ferguson M, Owen S. Description and process evaluation of a physical training program for obese children. *Res Q Exerc Sport* 1999; 70: 65–9.
24. Sallis J, Prochaska J, Taylor W. A review of correlates of physical activity of children and adolescents. *Med Sci Sports Exerc* 2000; 32: 963–75.
25. Wilkens SC, Kendrick OW, Stitt KR, Stinett N, Hammarlund VA. Family functioning is related to overweight in children. *J Am Diet Assoc* 1998; 98: 572–4.
26. Golan M, Fainaru M, Weizman A. Role of behaviour modification in the treatment of childhood obesity with the parents as the exclusive agents of change. *Int J Obes Relat Metab Disord* 1998; 22: 1217–24.
27. Golan M, Weizman A, Apter A, Fainaru M. Parents as the exclusive agents of change in the treatment of childhood obesity. *Am J Clin Nutr* 1998; 67: 1130–5.
28. Fairburn CG, Doll HA, Welch SL, Hay PJ, Davies BA, O'Connor ME. Risk factors for binge eating disorder: a community based, case control study. *Arch Gen Psychiatry* 1999; 55: 425–32.
29. Taylor RW, Jones IE, Williams SM, Goulding A. Evaluation of waist circumference, waist-to-hip ratio, and the conicity index as screening tools for high trunk fat mass, as measured by dual-energy X-ray absorptiometry, in children aged 3–19 y. *Am J Clin Nutr* 2000; 72: 490–5.
30. Sasaki J, Shindo M, Tanaka H, Ando M, Arakawa K. A long-term aerobic exercise program decreases the obesity index and increase the high density lipoprotein cholesterol concentration in obese children. *Int J Obes* 1987; 11: 339–45.

DISCUSSION

Dr. Srivastava: There are situations where the whole family is obese. It's difficult to tackle these situations. What is your approach in such cases?

Dr. Steinbeck: I agree this is very difficult, especially because in our experience not every family member will identify themselves as obese. We first ask them to state whether they consider themselves to be underweight, of normal weight, or overweight, and it's surprising how often only one child is identified as overweight. I think that by and large those families do poorly unless you can change their outlook. What we generally do under those circumstances is to aim for weight management in the family. We also work with a family therapist who is often useful in reframing the family's outlook.

Dr. Moore: I have a comment on the failure to recognize obesity. We have recently completed a study in obese and overweight children where we used two scales: a visual scale and a verbal scale. Both the children and the parents did much better on visual analog scale recognition of obesity than on the verbal scale. Using the visual scale, only one-third of the parents and children weren't prepared to acknowledge that the child was obese, whereas on the verbal scale, two-thirds of the children and two-thirds of the parents did not acknowledge that the child was overweight or obese. I think that has implications with regard to motivation. Do you have any comment about that?

Dr. Steinbeck: That's congruent with other observations. It is quite difficult to know how to address this issue without losing your patient before you've even started. If there seems to be a degree of "fat blindness" in our patients, we initially choose not to do too much about it and simply try to work with the presenting child, and through that child with the rest of the family. But this does raise a question about how we identify obese children, because I'm not certain that all members of the health profession are as eager as we are to do something about obesity. If the patients are not interested, then they are unlikely to raise the topic, and that's an important concept.

Dr. Birch: We have been presented with a lot of evidence about sex differences in relation to prevalence and so on. Do you have any comments about sex differences with respect to treatment?

Dr. Steinbeck: I have no comments at the pediatric level, but we run sex-specific programs for male and female adult patients and that is certainly effective. We haven't at this stage introduced pediatric sex-specific programs, though I think it would be desirable if resource intensive. Mixed groups are probably suitable for primary school children, but in adolescents one does need separate agendas—girls need more talking and boys need more action.

Dr. Rütishauser: In obese adolescents, what is the benefit of counseling both the adolescent and the parents? Is there any evidence about whether it is better to counsel them separately or to have joint sessions?

Dr. Steinbeck: I think the evidence is that you don't actually counsel them together. In my own view, weight management in adolescents is almost too late! It is an extremely difficult time for young people to lose weight—you need a degree of psychological energy for this that most adolescents don't have. I would go for separate counseling, and we try to have one person for the adolescent and one for the parents, so that there is a perception of confidentiality. One also needs to do what one can to support parenting skills.

Dr. Bar-Or: I would like to reemphasize two points that you made. One is regarding the studies of Epstein about long-term adherence to weight reduction programs and their benefits (1,2). I think we need to be very careful when interpreting these studies because of Epstein's approach to selecting the subjects. They excluded *a priori* children who seemed likely not to be compliant. Thus this was obviously a very highly selected group. I think it is important that other investigators repeat these studies. My other comment is regarding the possible danger of generating eating disorders when treating obese children. In our experience of nearly 2,000 children going through our program in the last 15 years, we had only two girls who became anorexic within 2 years. Thus I agree with you that the risk of this happening is really quite minuscule.

Dr. Steinbeck: Thank you for those two comments. I agree there are a lot of exclusions in Epstein's study groups, but I think it would be unwise to dismiss those studies. As you say, we need to try and replicate them in other settings. In relation to eating disorders, we have never had a patient develop anorexia nervosa. On testing, at least 20% of our children and adolescents have some form of binge eating, or secretive eating, and this starts quite young, from about 8 years onward.

Dr. Maffeis: Do you have any information about techniques to improve motivation in children and adolescents? How can one maintain motivation to continue with treatment?

Dr. Steinbeck: I don't have a magic answer and I don't think there is one. There are several things to consider. First, you need to have the involvement of somebody who is truly interested in being with adolescents. Second, as health professionals, we tend to try to do everything at once to solve the issue. Motivation appears to be greater in adolescents if you take time to find out what is most important and meaningful to them. This may not be what is most important and meaningful to you. You then need to tackle one goal or objective at a time. Nevertheless, this does not stop our dropout rate for adolescents being close to 50% at 12 months.

Dr. Koletzko: I thank the organizers for the opportunity to present a concept we developed in Munich in response to the large numbers of obese children there—some 12% in primary schools and 15% to 16% in secondary schools. It is very difficult to have physician-based treatment for such large numbers of children. We therefore developed a child-based behavioral intervention with attractive modern media, the Power Kids program. It is like a game—played like Monopoly if you like—and the emphasis is on children learning self-control to moderate their fat intake and physical activity, using token economy concepts. There are points for fat consumption, called Fatsy points (the child does not really need to understand that this is about fat consumption), there are points for physical activity, and points for inactivity, and there are reinforcement points (Winnie points). Of importance, there are no external (parental or physician) restrictions, and we have placed a lot of emphasis on building self-confidence and achieving success.

It is a structured program lasting 12 weeks. It looks difficult to the parents, but the children find it easy because it's already part of their way of life—a gamelike concept designed for children 8 to 12 years of age in which they need to read and calculate. The emphasis is on behavior and not on cognition, and participating children are selected by the recommendation of a pediatrician, GP, or other health professional. The program is actively performed by the child alone and there is no involvement of external people. It is described in detail on the Internet.

The child gets a box which is worth about 30 Euros or $US30. That is the price the family pays for it, and it's also the price of the game. The box contains a lot of media, including a videotape with 12 short clips that introduces the program, showing each task for the week, and various other program details that I cannot explain in the time available. Basically, the children learn, using with cards and games, which foods have high or low fat contents, and then they monitor their own fat consumption using a food frequency questionnaire. They can modulate this and have Fatsy points to spend each day.

We evaluated the program in a group of 141 obese children recruited from newspaper advertisements. Their weight-for-height was at least 120% of normal. The program was presented in a 30-minute group session, and the children were sent home without any further support. With conventional treatment we would not expect many children to return, but with this program 70% of the children returned after 3 months, again without any further support. We also tried out the program in a pediatric practice, where a pediatrician motivated the child, and there we had an even greater success rate of 84%.

Body mass index decreased over the 3 months of this very nonintense program by almost half a standard deviation score, and on follow-up 1 year after the end of the program, there was a further 0.5-SD reduction in BMI. About 90% of the children completed the program and were followed up after another year.

Our conclusion is that this self-directed behavioral program is effective in a large portion of schoolchildren with uncomplicated overweight. It is unlikely to be adequate for children with severe psychosocial or other problems. It is low in cost and economical of personnel, so it can be widely applied. Nine thousand children are already using it in Germany.

Dr. Endres: Does the Power Kids program aim to increase knowledge about food or nutrition?

Dr. Koletzko: There is no real increase in knowledge. In the material we provided there was a little booklet with questions and answers on nutrition, but in the questionnaires we got back from the children who used the program it appeared that most of them did not read it, though their parents did. The concept of the program doesn't really involve cognition, because we feel that knowledge of nutrition does not translate into behavior. Many children tell their parents that they mustn't buy all these foods that are high in Fatsies, that these are not good; they need foods that are low in Fatsies. But they had not understood that a Fatsie is 3 grams of fat, and in the younger age group of around 8 years they did not have much understanding of what fat really is. However, the program still worked because it involved a positive selection of foods.

Dr. Freedman: In the small amount of data you showed there was no control group, and I wonder to what extent a simple regression to the mean could explain the results you found?

Dr. Koletzko: I don't think it is a reasonable assumption that in 8- to 12-year-old overweight children with a mean weight-for-height standard deviation of 4 there would be a 1 SD regression to the mean in the course of 1 year. We had some difficulties with a control group. We had applied to our ethics committee to randomize the children to intervention and nonintervention, but the ethical review board said that as it was our practice to intervene in overweight children of more than 120% weight-for-height, we should not have a control group without intervention. We therefore compared the data with our other interventions, which were intensely physician based, and even if we were not doing any better with Power Kids, we certainly weren't doing any worse!

REFERENCES

1. Epstein LH. Methodological issues and ten-year outcomes for obese children. *Ann NY Acad Sci* 1993: 699; 237–49.
2. Epstein LH, Mc Curley J, Wing RR, *et al.* A five-year follow-up of family-based behavioral treatments for childhood obesity. *J Consult Clin Psychol* 1990: 58; 661–64.

Obesity in Childhood and Adolescence, edited by
Chunming Chen and William H. Dietz. Nestlé
Nutrition Workshop Series, Pediatric Program,
Vol. 49. Nestec Ltd., Vevey/Lippincott
Williams & Wilkins, Philadelphia © 2002.

Aggressive Therapy for Childhood and Adolescent Obesity

Jack A Yanovski

*Unit on Growth and Obesity, Developmental Endocrinology Branch, National Institute of
Child Health and Human Development, National Institutes of Health, Bethesda,
Maryland, USA*

For obese children and adolescents, treatments to minimize future weight gain and
induce weight loss are necessary to prevent the development of long-term complications of obesity. Programs prescribing moderate energy restriction, increased physical activity, and decreased sedentary behavior should always be the first line of approach for the overweight child (1). At least one such program has shown long-term
efficacy of weight control in a substantial portion of the 6- to 12-year-old children
participating (2,3). Unfortunately, many children and adolescents—especially those
with severe obesity—may not respond to such programs. As a result, various, more
aggressive therapeutic approaches have been proposed for obese children who have
failed conservative treatment. Aggressive approaches include restriction of energy
intake below 1,000 kcal/d, pharmacotherapy, and bariatric surgery. In this paper I
will review the limited data on these aggressive treatment regimens in childhood obesity and detail their potential benefits and risks.

INDICATIONS AND CONSIDERATIONS FOR AGGRESSIVE
TREATMENT OF PEDIATRIC OBESITY

In general, only those children and adolescents who have a body mass index (BMI)
greater than the 95th centile for age and sex and who also have developed a demon-
strable obesity-related comorbid condition that may be remediable by weight reduction should be considered for aggressive treatment. All overweight children and adolescents should have their BMI plotted on a sex-appropriate BMI chart (Figs. 1 and
2) to determine the severity of their obesity. Many complications of obesity are ob-
servable during childhood, including dyslipidemia (high total cholesterol, low-density lipoprotein cholesterol and triglycerides, and reduced high-density lipoprotein
cholesterol), disorders of glucose metabolism ranging from hyperinsulinemia
through glucose intolerance to frank type 2 diabetes, hepatic steatosis, systolic and
diastolic hypertension, pseudotumor cerebri, sleep apnea, and orthopedic complications such as Blount disease and slipped capital femoral epiphysis (4).

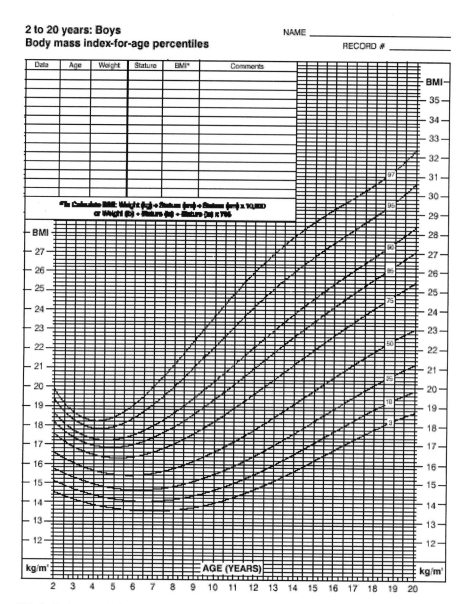

FIG. 1. Body mass index for boys 2 to 20 years of age. Developed by the National Center for Health Statistics in collaboration with the National Center for Chronic Disease Prevention and Health Promotion.

2 to 20 years: Girls
Body mass index-for-age percentiles

NAME _____

RECORD # _____

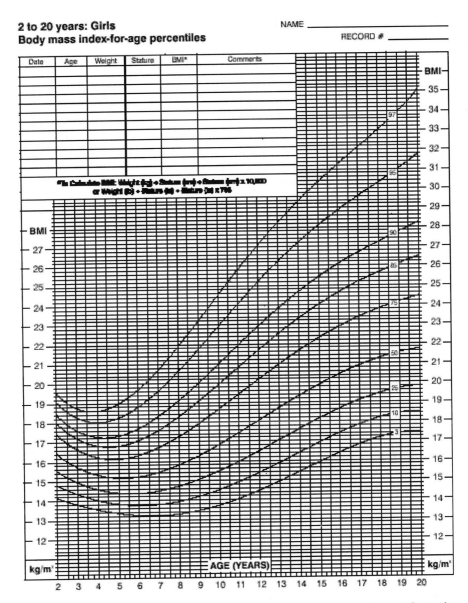

FIG. 2. Body mass index for girls 2 to 20 years of age. Developed by the National Center for Health Statistics in collaboration with the National Center for Chronic Disease Prevention and Health Promotion.

Most obesity specialists recommend that the intensity of the proposed treatment match the severity of the obesity. For this severity–intensity matching, many investigators describe pediatric body weight relative to the subject's "ideal body weight" (IBW), defined as the 50th centile weight-for-height for a child of the same age and sex. Any child who is more than 120% of IBW (equivalent to a BMI greater than the 95th centile) may be a candidate for a standard program of behavior modification, a 500-kcal/d-deficit diet, and increased activity. Very-low-energy diet programs are generally employed only for those more than 140% of IBW (5), and bariatric surgery is usually restricted only to those weighing at least double their IBW (6).

All aggressive treatments for pediatric obesity—whether they involve dietary restriction, pharmacotherapy, or surgery—should be considered as adjuncts to behavioral treatment designed to improve diet, increase physical activity, and decrease inactivity. Because the best results seem to be found in programs using multidisciplinary teams not readily available to the individual practitioner, aggressive treatments for pediatric obesity should whenever possible be carried out in specialized centers that have experience with such treatments.

Finally, as many of the aggressive treatment regimens for obesity are considered investigational when used in children, it may be advisable to obtain written informed consent from parents before initiating such treatments.

AGGRESSIVE REGIMENS TO RESTRICT INTAKE

The conventional pediatric dietary prescription for weight loss typically aims to reduce intake by approximately 500 to 700 kcal/d (to induce a 0.5-kg weight loss each week). Except for the youngest children, this generally results in total energy intakes of more than 1,000 kcal/d. More restrictive diet prescriptions are termed *very-low-energy diets.* The most common version of the very-low-energy diet is the protein-sparing modified fast (PSMF). Currently employed PSMF regimens supply a daily intake of between 600 and 800 kcal and 1.5 to 2.5 g of high-quality protein per kilogram of ideal body weight. They also usually restrict carbohydrate intake to 20 to 40 g/d. Such formulations do not cause cardiac arrhythmias or sudden death, as was observed in the 1970s, when liquid protein diets containing only hydrolyzed collagen as a protein source were used (7,8). Many PSMF programs use readily available lean meats, poultry, and fish as protein sources (9), although commercially available formula diets consumed as liquids may induce a PSMF. Patients using a PSMF are recommended to take a daily vitamin and mineral supplement and consume more than 1,500 ml of free water daily. In most programs, a PSMF is prescribed for no longer than 12 weeks, and is conducted under medical supervision. Figueroa-Colon *et al.* (5) found that 12 third to fifth graders weighing more than 140% of IBW enrolled in a comprehensive 6-month school-based program that included a 10-week PSMF lost 5.6 ± 7.6 kg, versus a weight gain of +2.8 ± 3.1 kg in seven untreated control children. Some uncontrolled trials suggest at least some weight loss can be found up to 1 year after a PSMF. Stallings *et al.* (10) treated 17 obese adolescents with a PSMF for 3 months, along with diet and activity counseling, and found that at follow-up 1 year later, 48% had maintained at least some weight loss. Sothern *et al.* (9) reported that among 87 children weighing more than 120% of IBW who remained enrolled in a 1-year multidisciplinary weight reduction program that included 10 weeks of PSMF, an exercise program, and behavior modification sessions, weight was 8.4 kg less after 1 year of treatment than at baseline. However, no information about dropouts was presented, and no control groups using a higher-energy diet were studied. Some investigators have employed PSMFs for longer periods. Suskind *et al.* (11) reported results from 50 obese children and adolescents 7 to 17 years of age who enrolled in a 10-week nutrition, activity, and behavior modification education program plus a PSMF. They allowed those who were still more than 150% of IBW to continue, taking the PSMF for as long as 30 weeks. Whenever they stopped the PSMF, all subjects were offered a 1,200-kcal/d balanced diet maintenance program consisting of weekly exercise sessions and bimonthly educational programs. Fifteen subjects (30%) took the PSMF for more than 15 weeks. While 80% completed the 10-week program, only 60% were reported to have entered the weight maintenance program, and only 40% were reported as having a 26-week follow-up. However, those subjects with the 26-week follow-up reduced their body weight by approximately 9 kg and had improvements in plasma lipids. Whether these results are better than those achievable with conventional dietary interventions has not been proven.

In children aged 7 to 17 years randomized to participate in a PSMF (600 to 800 kcal/d) or a hypocaloric balanced diet (800 to 1,000 kcal/d) plus a behavior modification program for 10 weeks, who were then placed on a 1,000- to 1,200-kcal/d balanced diet, Figueroa-Colon *et al.* (12) reported greater weight losses in children taking the PSMF (-11.2 versus -5.1 kg, $p < 0.01$) at the 10-week time point. However, follow-up 1 year later revealed similar mean weights in both groups (12), suggesting no long-lasting benefit of the PSMF relative to a balanced hypocaloric diet.

The potential risks of PSMF regimens include cholelithiasis, hyperuricemia (13), decreases in serum proteins including transferrin, retinol-binding protein, and complement β_1C (14), orthostatic hypotension, halitosis, and diarrhea (15). Serious complications in patients treated with modern PSMFs appear to be rare.

In sum, PSMF programs seem to be reasonably safe when carried out under medical supervision, and produce more rapid weight losses in the short term than conventional diets. However, they have not been shown to offer significant improvements in long-term outcome compared with less restrictive diets offered in the context of a comprehensive program. Although selected patients may benefit from a PSMF, particularly when rapid short-term weight loss is desirable (e.g., those who must lose weight before a surgical procedure can be performed, or who have life-threatening complications of obesity), it remains unclear whether programs employing a PSMF are better at inducing the long-lasting significant weight changes desired for treatment of pediatric obesity than long-term programs using moderate energy restriction.

PHARMACOTHERAPY

Because obesity is now believed to be a chronic disease best treated using a long-term medical treatment model (16), drugs that might be prescribed for long periods have been investigated. Although adverse effects have led to some anorectic agents being withdrawn from use, in the interests of completeness I will review in the following section all drug treatments for obesity that have been studied in children or adolescents, as identified by a MEDLINE search and manual review of published reports, even if the drug is no longer available (Table 1). As will be seen, there have been no long-term (≥ 1 year), randomized, double-blind, placebo-controlled trials in which the efficacy of drug treatment has been compared against that of a program including diet, exercise, and behavior modification.

Drugs Reducing Energy Intake

A few pediatric studies have examined the efficacy of drugs that reduce food intake by decreasing appetite or increasing satiety.

Fenfluramine decreases appetite by stimulating the release of both serotonin and dopamine from nerve terminals and selectively inhibiting their reuptake, and, particularly when combined with phentermine, appeared to decrease body weight in adults (16,17). One randomized, double-blind, placebo-controlled trial of the effects of fenfluramine on the weight of 5- to 18-year-old children found no difference in short-term weight loss between those taking placebo and those taking fenfluramine (18). Similar results were reported in a nonrandomized study with an untreated control group (19). Pedrinola *et al.* (20) performed a nonrandomized, placebo-controlled trial of fenfluramine in 11- to 17-year-old overweight Brazilian children who were given a minimal diet and exercise intervention (visits every 2 months). When examined after 12 months, the fenfluramine-treated children who remained in the study decreased BMI by -5.1 kg/m^2, whereas in placebo-treated children the change in BMI was -1.3 kg/m^2 ($p < 0.05$) (20). Because this study was not reported as randomized or double blind, did not report results from a substantial portion of enrolled subjects, and did not include a significant behavioral modification, diet, or exercise program, it is not possible to interpret the results as indicating an advantage of fenfluramine treatment over conventional programs. The potential risks of fenfluramine treatment led to its being withdrawn from use by its manufacturer in 1998, when cardiac valvopathies similar to those seen in the carcinoid syndrome were found to follow its use (21,22).

Phentermine is an orally active, DEA schedule C-IV-controlled substance that affects appetite by increasing the release of norepinephrine and dopamine from nerve terminals and inhibiting their reuptake. Two studies lasting 4 weeks using phentermine resin, 5 to 15 mg, versus placebo have reached contradictory conclusions about its efficacy in children and adolescents (23,24). Rauh and Lipp (25) compared weight change in 28 adolescent girls enrolled in a randomized controlled trial to receive either chlorphentermine 65 mg/d or placebo. Subjects were seen every 2 weeks, but not given an exercise or diet intervention. During the 12-week trial, those receiving chlorphentermine lost significantly more weight (-6.7 kg) than those taking placebo ($+0.55$ kg). Longer-term follow-up was not performed.

Diethylpropion and *mazindol* are other orally active DEA schedule C-IV controlled substances, with a mechanism of action similar to that of phentermine that have been evaluated as anorectic agents in children and adolescents. Two randomized controlled trials (26,27) studied diethylpropion hydrochloride 65 mg/d given for 8 to 12 weeks, in conjunction with minimal dietary interventions, and found that subjects taking diethylpropion lost 2 to 5 kg more than those taking placebo. Longerterm follow-up was not done. Short-term studies with mazindol suggest similar shortterm improvements in weight loss (28–30).

The side effect profiles of phentermine, diethylpropion, and mazindol in adults include insomnia, restlessness, euphoria, palpitations, hypertension, cardiac arrhythmias, dizziness, blurred vision, and ocular irritation. Sympathomimetic agents such as phentermine, mazindol, or diethylpropion cannot be used concurrently with monoamine oxidase inhibitors.

Sibutramine, an inhibitor of the synaptic reuptake of norepinephrine, serotonin, and dopamine, has been found in adults to decrease weight in 6-month to 1-year randomized, double-blind, placebo-controlled studies (31). Side effects have included increases in blood pressure and pulse, which are usually mild but which may be substantial in some patients. Other adverse reactions include headache, insomnia, anxiety, nervousness, depression, somnolence or drowsiness, edema, palpitations, diaphoresis, xerostomia, constipation, dizziness, paresthesias, mydriasis, and nausea. Sibutramine cannot be given in conjunction with monoamine oxidase inhibitors or selective serotonin reuptake inhibitors. Clinical trials evaluating the safety and efficacy of sibutramine in adolescents are ongoing, but no data from children or adolescents are currently available.

Drugs Reducing Absorption of Nutrients

There have been no published randomized, placebo-controlled trials of drugs that affect absorption of nutrients from the gastrointestinal tract in children or adolescents.

Orlistat, an inhibitor of gastrointestinal lipases, has been shown in placebo-controlled trials to have modest efficacy in adults for periods as long as 2 years (32–34). A 3-month open-label trial of orlistat reporting a 4.6% decrease in body fat in a small number of very overweight adolescents (initial BMI 43.8 ± 12.4 kg/m^2) has been published in abstract form (35). Side effects include decreases in fat-soluble vitamin levels (primarily vitamin D), flatulence with discharge, fecal urgency, fecal incontinence, steatorrhea, oily spotting, and increased frequency of defecation. These side effects are usually mild to moderate, and generally decrease in frequency with continued treatment. Placebo-controlled, randomized, double-blind clinical trials evaluating the safety and efficacy of orlistat in adolescents are ongoing.

Other Drugs

Leptin

Leptin is a hormone secreted by adipocytes, the level of which, under nonfasted conditions, reflects total body lipid content (36,37). Serum leptin concentrations fall precipitously during fasting, and it appears likely that its intended function is primarily

TABLE 1. *Obesity pharmacotherapy trials in children and adolescents*

Study	Type of study	Subjects	Treatment duration	Nondrug intervention	Study groups
Bacon and Lowrey, 1967 (18)	RCT	71% F, 5–17 y >97th weight centile	1 month, then crossover to other treatment for 1 month	1,000–1,2000 kcal diet prescription	d,l-fenfluramine 10–20 mg bid or tid Placebo
Pedrinola *et al.*, 1994 (20)	Not clear if randomized but had placebo control group	55% F Brazilian children 11–17 y, 120% to 260% IBW	12 months	800–1000 kcal/d diet, instructed to increase activity. Visits q2 mo	d,l-fenfluramine 30–60 mg bid Placebo
Malecka-Tendera *et al.*, 1996 (19)	Non-randomized untreated control group	71% F Polish children 16 ± 2 y, unre-sponsive to out-patient program	6 weeks	Inpatient admission for 3 weeks 600 kcal/d diet, out-patient for 3 weeks 600 kcal/d diet	D,l-fenfluramine 15 mg bid No medication
Komorowski *et al.*, 1982 (30)	RCT	43% F Polish children age 9–15 y	8 weeks	Low-calorie diet	Mazindol 1 mg/d Placebo
Golebiowska *et al.*, 1981 (28,29)	Not clear if randomized but had placebo control group	44% F Polish children age 9–16y	8 weeks	2-week residential 1,600–1,800 kcal/d, with supervised activity, then outpatient	Mazindol 1 mg/d Placebo
Rauh and Lipp, 1968 (25)	RCT with last observation carried forward	100% F Tanner IV or V pubertal develop-ment age 10–19 y	12 weeks	None, visits q2 weeks	Chlorphenter mine 65 mg/d Placebo
Von Spranger, 1965 (23)	Placebo controlled, unclear if randomized	Children, 5–15 y	1 month	Diet prescription, 1 visit	Phentermine 5–15 mg/d Placebo Diet alone
Lorber 1966 (24)	RCT	62% F age 3–15 y >120% of IBW	1 month, then crossover for 1 month, then crossover for 1 month	No snacks between meals, no sweets, to canned fruits	Phentermine 15 mg/d Amphetamine resinate 12.5 mg/d Placebo

No. of subjects	Final number of subjects (% completing study)	BMI (kg/m^2) or % IBW or weight (kg) at baseline	Change in weight (kg) or BMI (kg/m^2) at endpoint	% Reduction in weight at endpoint	Side effects in treated subjects
10	5 (50%)	NR	−3.0 kg	NR	Weakness, dizziness, fainting,
10	9 (90%)	NR	−1.5 kg	NR	disorientation
90	68 (76%)	29 ± 5 kg/m^2 (154 ± 24%)	−5.1 kg/m^{2*}	NR	Drowsiness (18%), dry mouth,
40	17 (42%)	30 ± 4 kg/m^2 (161 ± 28%)	−1.3 kg/m^2	NR	nausea, diarrhea
19	19 (100%)	31 ± 5 kg/m^2 85 ± 19 kg	−3.9 kg/m^2	NR	Dry mouth (58%), sleep disorders (21%)
19	19 (100%)	34 ± 12 kg/m^2 80 ± 19 kg	−5.7 kg/m^2	NR	
8	8 (100%)	66 ± 10 kg	−5.7 ± 1.5 kg*	−11.7%*	NR
6	6 (100%)	59 ± 8 kg	−3.0 ± 2.2 kg	−6.9%	
21	21 (100%)	71 kg	−5.4 kg*	−7.6%*	Palpitations (9.5%), dry
20	20 (100%)	90 kg	−3.4 kg	−4.9%	mouth (33%), skin eruption (4.7%)
15	13 (93%)	95 kg	−6.7 kg**	NR	None
13	10 (77%)	96 kg	+0.55 kg	NR	
41	41 (100%)	23 kg	−3.5 ± 1.5 kg	NR	NR
31	31 (100%)	21 kg	−19 ± 1.8 kg	NR	
20	10 (100%)	24 kg	−1.9 ± 1.4 kg	NR	
	80% total				Insomnia, irritability
84	24	NR	−3.4 kg	NR	
total	22	NR	−2.2 kg	NR	
	22	NR	−2.1 kg	NR	

(continued)

TABLE 1. Continued

Study	Type of study	Subjects	Treatment duration	Nondrug intervention	Study groups
Stewart et al., 1970 (27)	RT with last observation carried forward	58% F age 5–16 y >97th centile for weight	8 weeks, then crossover for 8 weeks	1,200 kcal/d diet prescription	Diethylpropion 75 mg qd Placebo
Andelman et al., 1967 (26)	RCT	84% F age 12–18 y >120% of IBW	11 weeks	No snacks between meals	Diethylpropion 75 mg qd Placebo
Lustig et al., 1999 (45)	Open label	56% F children 8–18 y with hypo-thalamic obesity	6 months	Dietary counseling	Octreotide 5 μg/kg/d ÷ tid
Lustig et al., 2001 (46)	RCT	39% F children 10–18 y hypo-thalamic obesity	6 months	NR	Octreotide 5–15 μg/kg/d ÷ tid Placebo
McCann et al., 2000 (35)	Open label	50% F black and white children 12–17 y	3 months	Psycho educational program; 12 weekly meetings 500 kcal/d deficit diet	Orlistat 120 mg tid
Farooqi et al., 1999 (40)	Open label	100% F leptin deficient	12 months	None	Recombinant leptin
Lutjens and Smith 1977 (53)	Open label	8–14 y children	3 months	Diet prescription	Metformin 500 mg tid Diet alone
Lustig et al., 1999 (54)	Open label	100% F 1.3–17 y	28 weeks	Diet prescription	Metformin 500 mg tid
Freemark and Bursey, 2000 (55)	RCT	Obese adoles-cents M and F	6 months	None reported	Metformin 500 bid Placebo

Abbreviations: RCT, randomized, double-blind, placebo-controlled trial; NR, not reported. For crossover studies, results from first treatment period are reported.
* $p < 0.05$.
** $p < 0.01$ vs. control.

No. of subjects	Final number of subjects (%) completing study)	BMI (kg/m^2) or % IBW or weight (kg) at baseline	Change in weight (kg) or BMI (kg/m^2) at endpoint	% Reduction in weight at endpoint	Side effects in treated subjects
24	NR	NR	−2.1 kg*	NR	Headache, abdominal pain, increased activity
14	NR	NR	+0.36	NR	
51	37 (73%)	154%	−5.1 kg	−16.9%	Drowsiness, jitteriness, nervousness, insomnia, dry mouth, irritability, headache
46	10 (22%)	154%	+0.3 kg	NR	
9	8 (89%)	36 ± 2 kg/m^2	−4.8 ± 1.8 kg −2.0 ± 0.7 kg/m^2	−4.6%	Edema (11%) abdominal discomfort, flatulence, or loose stools (78%), increased thyroid hormone requirements (67%), gall bladder sludging (44%)
9	NR	All subjects 99 ± 6 kg 36 ± 1.3 kg/m^2	+1.6 ± 0.6 kg** −0.2 ± 0.2 kg/m^2	NR	Diarrhea (100%), glucose intolerance (22%), bile sludging/gall stones (44%)
9			+9.2 ± 1.5 kg +2.2 ± 0.5 kg/m^2		
20	17 (85%)	44 ± 12 kg/m^2	−2.9 ± 4.8 kg −1.4 ± 1.8 kg/m^2	−2.6%	Low vitamin D (3/20); oily stools (20/20)
1	1 (100%)	48 kg/m^2	−16.4 kg −10.1 kg/m^2	−17.4%	None
9	9 (100%)	29 ± 4 kg/m^2 68 ± 19 kg/m	−4.8 ± 1.6 kg/m^2 −10.9 ± 4.1 kg	−16 ± 6%**	None
9	9 (100%)	30 ± 4 kg/m^2 70 ± 20 kg	+0.3 ± 1 kg/m^{2}** +1.1 ± 2.5 kg**	+1.6 ± 3.5%	
8	8 (100%)	39 ± 2 kg/m^2 116 ± 9 kg	−1.2 ± 0.7 kg/m^2	−3.4 ± 1.9%	None
16	15 (94%)	42 ± 4 kg/m^2	−0.5 kg/m^2	−1.3%*	Intermittent nausea (6%)
16	14 (88%)	39 ± 5 kg/m^2	+0.9 kg/m^2	+2.3%	Abdominal discomfort (19%) exacerbation of migraine (6%)

as a peripheral signal to the hypothalamus of an inadequate food intake (38) rather than as a satiety signal. A few children have been identified who are unable to make functional leptin protein (39). Such individuals have severe early-onset obesity. Treatment of a leptin-deficient girl with recombinant leptin has been reported to induce a dramatic effect on body weight (40). Over a 12-month treatment period she lost weight at a rate of approximately 1 to 2 kg a month, with a total weight loss of 16.4 kg, of which 95% was due to reduction in adipose tissue mass. Considerably less dramatic changes in body weight have been observed in leptin-sufficient adults treated with differing regimens of recombinant leptin (41,42). It remains unknown whether leptin treatment of obese children or adolescents who do not have mutations in the leptin gene will be of benefit.

Octreotide

Among its many effects, the somatostatin receptor agonist octreotide can suppress pancreatic secretion of insulin by inhibiting G_0 protein effects on voltage-dependent calcium channels. Octreotide has therefore been evaluated for its ability to affect body weight in patients believed to have obesity resulting from primary hyperinsulinemia, particularly those who have suffered cranial insults. In rodents and humans, damage to the ventromedial hypothalamus (VMH) can cause considerable obesity and significant hyperinsulinemia. Although the observed hyperinsulinemia may in part be a response to insulin resistance induced by weight gain, there is evidence that VMH damage induces neurally mediated hyperinsulinemia, acting through the autonomic supply to the pancreas. In rats, hyperinsulinemia is found shortly after surgical disruption of the VMH, and either vagotomy or denervation of the pancreas can prevent the weight gain that follows such hypothalamic lesions (43,44).

Lustig *et al.* (45) proposed the hypothesis that neurally mediated hyperinsulinemia could be one of the primary stimuli for overeating in children who have sustained damage in the region of the hypothalamus. To test this hypothesis, they examined the effects of suppressing insulin secretion with octreotide in a pilot study of children who had intractable obesity following intracranial treatment for brain tumors or leukemia (45). Whereas before starting treatment, these children were gaining an average of 6.0 ± 0.7 kg every 6 months, while taking octreotide they lost 4.8 ± 1.8 kg over a 6-month interval. Because these data were collected in an open-label fashion, the true magnitude of the benefit cannot be determined. A recent report in abstract form of a 6-month randomized controlled trial using octreotide or placebo in 18 children with hypothalamic obesity found weight stabilization in treated subjects ($+1.6 \pm 0.6$ kg in 6 months), in contrast to significant weight gains ($+9.2 \pm 1.5$ kg in 6 months) in those receiving placebo (46). Because somatostatin has many actions, it is also unknown whether the effects of octreotide at the pancreatic level are the explanation for these children's weight loss.

There are many known complications of octreotide treatment, such as pain at injection sites, gallstones, diarrhea, abdominal pain, nausea, vitamin B-12 deficiency (47), hypothyroidism, suppression of growth hormone secretion, frank type 1 diabetes, and abnormalities of cardiac function. As a result, larger studies with longer treatment duration are needed to determine whether this drug provides sufficient benefit for children with intractable obesity related to hypothalamic injury. Octreotide offers a novel approach to the treatment of hypothalamic obesity in children and continues to be studied in placebo controlled trials.

Metformin

Metformin is a drug that inhibits hepatic glucose production and is used for the treatment of type 2 diabetes. It not only improves hyperglycemic indices, but also decreases weight gain and promotes weight loss in adults (48–52). It has been used in a limited number of school-aged children and adolescents with obesity. In one open-label study, metformin 500 mg three times daily was given to nine obese children 8 to 14 years of age, who were also given dietary instruction (53). There was an impressive reduction in weight over a 3-month period of -10.9 ± 4.1 kg (range -4.0 to -15.0 kg). More recently, two small studies of metformin have been reported. Lustig *et al.* (54) treated eight obese, hyperinsulinemic adolescent girls with open-label metformin (2,000 mg/day) for 28 weeks and reported a mean decrease in weight of 0.53 ± 0.69 kg per month. Freemark and Bursey randomized 29 obese adolescents with hyperinsulinemia to metformin 500 mg twice daily or placebo without any dietary treatment, and found a 1.3% decrease in BMI following use of metformin for 6 months versus a 2.3% increase in BMI for those taking placebo ($p < 0.05$) (55). Because such studies have not examined subjects in comprehensive weight management programs, it is unclear whether metformin treatment improves the outcome found with such programs.

Metformin may cause nausea, flatulence, bloating, and diarrhea at the start of treatment, and approximately 5% of adults cannot take it at any dose because of these symptoms. Vitamin B-12 deficiency has also been reported in as many as 9% of patients using metformin. The most feared complication of metformin is lactic acidosis, which is estimated to occur at a rate of 3/100,000 patient-exposure years, primarily in patients with contraindications to the use of metformin. These contraindications include renal insufficiency, defined as a serum creatinine of ≥ 124 μmol/l in women and ≥ 133 μmol/l in men, congestive heart failure requiring drug treatment, any cardiac or pulmonary insufficiency severe enough to result in hypoxia and reduced peripheral perfusion, liver disease, and alcohol use sufficient to cause acute hepatic toxicity. Metformin should also be withheld when patients are admitted to hospital with any severe illnesses, with any condition that may cause decreased systemic perfusion, or when the use of contrast agents is anticipated. Randomized controlled trials testing the efficacy of metformin for control of weight in children and adolescents with hyperinsulinemia are ongoing.

Drug Treatment Summary

At present, none of the currently approved drugs for the amelioration of obesity can be recommended for obese children and adolescents, except in the context of clinical trials. Given its efficacy (40), leptin replacement therapy for leptin-deficient children does appear justified. It is possible that ongoing clinical trials will provide the necessary data within the next few years to support the use of pharmacotherapy for other causes of childhood obesity. Because obesity is a chronic condition that requires continuous treatment, both the immediate and long-term risks and benefits of pharmacotherapy must be carefully weighed before drugs are prescribed for obese children or adolescents.

BARIATRIC SURGERY

There are limited data regarding surgical procedures to induce weight loss in severely obese children and adolescents (6,56–62). Water-filled balloons placed within the stomach to induce a sense of fullness have recently been shown not to be effective at decreasing BMI in morbidly obese children (61). Silber *et al.* (60) described 11 morbidly obese adolescents who underwent jejunoileal bypass. Ten years later, they had maintained weight losses ranging from 45 to 90 kg. Unfortunately, each patient had at least one complication of the procedure. These complications included encephalopathy, cholelithiasis, nephrolithiasis, renal cortical nephropathy, hypoproteinemia, and other nutritional deficiencies. More than 25% had complications that required reversal of the operations. Other studies of jejunoileal bypass have shown similar results (59).

Because of the severity of the complications from jejunoileal bypass, this procedure is now rarely performed. Instead, the Roux-en-Y gastric bypass (RYGB) has become the most commonly performed type of bariatric surgery. RYGB involves dividing the stomach to create a small (15- to 30-ml) stomach pouch into which a segment of jejunum—around 15 to 60 cm below the ligament of Treitz—is inserted, while the proximal portion of the jejunum that drains the bypassed lower stomach and duodenum is reanastomosed 40 to 75 cm below the gastrojejunostomy (Fig. 3). In adults, rapid weight loss is usually observed, and with it improvement of comorbid conditions, including resolution of type 2 diabetes in more than 80% of cases (63) and improvements in hepatic steatosis (64). Early postoperative complications include staple line leaks, wound dehiscence, subhepatic abscess, small bowel obstruction, thrombophlebitis, and pulmonary embolus. Late postoperative complications include stomal stenosis, incisional hernia, volvulus, gastrointestinal bleeding, marginal ulcers, cholelithiasis, and nutritional deficiencies (65). The perioperative mortality and complication rates in one very large adult series were 1.5% and 8.5%, respectively (66).

Older adolescents who have undergone RYGB have been included in various case series of adults (65,67,68), but their results have not usually been reported separately. One group has reported results of obesity surgery, primarily RYGB, in genetically normal adolescents and in adolescents with the Prader–Willi syndrome, all of whom weighed more than twice their IBW (6,58). In the later, more complete report (6), 30 karyotypically normal adolescents decreased their weight from 238% of IBW before RYGB to 187% of IBW 5 years later, whereas those with Prader–Willi syndrome decreased weight from 231% of IBW to 175% of IBW 5 years later. Complications

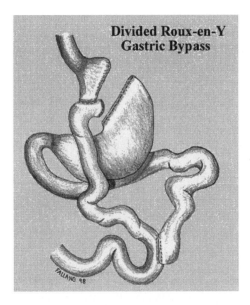

FIG. 3. Roux-en-Y gastric bypass. First, a small stomach pouch is created by stapling or by vertical banding. This causes restriction in food intake. Next, a Y-shaped section of the small intestine is attached to the pouch to allow food to bypass the duodenum as well as the first portion of the jejunum. This causes reduced calorie and nutrient absorption. (Original drawing by David Fallang, MD.)

included wound infections and dehiscence (10%), stomal obstruction (5%), atelectasis and pneumonia (12%), subphrenic abscess (2%), and death (5%). Ten patients, four who were karyotypically normal and six with Prader–Willi syndrome (amounting to around half of their patients with Prader–Willi syndrome) required surgical revisions for failure to lose weight. Three developed incisional hernias requiring further surgery. More recently, Strauss *et al.* (62) reviewed a separate case series of 10 obese adolescents (BMI 52.5 $\pm$ 10.0 kg/m^2) who underwent bariatric procedures, mostly RYGB, and were followed for a mean of 69 months (range, 8 to 144 months). After bariatric surgery, 90% had weight losses of more than 30 kg (the mean weight loss was 53.6 $\pm$ 25.6 kg), comprising 65% of their excess body weight; patients also had improvements in comorbid conditions. Complications included iron deficiency anemia (50%), transient folate deficiency (30%), and events requiring operative interventions (40%) (cholecystectomy in 20%, small bowel obstruction in 10%, incisional hernia in 10%).

Greenstein and Rabner (69) studied the long-term effects of vertical banded gastroplasty in 18 adolescents, 14 of whom (three boys and 11 girls) were willing to be interviewed an average of 5.1 years after surgery. All but one child had a significant decrease in BMI (on average by 14.6 kg/m^2). As a group, these children lost 55.9% of their excess body weight, and 79% lost more than 25%. The major morbidity described in this case series of vertical banded gastroplasty was the development of recurrent gastric ulceration in two patients (70). Comparison studies in adults suggest that the efficacy in terms of long-term weight reduction and improvement in quality of life following RYGB is greater than that seen with restrictive procedures such as vertical banded gastroplasty (71–74), although there are no such studies in children or adolescents.

These case series suggest that patients in the pediatric age group who undergo RYGB trade the disorders associated with obesity for lifelong medical care for nutritional deficiencies but do have large sustained weight reductions following the procedures. Although bariatric surgery is the only treatment for which there is any evidence of significant and long-lasting weight-reducing effects in severely obese adolescents, such interventions cannot be recommended for any but those at the highest risk of mortality from their obesity. We agree with Strauss *et al.*, who concluded that "gastric bypass remains a last resort option for severely obese adolescents" (62).

SUMMARY AND CONCLUSIONS

The aggressive treatments that have been used for pediatric and adolescent obesity include very-low-energy diets, pharmacotherapy, and bariatric surgery. None of these approaches has been reported in large enough numbers of subjects who have taken part in well-designed experiments with long-term follow-up to demonstrate convincingly their true value in the treatment of pediatric obesity. As the potency of the treatment increases, so does its possible adverse consequences. Of the aggressive approaches, only in the case of bariatric surgery are there even small studies supporting its ability to induce long-lasting effects (more than 1 year) on body weight in severely obese adolescents without a defined syndrome. Leptin treatment of those rare children who have genetic mutations of the leptin gene also appears justified.

Future studies of aggressive treatments in children and adolescents should in general be carried out in large, diverse samples; be designed as randomized controlled trials; be carried out for 6 months or longer; and include a comprehensive weight management program offered to all participants. They should systematically evaluate adverse events and include follow-up of most, if not all, subjects. It would also be useful if such studies reached conclusions regarding appropriate subject selection, or offered a risk–benefit calculation so that the value of aggressive treatments for individual subjects could be judged. Studies examining prevention of weight regain after aggressive treatments are also lacking for the pediatric population. In particular, the use of pharmacotherapy for preventing weight regain in children and adolescents has received little attention. Systematic trials of the efficacy of differing bariatric surgical approaches are also lacking in children and adolescents.

The risks and benefits of aggressive weight management treatments should be carefully weighed before they are used in patients in the pediatric age group. Until further controlled trials become available, aggressive treatments for pediatric obesity should be considered only for those who have not responded to conventional weight management programs but have significant complications of their obesity. Aggressive approaches should generally be restricted to specialized centers that have experience with those treatments and should be carried out in the context of a comprehensive weight management program.

REFERENCES

1. Barlow SE, Dietz WH. Obesity evaluation and treatment: Expert Committee recommendations. The Maternal and Child Health Bureau, Health Resources and Services Administration and the Department of Health and Human Services. *Pediatrics* 1998; 102: 29.
2. Epstein LH, Valoski A, Wing RR, McCurley J. Ten-year follow-up of behavioral, family-based treatment for obese children. *JAMA* 1990; 264: 2519–23.
3. Epstein LH, Valoski A, Wing RR, McCurley J. Ten-year outcomes of behavioral family-based treatment for childhood obesity. *Health Psychol* 1994; 13: 373–83.
4. Must A, Strauss RS. Risks and consequences of childhood and adolescent obesity. *Int J Obes Relat Metab Disord* 1999; 23: 2–11.
5. Figueroa-Colon R, Franklin FA, Lee JY, von Almen TK, Suskind RM. Feasibility of a clinic-based hypocaloric dietary intervention implemented in a school setting for obese children. *Obes Res* 1996; 4: 419–29.
6. Anderson AE, Soper RT, Scott DH. Gastric bypass for morbid obesity in children and adolescents. *J Pediatr Surg* 1980; 15: 876–81.
7. Michiel RR, Sneider JS, Dickstein RA, Hayman H, Eich RH. Sudden death in a patient on a liquid protein diet. *N Engl J Med* 1978; 298: 1005–7.
8. Anon. *Liquid protein diets.* Atlanta: Centers for Disease Control, 1979.
9. Sothern MS, von Almen TK, Schumacher HD, Suskind RM, Blecker U. A multidisciplinary approach to the treatment of childhood obesity. *Del Med J* 1999; 71: 255–61.
10. Stallings VA, Archibald EH, Pencharz PB, Harrison JE, Bell LE. One-year follow-up of weight, total body potassium, and total body nitrogen in obese adolescents treated with the protein-sparing modified fast. *Am J Clin Nutr* 1988; 48: 91–4.
11. Suskind RM, Sothern Ms, Farris RP, *et al.* Recent advances in the treatment of childhood obesity. *Ann N Y Acad Sci* 1993; 699: 181–99.
12. Figueroa-Colon R, von Almen TK, Franklin FA, Schuftan C, Suskind RM. Comparison of two hypocaloric diets in obese children. *Am J Dis Child* 1993; 147: 160–6.
13. Mathew G, Lifshitz F. Hyperuricemia in a child: a complication of treatment of obesity. *Pediatrics* 1974; 54: 370–1.
14. Merritt RJ, Blackburn GL, Bistrian BR, Palombo J, Suskind RM. Consequences of modified fasting in obese pediatric and adolescent patients: effect of a carbohydrate-free diet on serum proteins. *Am J Clin Nutr* 1981; 34: 2752–5.
15. Brown MR, Klish WJ, Hollander J, Campbell MA, Forbes GB. A high protein, low calorie liquid diet in the treatment of very obese adolescents: long-term effect on lean body mass. *Am J Clin Nutr* 1983; 38: 20–31.
16. Anon. Long-term pharmacotherapy in the management of obesity. National Task Force on the Prevention and Treatment of Obesity. *JAMA* 1996; 276: 1907–15.
17. Weintraub M, Hasday JD, Mushlin AI, Lockwood DH. A double-blind clinical trial in weight control. Use of fenfluramine and phentermine alone and in combination. *Arch Intern Med* 1984; 144: 1143–8.
18. Bacon GE, Lowrey GH. A clinical trial of fenfluramine in obese children. *Curr Ther Res Clin Exp* 1967; 9: 626–30.
19. Malecka-Tendera E, Koehler B, Muchacka M, Wazowski R, Trzciakowska A. Efficacy and safety of dexfenfluramine treatment in obese adolescents. *Pediatr Pol* 1996; 71: 431–6.
20. Pedrinola F, Cavaliere H, Lima N, Nedeiros-Neto G. Is D,L-Fenfluramine a potentially helpful drug therapy in overweight adolescent subjects. *Obes Res* 1994; 2: 1–4.
21. Anon. Cardiac valvulopathy associated with exposure to fenfluramine or dexfenfluramine. Interim public health recommendations, November 1997. Washington DC: US Department of Health and Human Services, 1997.
22. Connolly HM, Crary JL, McGoon MD, *et al.* Valvular heart disease associated with fenfluramine-phentermine [see comments]. *N Engl J Med* 1997; 337: 581–8. [Published erratum appears in *N Engl J Med* 1997; 337: 1783.]
23. von Spranger J. Phentermine resinate in obesity. Clinical trial of Mirapront in adipose children. *Munch Med Wochenschr* 1965; 107: 1833–4.

24. Lorber J. Obesity in childhood. A controlled trial of anorectic drugs. *Arch Dis Child* 1966; 41: 309–12.
25. Rauh JL, Lipp R. Chlorphentermine as an anorexigenic agent in adolescent obesity. Report of its efficacy in a double-blind study of 30 teenagers. *Clin Pediatr (Phila)* 1968; 7: 138–40.
26. Andelman MB, Jones C, Nathan S. Treatment of obesity in underprivileged adolescents. Comparison of diethylpropion hydrochloride with placebo in a double-blind study. *Clin Pediatr (Phila)* 1967; 6: 327–30.
27. Stewart DA, Bailey JD, Patell H. Tenuate dospan as an appetite suppressant in the treatment of obese children. *Appl Ther* 1970; 12: 34–6.
28. Golebiowska M, Chlebna-Sokol D, Kobierska I, *et al.* Clinical evaluation of Teronac (mazindol) in the treatment of obesity in children. Part II. Anorectic properties and side effects [author's translation]. *Przegl Lek* 1981; 38: 355–8.
29. Golebiowska M, Chlebna-Sokol D, Mastalska A, Zwaigzne-Raczynska J. The clinical evaluation of teronac (Mazindol) in the treatment of children with obesity. Part I. Effect of the drug on somatic patterns and exercise capacity [author's translation]. *Przegl Lek* 1981; 38: 311–4.
30. Komorowski JM, Zwaigzne-Raczynska J, Owczarczyk I, Golebiowska M, Zarzycki J. Effect of mazindol (teronac) on various hormonal indicators in children with simple obesity. *Pediatr Pol* 1982; 57: 241–6.
31. Bray GA, Blackburn GL, Ferguson JM, *et al.* Sibutramine produces dose-related weight loss. *Obes Res* 1999; 7: 189–98.
32. Davidson MH, Hauptman J, DiGirolamo M, *et al.* Weight control and risk factor reduction in obese subjects treated for 2 years with orlistat: a randomized controlled trial [see comments]. *JAMA* 1999; 281: 235–42.
33. Rossner S, Sjostrom L, Noack R, Meinders AE, Noseda G. Weight loss, weight maintenance, and improved cardiovascular risk factors after 2 years treatment with orlistat for obesity. European Orlistat Obesity Study Group. *Obes Res* 2000; 8: 49–61.
34. Hauptman J, Lucas C, Boldrin MN, Collins H, Segal KR. Orlistat in the long-term treatment of obesity in primary care settings. *Arch Fam Med* 2000; 9: 160–7.
35. McCann S, McDuffie J, Nicholson J, *et al.* A pilot study of the efficacy of orlistat in overweight adolescents. *Obese Res* 2000; 8: 58.
36. Maffei M, Halaas J, Ravussin E, *et al.* Leptin levels in human and rodent: measurement of plasma leptin and ob RNA in obese and weight-reduced subjects. *Nat Med* 1995; 1: 1155–61.
37. Hassink SG, Sheslow DV, de Lancey E, *et al.* Serum leptin in children with obesity: relationship to gender and development. *Pediatrics* 1996; 98: 201–3.
38. Ahima RS, Prabakaran D, Mantzoros C, *et al.* Role of leptin in the neuroendocrine response to fasting. *Nature* 1996; 382: 250–2.
39. Montague CT, Farooqi IS, Whitehead JP, *et al.* Congenital leptin deficiency is associated with severe early-onset obesity in humans. *Nature* 1997; 387: 903–8.
40. Farooqi IS, Jebb SA, Langmack G, *et al.* Effects of recombinant leptin therapy in a child with congenital leptin deficiency. *N Engl J Med* 1999; 341: 879–84.
41. Heymsfield SB, Greenberg AS, Fujioka K, *et al.* Recombinant leptin for weight loss in obese and lean adults: a randomized, controlled, dose-escalation trial [see comments]. *JAMA* 1999; 282: 1568–75.
42. Hukshorn CJ, Saris WH, Westerterp-Plantenga MS, *et al.* Weekly subcutaneous pegylated recombinant native human leptin (PEG-OB) administration in obese men. *J Clin Endocrinol Metab* 2000; 85: 4003–9.
43. Inoue S, Bray GA, Mullen YS. Transplantation of pancreatic beta-cells prevents development of hypothalamic obesity in rats. *Am J Physiol* 1978; 235: 266–71.
44. Cox JE, Powley TL. Prior vagotomy blocks VMH obesity in pair-fed rats. *Am J Physiol* 1981; 240: 573–83.
45. Lustig RH, Rose SR, Burghen GA, *et al.* Hypothalamic obesity caused by cranial insult in children: altered glucose and insulin dynamics and reversal by a somatostatin agonist [see comments]. *J Pediatr* 1999; 135: 162–8.
46. Lustig RH, Hinds PS, Smith KR, *et al.* A double-blind, placebo-controlled trial of octreotide in pediatric hypothalamic obesity. LWPES/ESPE 6th Joint Meeting, Montreal, Canada, 2001.
47. Flogstad AK, Halse J, Bakke S, *et al.* Sandostatin LAR in acromegalic patients: long-term treatment [see comments]. *J Clin Endocrinol Metab* 1997; 82: 23–8.
48. DeFronzo RA, Goodman AM. Efficacy of metformin in patients with non-insulin-dependent diabetes mellitus. The Multicenter Metformin Study Group [see comments]. *N Engl J Med* 1995; 333: 541–9.

49. Lee A, Morley JE. Metformin decreases food consumption and induces weight loss in subjects with obesity with type II non-insulin-dependent diabetes. *Obes Res* 1998; 6: 47–53.
50. Munro JF, MacCuish AC, Marshall A, Wilson EM, Duncan LJ. Weight-reducing effect of diguanides in obese non-diabetic women. *BMJ* 1969; ii: 13–5.
51. Fontbonne A, Charles MA, Juhan-Vague I, *et al.* The effect of metformin on the metabolic abnormalities associated with upper-body fat distribution. BIGPRO Study Group. *Diabetes Care* 1996; 19: 920–6.
52. Stumvoll M, Nurjhan N, Perriello G, Dailey G, Gerich JE. Metabolic effects of metformin in non-insulin-dependent diabetes mellitus [see comments]. *N Engl J Med* 1995; 333: 550–4.
53. Lutjens A, Smit JL. Effect of biguanide treatment in obese children. *Helv Paediatr Acta* 1977; 31: 473–80.
54. Lustig R, Rose S, Pitukcheewanont P, *et al.* Metformin effects on weight and insulin secretion in adolescent females with obesity/hyperinsulinemia/acanthosis nigricans. 1999: Twelfth Annual Investigators Meeting of the National Cooperative Growth Study. Annual Investigators Meeting of the National Cooperative Growth Study, 1999; 12: 13.
55. Freemark M, Bursey D. The effects of metformin on body mass index and glucose tolerance in obese adolescents with fasting hyperinsulinemia and a family history of type 2 diabetes. *Pediatrics* 2001; 107: 55.
56. White JJ, Cheek D, Haller JA. Small bowel bypass is applicable for adolescents with morbid obesity. *Am Surg* 1974; 40: 704–8.
57. Randolph JG, Weintraub WH, Rigg A. Jejunoileal bypass for morbid obesity in adolescents. *J Pediatr Surg* 1974; 9: 341–5.
58. Soper RT, Mason EE, Printen KJ, Zellweger H. Gastric bypass for morbid obesity in children and adolescents. *J Pediatr Surg* 1975; 10: 51–8.
59. Organ CH, Kessler E, Lane M. Long-term results of jejunoileal bypass in the young. *Am Surg* 1984; 50: 589–93.
60. Silber T, Randolph J, Robbins S. Long-term morbidity and mortality in morbidly obese adolescents after jejunoileal bypass. *J Pediatr* 1986; 108: 318–22.
61. Vandenplas Y, Bollen P, De Langhe K, Vandemaele K, De Schepper J. Intragastric balloons in adolescents with morbid obesity. *Eur J Gastroenterol Hepatol* 1999; 11: 243–5.
62. Strauss RS, Bradley LJ, Brolin RE. Gastric bypass surgery in adolescents with morbid obesity. *J Pediatr* 2001; 138: 499–504.
63. Pories WJ, MacDonald KG, Flickinger EG, *et al.* Is type II diabetes mellitus (NIDDM) a surgical disease? *Ann Surg* 1992; 215: 633–42; discussion, 643.
64. Silverman EM, Sapala JA, Appelman HD. Regression of hepatic steatosis in morbidly obese persons after gastric bypass. *Am J Clin Pathol* 1995; 104: 23–31.
65. Brolin RE, Kenler HA, Gorman RC, Cody RP. The dilemma of outcome assessment after operations for morbid obesity. *Surgery* 1989; 105: 337–46.
66. Pories WJ, Swanson MS, MacDonald KG, *et al.* Who would have thought it? An operation proves to be the most effective therapy for adult-onset diabetes mellitus. *Ann Surg* 1995; 222: 339–50; discussion, 350–2.
67. Yale CE. Gastric surgery for morbid obesity: complications and long-term weight control. *Arch Surg* 1989; 124: 941–6.
68. Higa KD, Boone KB, Ho T, Davies OG. Laparoscopic Roux-en-Y gastric bypass for morbid obesity: technique and preliminary results of our first 400 patients. *Arch Surg* 2000; 135: 1029–33; discussion, 1033–4.
69. Greenstein RJ, Rabner JG. Is adolescent gastric-restrictive antiobesity surgery warranted? *Obes Surg* 1995; 5: 138–44.
70. Greenstein RJ. Reexploration following vertical banded gastroplasty: technical observations, and co-morbidity from dentition, smoking and esophageal pathology. *Obes Surg* 1993; 3: 265–9.
71. Fobi MA. Vertical banded gastroplasty vs gastric bypass: 10 years follow-up. *Obes Surg* 1993; 3: 161–4.
72. Brolin RL, Robertson LB, Kenler HA, Cody RP. Weight loss and dietary intake after vertical banded gastroplasty and Roux-en-Y gastric bypass. *Ann Surg* 1994; 220: 782–90.
73. Howard L, Malone M, Michalek A, *et al.* Gastric bypass and vertical banded gastroplasty: a prospective randomized comparison and 5-year follow-up. *Obes Surg* 1995; 5: 55–60.
74. Hell E, Miller KA, Moorehead MK, Norman S. Evaluation of health status and quality of life after bariatric surgery: comparison of standard Roux-en-Y gastric bypass, vertical banded gastroplasty and laparoscopic adjustable silicone gastric banding. *Obes Surg* 2000; 10: 214–19.

DISCUSSION

Dr. Dietz: I have a couple of comments. The claims of safety that Suskind and his coworkers made about the protein-sparing modified fast were only based on 50 patients. One of our findings that we never published was that in our inpatients who were either on the protein-modified fast—which is what I call it, because I'm not sure that it is actually protein sparing—and/or on an isocaloric, isonitrogenous diet containing carbohydrate, we regularly saw ventricular arrhythmias that disappeared when the diet was normalized. We never were able to replicate this finding when we used the diets in outpatient centers. The reason may have been that when we were studying the patients as inpatients, we had them on a very restricted diet, whereas in the outpatient situation there was more diversity. I think you were properly cautious in saying that informed consent is still required. I'm not sure that we have put the issue of cardiac arrhythmias properly to rest in this population, where the myocardium may be more sensitive.

My second comment is that a couple of months ago I calculated the cost of putting every patient in the United States with a BMI of more than 30 on drug treatment, based on the local cost of Sibutramine in Atlanta. The direct costs of obesity in the United States are known to be of the order of 50 billion dollars a year, while the cost of putting every obese person in the United States on Sibutramine worked out at about 35 billion dollars a year. This puts us in a peculiar situation—we have a problem we cannot afford to treat, and one that we cannot afford not to treat!

Dr. Campos: We heard Dr. Steinbeck say that growth requires very few calories. But we also heard Dr. Uauy and Dr. Chen say that in the developing countries, when they switch from malnutrition to obesity, there is a lack of linear growth. Furthermore, those children apparently have some form of dyslipidemia. In view of the delay in catch-up growth, the dyslipidemia, and the obesity, and also the fact that obese children enter puberty earlier, might there not be a place for thyroid hormone supplementation? It is known that the malnourished population tends to have a low T4 with a normal TSH. Although this is probably mainly an adaptive response, might it not also be a mechanism contributing to the delay in catch-up linear growth?

Dr. Yanovski: I don't believe there is any place for thyroid hormone treatment in anyone for the treatment of obesity, except where there is clear evidence of significant hypothyroidism.

Dr. Maffeis: I am concerned about the high mortality from obesity surgery. I think a 5% mortality is very high. Do you have any views about criteria for surgery other than ideal body weight?

Dr. Yanovski: The 5% mortality was from a fairly early paper. I think the mortality is lower than that in more recent series, and the laparoscopic approach decreases it even more so, though I have seen no laparoscopic series in children. Dr. Strauss, do you want to comment on this?

Dr. Strauss: I can make a quick comment on each of the aggressive treatments because we use them all in some form or other. Protein-sparing modified fast in a child of less than 14 or 15 years of age is punitive, so we only use it in selected children who demonstrated motivation and who have been in our program for at least 2 to 3 months. In that setting, where the harder changes are made first, you may have some long-term weight loss, but only one in 20 or 30 of the children we see are qualified for that diet. Even the best drug treatments only produce a 10- to 12-kg weight loss compared with placebo, and in most cases less. In children who are 100 kg overweight, this won't do anything to reduce their morbidity, while children who need to lose 10 to 12 kg should exercise and eat properly and shouldn't be on medicines. As far as surgery is concerned, I have only referred a handful. Generally these have had severe sleep apnea and ventricular arrhythmias and are at high medical risk. They have all been on other types of treatment. Other children selected for surgical treatment are those with severe orthopedic problems and also the most difficult group with serious psychological disturbances—children who are missing school, who are frankly depressed, and who can't face their peers because of their weight. Some of those did have surgery and tended to be referred through the parents, who also had the surgery. Everyone I tracked down up to 10 years later was extremely happy with the results of their surgery.

I don't know who needs surgery. The children who you think may need to have it don't want it, and the ones who ask for it shouldn't have it. The published mortality figures were on some of the initial patients done in the 1960s and reported in the 1980s.

Dr. Yanovski: I believe you still need to think very hard before you decide to refer an adolescent for a gastric bypass, given the fact that you are going to be trading one set of disorders for another. Although the nutritional deficiencies are manageable, they are real and can be significant.

Dr. Uauy: In relation to the hypothalamic syndrome, the craniopharyngiomas also fit into that category. Immediately after surgery, there is usually an acute increase in weight. Is there anything that can be done before they get to be massively obese?

Dr. Yanovski: I think this may be a matter of keeping a close eye on how fast they are crossing the centiles, to decide when they are getting into trouble. In general, I think that right after surgery for craniopharyngioma the most important thing is probably to ensure adequate hormone replacement therapy with thyroid hormone and growth hormone. If in spite of that you see a rapid increase in weight, the chances are that the child is going to develop this full-blown syndrome. The question then is whether octreotide therapy is good enough to use at this point. I'm not convinced of that and I think we need some longer-term data. The side effects are real. Even though we can control gallstones with ursodeoxycholic acid, that is a complication that could lead to surgical intervention. The other side effects such as diarrhea are also major problems. Also, in any individual who does not have growth hormone deficiency and who is not being treated with growth hormone, the expectation is that the child is going to become growth hormone deficient because of the treatment. Second, the way this drug works is by inducing a relative insulinopenia in the blood. This means that at some point at least there is bound to be hyperglycemia, which could, in the long term, lead to the complications associated with diabetes—and the avoidance of diabetes is of course one of the reasons why we might want to protect these children from massive weight gain. So I think there are a lot of issues to be clarified before octreotide treatment should be used as a routine approach.

Dr. Bar-Or: Just a comment regarding craniopharyngioma. We have five or six girls who are being followed up after surgery for this condition. We have managed them quite well with a multidisciplinary behavioral approach, so at least in our hands we felt that there was no need for anything drastic. Obviously, they were getting their hormone replacement therapy, but as far as their obesity was concerned they responded quite nicely to behavioral changes.

Dr. Yanovski: I think there is no question that the first step in any individual who is overweight has to be conventional management. I am also equally convinced that there are individuals who have lost their capacity to respond to leptin who will develop significant obesity that will not be controlled by conventional approaches.

Unidentified participant: Is it better to use single therapy or a combination of treatments?

Dr. Yanovski: By the time you've got as far as surgery I'd be very loathe to combine that with drug treatment, but conventional dietary management is certainly part of the postoperative care of anyone who has had surgery. There is significant interest in combination pharmacotherapy in any situation, and we will certainly have more information relating to Sibutramine, which seems to have more than one mechanism of action. Caffeine and ephedrine is a combination therapy that has been tried. One of the areas that would be interesting to look at is the prevention of weight regain by pharmacotherapy after a very-low-energy diet. To the best of my knowledge that has not been studied in the pediatric population.

Unidentified participant: Are there some new drugs on the horizon?

Dr. Yanovski: I have restricted my remarks to those drugs that have had some clinical trials in pediatric populations. There are various compounds under development that may be of interest to us in the future, but I'd rather not speculate on which of these will ever get out of the drug companies' hands and into ours.

Dr. Steinbeck: Apart from leptin, none of the drugs that have been discussed are well targeted. That is a significant problem. Leptin works very well because it is targeted at the etiology of a particular form of obesity. Until we have drugs that are more effectively targeted, including those for hypothalamic obesity, we will continue to have the sort of results that you've talked about today.

Dr. Yanovski: That's very true. One of our jobs as clinicians has to be the development of a nosology of obesity that allows us to determine which groups might respond to different therapeutic approaches.

Dr. Anantharaman: Have you studied the eating habits of these very overweight children at all? I assume that they must be consuming massive amounts of food in order to continue to gain so much weight? Is this associated with any particular eating pattern?

Dr. Yanovski: The general answer is that a fair number of these children do have evidence of binge eating, although surprisingly few will meet the criteria for the binge eating disorder. Depression is present in about a third of cases. We haven't looked carefully at whether the night eating syndrome is present or not. There is not as much secretive eating in the younger children as you might imagine. Once they are adolescents, though, there is often a lot of the same type of disordered eating you see in adults.

Dr. Jiang: What is the compliance with a very-low-calorie diet, and is it damaging to development and growth?

Dr. Yanovski: Compliance with a very-low-calorie diet is quite variable, and children under 13 or 14 years of age don't have the maturity to be on such a restricted diet. I wouldn't try it unless there is a really severe medical indication. The compliance issue is certainly substantial. Various programs have insisted on ketosis and measurable ketones in the urine as a measure of compliance, and even when you do that the best programs probably get around 70% compliance at best—and that's after everyone who does not comply has dropped out.

In terms of growth and development, there are some data from Figueroa-Colon's paper (1) suggesting that at least over a period of a year there are no adverse consequences on growth, although short term there did appear to be a deceleration of growth velocity in the protein-sparing modified fast group. In contrast, Epstein's studies of conventional dietary management have not shown any decrements in growth velocity and final height attainment (2).

Dr. Rusli Sjarif: Do you have any experience with aggressive treatments for obesity in children under 10 years old?

Dr. Yanovski: There are very few published trials that have included children under the age of 10. I don't believe there are any good data that I can point to that would recommend the use of aggressive therapy in such young children. One should be very cautious in young children to avoid problems with growth and development.

REFERENCES

1. Figueroa-Colon R, von Almen TK, Franklin FA, *et al.* Comparison of two hypocaloric diets in obese children. *Am J Dis Child* 1993; 147: 160–6.
2. Epstein LH, McCurley J, Valoski A, *et al.* Growth in obese children treated for obesity. *Am J Dis Child* 1990; 144: 1360–4.

Obesity in Childhood and Adolescence, edited by
Chunming Chen and William H. Dietz. Nestlé
Nutrition Workshop Series, Pediatric Program,
Vol. 49. Nestec Ltd., Vevey/Lippincott
Williams & Wilkins, Philadelphia © 2002.

Obesity Prevention

Thomas N. Robinson

*Division of General Pediatrics, Department of Pediatrics and Center for Research in
Disease Prevention, Stanford University School of Medicine, Palo Alto, California, USA*

WHY PREVENTION?

Obesity has become one of the most important public health problems facing both developed and developing countries throughout the world (1). Recent surveys suggest a rapidly increasing rate of obesity among children and adolescents (1,2). In the United States, more than 50% of adults are overweight, defined as a body mass index (BMI) of 25 or greater (3). Therefore at least half of American children can already be considered at risk of future overweight and its associated morbidities. However, known risk factors—such as child overweight, parental overweight, parental morbidity, and the timing of the adiposity rebound—are not sufficiently sensitive or specific to identify which children will go on to develop obesity-related clinical complications, persistent obesity into adulthood, or adult-onset obesity (4).

There is also evidence of substantial undetected obesity-associated morbidity in children. Data from the Bogalusa (Louisiana, USA) Heart Study suggest that about 60% of overweight children already manifest at least one additional physiologic cardiovascular disease risk factor—hypertension, hyperlipidemia, or hyperinsulinemia (5)—and are at increased risk of early atherosclerotic lesions in the aorta and coronary arteries (6). Finally, although some intensive behavioral obesity treatment programs have shown long-term success in up to one-third of obese children (7), most available treatments have produced disappointing long-term results, including some significant adverse effects (7–9), and we are unable to identify accurately which children are most likely to benefit from treatment (4). Adult treatment results have generally been even more disappointing (10). Therefore a population-based prevention approach—one that targets the entire population of children and adolescents—is likely to hold the greatest promise in addressing the current worldwide epidemic of obesity.

PREVENTION APPROACHES

In theory, obesity prevention may be achieved by any intervention that results in a balance between energy intake and energy expenditure. Of course there are many

245

possible ways to achieve such a goal. Examples of some different approaches are included in Fig. 1. Simple thermodynamics would suggest that only small changes in diet or activity levels are needed to achieve a balance for most children. For example, if all else is held constant, adding or subtracting a single small 10 kcal piece of hard candy in the diet every day would result in a weight difference of approximately ± 1 lb (about 0.5 kg) over the course of a year. Similarly, a single 12 oz (355 ml) soft drink usually contains about 150 kcal, or the equivalent of about 15 lb (7 kg) when consumed daily over the course of a year. Thus prevention programs should only need to promote small shifts in behavior to produce substantial effects on the prevalence of obesity in the population. Despite this, however, producing sufficient behavior changes to prevent excessive weight gain has proven to be a formidable challenge. Many questions remain over how and where to deliver prevention programs to maximize their effectiveness. The three main venues suggested for childhood obesity

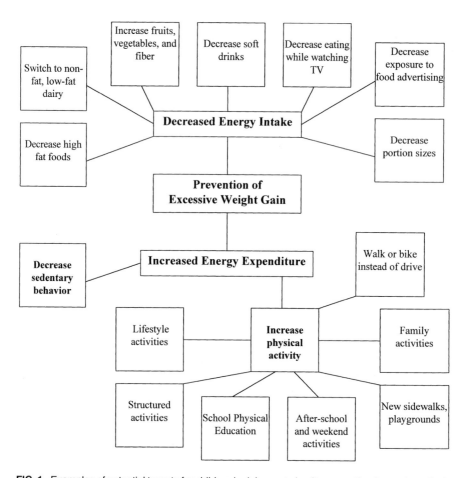

FIG. 1. Examples of potential targets for child and adolescent obesity prevention (nonexhaustive).

prevention programs are primary care clinical settings, community settings, and schools.

PRIMARY CARE–BASED PREVENTION PROGRAMS

Primary care settings include primary care physicians' offices, public health clinics, public hospitals, and school-based clinics. Primary care–based assessment and counseling about obesity, nutrition, and physical activity have been widely endorsed (11). Because primary care encounters provide attractive opportunities for such counseling, recent interest has increased in designing and implementing clinical preventive interventions. However, research is lacking on the current prevalence and efficacy of diet and activity counseling for preventing obesity in children and adolescents. Data from other areas of prevention suggest that primary care clinicians often do not provide the recommended preventive services. Identified barriers include inadequate reimbursement, insufficient time, lack of clinical skills, lack of clinician or patient interest, uncertainty or doubt about efficacy, and lack of organizational or medical care system support to facilitate the delivery of preventive care (12). In addition, primary care encounters may not be of sufficient duration and frequency to deliver an adequate "dose" of an intervention to produce sustained changes in behavior.

One recent example of a primary care intervention is the patient-centered assessment and counseling for exercise plus nutrition (PACE+) project from San Diego State University, California (Patrick K, Sallis JF, personal communication). This project was designed to address many of the previously identified barriers to improving primary care–based preventive counseling about diet and physical activity for adolescents. It uses an interactive computer-based assessment, primary care provider counseling at the time of the medical visit, and extended follow-up phone and mail counseling from nonclinician staff. The preliminary evaluation of PACE+ suggested the feasibility of this approach in several primary care offices. However, the efficacy of the approach is still unknown because it has not yet been tested against a control group.

Although the existing research does not yet support the efficacy of primary care interventions for preventing obesity, it may be possible to suggest appropriate strategies for preventive counseling based on research from other settings. Effective behavioral interventions for children have generally included the following: frequent counseling over a prolonged period, including parents in the process; simple and explicit behavioral targets (e.g., targeting single foods or types of food, physical activities, and sedentary behaviors that are easy to identify, count, and track over time); short- and long-term self-monitoring; goal setting and contracting with appropriate rewards; providing children with some input and choice regarding their targeted behaviors; altering the home and family environment to support the child's changes (e.g., removing targeted foods from the home, decreasing eating out, instituting family walks every morning or after dinner); strategies for dealing with lapses; and training of parents in basic parenting skills to promote and reward their children's behavior change (13).

COMMUNITY-BASED PREVENTION PROGRAMS

Community settings—such as churches, community centers, parks and recreation programs, and after-school and weekend athletic leagues—have also been receiving increased interest as potential venues for obesity prevention programs. As with primary care–based programs, however, research is lacking on what types of program are effective in these settings. One of the few examples of a community-based program that has been evaluated was a 12-week, culturally specific obesity prevention program for low-income African-American mothers and daughters living in public housing. However, while the intervention resulted in statistically significant improvements in mothers' self-reported diets, daughters' self-reported behaviors changed "only minimally" and there were no significant changes in body weight (14).

We have recently started a randomized controlled pilot study of a community-based intervention for 8- to 10-year-old African-American girls. In this pilot study we are comparing two 12-week interventions: (a) a traditional health education intervention promoting a low-fat diet and increased physical activity, through monthly community meetings and weekly newsletters for girls and their parents; and (b) after-school dance classes at community centers and a family-based intervention to reduce television viewing. The goal of the dance and television reduction intervention is to provide activities that increase activity and decrease sedentary behavior sufficiently to produce meaningful changes in energy balance and adiposity. In this project we are also working with three other sites across the United States, each with its own interventions, to test a variety of approaches to community-based obesity prevention for African-American girls. Despite the recent interest in community-based programs, there are as yet few data to support the feasibility and efficacy of these approaches.

SCHOOL-BASED PREVENTION PROGRAMS

The vast majority of prevention programs have been implemented in schools, mainly because "that's where the kids are." In addition to providing a captive audience of children, however, many schools already include some form of health education and physical education in their standard curriculum, and provide meals or snacks during the school day, making them particularly appropriate settings for obesity prevention programs. Schools can also be a convenient avenue through which to reach parents, so as to try to influence the home environments of children.

To examine the overall efficacy of school-based obesity prevention programs we can look to the cardiovascular disease prevention literature. In a recent review, Resnicow and Robinson identified 19 controlled, school-based studies that were published from 1980 to 1997, assessed at least one major physiologic risk factor for cardiovascular disease (e.g., adiposity, blood lipids, blood pressure), and intervened on at least two different behaviors (e.g., physical activity and diet) (15). Of the 19 studies identified, 12 were from the United States, two were from Australia, and one each was from Greece, Russia, Israel, Finland, and Norway. Three intervened solely in either physical education classes or school lunch. When results were pooled across studies, there were varying success rates according to the targeted outcome. Across these 19 studies, there were statistically significant improvements in 80% of the smoking outcomes reported, 36% of the physical fitness outcomes, 34% of the diet outcomes, 31% of the blood lipid outcomes, 30% of the physical activity outcomes, 18% of the blood pressure outcomes, and only 16% of the adiposity outcomes (15). In other words, the success of school-based obesity prevention programs has been relatively modest. Although adiposity was not the primary outcome of most of these studies, it appears that obesity may be a more difficult problem to prevent than smoking and other risk factors. This is an important observation to acknowledge, because ineffective strategies should be avoided in the rush to provide prevention programs to address the obesity epidemic. However, those programs that have proven successful in the past—such as those reviewed below—can serve as useful models for the development of more effective future programs.

Classroom Curriculum Interventions

Most school-based prevention programs have included a classroom curriculum designed to help children and adolescents make more healthful diet and activity choices, and ultimately prevent obesity (15–17). Although many of these curricula have resulted in increased knowledge and improved attitudes about healthful behaviors, and many have successfully affected self-reported diet and activity behaviors, they have generally not been successful in reducing adiposity (15,17).

One exception to this was the Stanford Adolescent Heart Health program (18,19). This study involved all tenth graders in four high schools from two ethnically diverse school districts near San Jose, California. Within each district one school was randomly assigned to receive a 20-session cardiovascular disease risk reduction intervention (targeting smoking prevention/cessation, adoption of a low-fat diet, increased aerobic physical activity, and stress reduction) and the other school served as a control. The intervention was based on social cognitive theory (20) and social inoculation theory (21). Two months after the end of the intervention, the treatment group showed significant increases in regular aerobic activity and heart-healthy food choices, and significant reductions in experimental cigarette smoking, resting heart rate, body mass index (BMI), and triceps and subscapular skinfold thickness measurements compared with controls (19). What appears to differentiate this program from most other classroom-based programs is that it was conceived from the start as a "behavior change" intervention instead of a "health education" intervention. It was not designed by health education or nutrition education curriculum writers; instead, it was designed by behavioral scientists and physicians, and was strongly based in theory.

One of the major challenges in classroom curriculum interventions has been providing a sufficient "dose" of the intervention. School curricula are already crowded, and suggestions to squeeze in an additional 15 to 20 hours or more of new content are often met with resistance by teachers and administrators. A recent study attempted to address this by integrating its intervention content into existing major subject areas and physical education courses that were already being taught in the standard middle school curriculum. In a 10-school randomized controlled trial, Gortmaker and colleagues examined the effects of their intervention for sixth to eighth grade (11- to 13-year-old) children in Boston, Massachusetts (22). The 2-year intervention focused on decreasing television viewing as well as decreasing high-fat food intake, increasing fruit and vegetable intake, and increasing moderate and vigorous physical activity. Over the course of the study, boys and girls in the intervention schools reported reducing their television viewing more than controls, and girls in the intervention schools reported increasing their fruit and vegetable intakes more, and increasing their total energy intakes less, than girls in the control schools. The prevalence of obesity (defined by age- and sex-specific thresholds, using a combination of both BMI and triceps skinfold thickness) decreased significantly among intervention girls compared with control girls, but there were no significant effects on the prevalence of obesity among boys. There were also no effects on the entire sample distributions of BMI or triceps skinfold thickness. However, this study suggests that the integrated, interdisciplinary curriculum approach may be a useful strategy for increasing the intervention "dose" in school-based obesity prevention programs.

Classroom curriculum interventions generally attempt to create perceived incentive value for behavior change, alter social norms to favor healthful behaviors, teach skills to facilitate behavior change, and enhance self-efficacy for specific changes in behavior (19). As such, they require active individual behavior change. Another strategy has been to try to alter the school environment to promote behavior change passively. The two main environmental approaches have been changing the content of school meals and altering physical education.

School Food Service Interventions

Because many schools serve breakfast, lunch, and/or snacks to students during the school day, the content of school meals has been an attractive target for prevention programs. In fact, several interventions have successfully changed the content of school meals. These studies show that changes in the school food service can passively influence children's consumption of fat while at school (23–27). To date, however, these interventions have failed to show any beneficial effects on body fatness.

Physical Education Interventions

Physical education (PE) classes have been another environmental target for school-based obesity prevention efforts. Studies in the United States suggest that many standard PE classes may average as little as 10 minutes of moderate to vigorous physical activity a week (28,29). Alterations to standard PE have been somewhat effective at improving physical activity and fitness levels (26,30–32) but have not produced changes in adiposity (15). In contrast, the few PE interventions shown to have had significant effects on body fatness have made more radical changes to PE content itself. For example, in the Adelaide Heart Study in Australia, lengthening the standard

30- minute, 3-days-a-week PE to 75 minutes, 5 days a week did not improve fitness or reduce adiposity significantly. However, substituting endurance training for 75 minutes a day, 5 days a week produced significant improvements in cardiorespiratory fitness and decreased skinfold thickness measurements (33). Similarly, in our Dance for Health study—a small, randomized controlled pilot study—low-income Latino and African-American seventh-grade (12-year-old) children in northern California were randomized to either a hip-hop dance class or their usual physical education, for 40 to 50 minutes, 3 days a week. At the end of the 12-week intervention there were no significant differences between groups among the boys. However, the girls in the Dance for Health classes reduced their BMI and resting heart rates significantly compared with girls in regular PE classes (34). The main difference between these two successful PE interventions and most others appears to be the change in the content of the physical education lessons themselves. Traditional physical education activities may not lend themselves as well to the increases in intensity and duration required to prevent obesity. Compared with the traditional PE content, activities like dance and competitive sports may be more motivating for children.

"INDIRECT" INTERVENTIONS: REDUCING TELEVISION VIEWING

Most obesity prevention strategies have made a direct attempt to increase physical activity and improve the diet (Fig. 1). However, there has been recent interest in exploring other behavioral targets as well, particularly those that may indirectly influence physical activity levels and dietary intake. Examples are as varied as adding sidewalks to neighborhoods and building housing around local shopping areas to facilitate walking; slowing the speeds of elevators or escalators; enhancing stairwells with music and art (Dietz WH, personal communication); and taxing junk food (35).

Another target has been sedentary behavior, and television viewing in particular. Although all sedentary behaviors may displace more active behaviors with greater energy expenditures, television viewing may also influence energy intake through eating while watching, and through the effects of food advertising on food preferences and diets (36,37). To test the causal nature of the television and obesity link, and to examine the potential benefits of reducing children's television viewing in preventing obesity, we performed a small randomized controlled trial (37). It involved all third- and fourth-grade (8- to 10-year-old) children in two public elementary schools in San Jose, California. The schools were selected by school district personnel to be sociodemographically and scholastically comparable. One school was randomly selected to receive an 18-lesson social cognitive theory-based intervention to decrease television, videotape, and video game use, *without* specifically promoting other behaviors, to isolate the effects of reduced media use alone. The lessons were taught by the regular classroom teachers as part of their standard curriculum. The other school served as an assessments-only control. Assessments took place in the autumn and spring of a single school year. Over the course of the school year, children in the treatment group reported reducing their television, videotape, and video game use by about 8 hours a week, or about one third more than the controls. In addition, the intervention resulted in substantial and statistically significant relative reductions in body fatness. Over the course of the 7-month study, the children in the intervention school gained an average of 0.45 kg/m^2 less in BMI than the controls, the equivalent of nearly 2 lb (around 1 kg) less for a child of average height in the sample, an average of about 1.5 mm less in triceps skinfold thickness, and nearly 1 inch (2.3 cm) less in waist circumference. These results show that television viewing is a cause of increased adiposity in children and that reducing television viewing is a promising approach for obesity prevention—particularly because of the large changes seen in adiposity, larger than most interventions directly targeting physical activity and diet changes. These conclusions are also consistent with results from the Planet Health Study, in which reductions in television viewing were associated with changes in obesity (22), and from experimental studies of reducing sedentary behavior as part of weight control treatment for obese children (38,39).

CONCLUSIONS AND FUTURE DIRECTIONS

Dramatic increases in obesity have resulted in a rush to develop and disseminate obesity prevention programs. Facing a worldwide obesity epidemic, it will be difficult for medical and public health professionals to resist the urge to respond with traditional health and nutrition education interventions. Unfortunately, as illustrated previously, health status will suffer as a result. Instead, the successes and failures of past interventions should be used to help guide the development of more effective future programs. Based on the research to date, are there characteristics that help to define successful interventions?

Although sufficient detail about interventions is often lacking from published reports, it appears that the most successful interventions are those that are most strongly based in theories of behavior change. Faithful application of theory has been one of the major challenges in this field. The real-world concerns of primary care practices, community organizations, and schools present formidable obstacles to designing and implementing theoretically sound interventions that are also feasible. For example, classroom teachers may be more focused on teaching their students "facts" about diet and physical activity—things that can be assessed on a multiple-choice test—than providing opportunities for children to invent and practice strategies to overcome barriers to consuming low-fat foods and increasing physical activity. Primary care providers may not have sufficient training and may not believe they have the time to provide effective behavioral counseling with multiple follow-up visits. After-school programmers may feel compelled to focus only on homework and improving academic performance or violence prevention.

The most successful interventions appear to be those that focus on obesity as a *behavioral* problem, not just a nutritional one. Both eating and activity need to be targeted as behaviors rather than purely as energy values. Traditional nutrition education interventions—which teach children the importance of exercise and eating the proper number of servings from the food pyramid, foods high in vitamins and minerals, the energy content of foods, and so on—have never worked for preventing obesity. Unfortunately, that is still the model that is most commonly applied in health education programs. In contrast, the most successful interventions have focused more on the personal, social, and environmental contexts of eating and activity.

One of the key elements to address in intervention design is motivation—identifying intervention approaches and goal activities that are, in themselves, motivating to children. It sometimes appears that intervention developers assume that as soon as children, adolescents, and parents hear about the important health benefits of physical activity, a low-fat diet, and weight control, they will be sufficiently motivated to change their behavior. That is clearly not the case for most people. In fact, health benefits may be some of the weakest motivators for behavior change in well populations. In many of the successful prevention programs reviewed earlier, health and weight benefits were not promoted as the primary motivators for behavior change.

To produce behavior change, behavioral targets or their associated benefits must be sufficiently motivating for children to adopt them. For example, in our community-based intervention for African-American girls, instead of trying to persuade 8- to 10-year-old girls that they should be exercising at least 60 minutes a day because it is good for them or because it will make them feel good (the typical health education approach), we are establishing after-school African dance and hip-hop dance classes to help them become much more active, but without ever having to promote physical activity or health as a goal. The use of young adult African-American women as dance group leaders, a focus on African heritage and African-American culture, the promise of performing for their friends and family, the creation of a girls-only group, and the choice of dance as an activity make participation highly valued and enjoyable for the girls. As a result, they are excited about participating in an activity that they like (motivating for the girls), regardless of its potential health benefits (motivating for the investigators).

Once motivational strategies are identified, another key element of this approach is choosing target behaviors that are discrete and measurable, subject to monitoring and change. To make changes and track successes and failures, children must be able to recognize and count the target behavior they are attempting to change. For example, eating five fruits and/or vegetables each day (versus "servings," which are much more difficult to measure), switching to low-fat milk or nonfat milk, and reducing meals eaten at fast food restaurants are more discrete and measurable target behaviors than reducing dietary fat or energy intake, which is often the typical public health and health education message. Accumulating at least 5,000 steps a day on a pedometer, walking or biking to school each day, and going to dance class each day are more discrete and measurable target behaviors than being physically active for 60 minutes a day.

The biological and social sciences are making important advances toward understanding the etiologies and correlates of obesity. However, much less investment has been devoted to the translation of these findings into effective prevention interventions. To prevent obesity and significantly improve the health of our populations we need to focus much more attention on theory-based experimental intervention research. This includes development and testing of innovative methods of behavior change in small-scale "efficacy" trials, followed by large-scale "effectiveness" trials to translate efficacious methods into public health interventions.

ACKNOWLEDGMENTS

This work supported in part by grants from the National Heart, Lung, and Blood Institute, National Institutes of Health (R01 HL54102; R01 HL62224; U01 HL62663).

REFERENCES

1. World Health Organisation. *Obesity. Preventing and managing the global epidemic.* Report of a WHO consultation on obesity. Geneva: WHO, 1998.
2. Troiano RP, Flegal KM. Overweight children and adolescents: description, epidemiology, and demographics. *Pediatrics* 1998; 101: 497–504.
3. Holtzman D, Powell-Griner E, Bolen JC, Rhodes L. State- and sex-specific prevalence of selected characteristics—Behavioral Risk Factor Surveillance System, 1996 and 1997 (CDC surveillance summaries). MMWR 2000; 49 (No SS-6): 1–39.
4. Robinson TN. Defining obesity in children and adolescents: clinical approaches. *Crit Rev Food Sci Nutr* 1993; 33: 313–20.
5. Freedman DS, Dietz WH, Srinivasan SR, Berenson GS. The relation of overweight to cardiovascular risk factors among children and adolescents: the Bogalusa Heart Study. *Pediatrics* 1999; 103: 1175–82.
6. Berenson GS, Srinivasan SR, Bao W, *et al.* Association between multiple cardiovascular risk factors and atherosclerosis in children and young adults. *N Engl J Med* 1998; 338: 1650–6.
7. Epstein LH, Valoski A, Wing RR, McCurley J. Ten-year outcomes of behavioral family-based treatment for childhood obesity. *Health Psychol* 1994; 13: 373–83.
8. Epstein LH, Myers MD, Raynor HA, Saelens BE. Treatment of pediatric obesity. *Pediatrics* 1998; 101: 554–70.
9. Haddock CK, Shadish WR, Klesges RC, Stein R. Treatments for childhood and adolescent obesity. *Ann Behav Med* 1994; 16: 235–44.
10. National Institutes of Health Technology Assessment Conference Panel. Methods for voluntary weight loss and control. *Ann Intern Med* 1993; 119: 764–70.
11. Sallis JF, Patrick K, Frank E, Pratt M, Wechsler H, Galuska DA. Interventions in health care settings to promote healthful eating and physical activity in children and adolescents. *Prev Med* 2000; 31: 112–21.
12. US Preventive Services Task Force. *The guide to clinical preventive services.* Washington, DC: US Department of Health and Human Services, Office of Disease Prevention and Health Promotion, 1996.
13. Robinson TN. Behavioural treatment of childhood and adolescent obesity. *Int J Obes* 1999; 23: 52–7.
14. Stolley MR, Fitzgibbon ML. Effects of an obesity prevention program on the eating behavior of African American mothers and daughters. *Health Educ Behav* 1997; 24: 152–64.
15. Resnicow K, Robinson TN. School-based cardiovascular disease prevention studies: review and synthesis. *Ann Epidemiol* 1997; 7: 14–31.
16. Jackson MY, Proulx JM, Pelican S. Obesity prevention. *Am J Clin Nutr* 1991; 53: 1625–30.
17. Resnicow K. School-based obesity prevention. Population versus high-risk interventions. *Ann NY Acad Sci* 1993; 699: 154–66.
18. Killen JD, Robinson TN. School-based research on health behavior change: the Stanford adolescent heart health program as a model for cardiovascular disease risk reduction. In: Rothkopf E, ed. *Review of research in education* Washington, DC: American Educational Research Association, 1989: 171–200.
19. Killen JD, Telch MJ, Robinson TN, Maccoby N, Taylor CB, Farquhar JW. Cardiovascular disease risk reduction for tenth graders. *JAMA* 1988; 260: 1728–33.
20. Bandura A. *Social foundations of thought and action* Englewood Cliffs, NJ: Prentice-Hall, 1986.
21. McGuire W. Inducing resistance to persuasion. In: Berkowitz L, ed. *Advances in experimental social psychology.* New York: Academic Press, 1964: 191–229.
22. Gortmaker SL, Peterson K, Wiecha J, *et al.* Reducing obesity via a school-based interdisciplinary intervention among youth: Planet Health. *Arch Pediatr Adolesc Med* 1999; 153: 409–18.

23. Dwyer JT, Hewew LV, Mitchell PD, *et al.* Improving school breakfasts: effects of the CATCH Eat Smart program on the nutrient content of school breakfasts. *Prev Med* 1996; 25: 413–22.
24. Ellison RC, Capper AL, Goldberg RJ, Witschi JC, Stare FJ. The environmental component: changing school food service to promote cardiovascular health. *Health Educ Q* 1989; 16: 285–97.
25. Osganian SK, Ebzery MK, Montgomery DH, *et al.* Changes in nutrient content of school lunches: results from the CATCH Eat Smart foods service intervention. *Prev Med* 1996; 25: 400–12.
26. Luepker RV, Perry CL, McKinlay SM, *et al.* Outcomes of a field trial to improve children's dietary patterns and physical activity. The Child and Adolescent Trial for Cardiovascular Health (CATCH). *JAMA* 1996; 275: 768–76.
27. Whitaker RC, Wright JA, Finch AJ, Psaty BM. An environmental intervention to reduce dietary fat in school lunches. *Pediatrics* 1993; 91: 1107–11.
28. DeMarco T, Sidney K. Enhancing children's participation in physical activity. *J School Health* 1989; 59: 337–40.
29. Simons-Morton BG, Taylor WC, Snider SA, Huant IW. The physical activity of fifth-grade students during physical education classes. *Am J Public Health* 1993; 83: 262–4.
30. McKenzie TL, Nader PR, Strikmiller PK, *et al.* School physical education: effect of the Child and Adolescent Trial for Cardiovascular Health. *Prev Med* 1996; 25: 423–31.
31. Sallis JF, McKenzie TL, Alcaraz JE, Kolody B, Faucette N, Hovell MF. The effects of a 2-year physical education program (SPARK) on physical activity and fitness in elementary school students. *Am J Public Health* 1997; 87: 1328–34.
32. Simons-Morton BG, Parcel GS, Baranowski T, Forthofer R, O'Hara NM. Promoting physical activity and a healthful diet among children: results of a school-based intervention study. *Am J Public Health* 1991; 81: 986–91.
33. Dwyer T, Coonan WE, Leitch DR, Hetzel BS, Baghurst RA. An investigation of the effects of daily physical activity on the health of primary school students in South Australia. *Int J Epidemiol* 1983; 12: 308–13.
34. Flores R. Dance for health: improving fitness in African American and Hispanic adolescents. *Public Health Rep* 1995; 110: 189–93.
35. Jacobson MF, Brownell KD. Small taxes on soft drinks and snack foods to promote health. *Am J Public Health* 2000; 90: 854–7.
36. Borzekowski DLG, Robinson TN. The 30-second effect: an experiment revealing the impact of television commercials on food preferences of preschoolers. *J Am Diet Assoc* 2001; 101: 42–6.
37. Robinson TN. Reducing children's television viewing to prevent obesity: a randomized controlled trial. *JAMA* 1999; 282: 1561–7.
38. Epstein LH, Valoski AM, Vara LS, *et al.* Effects of decreasing sedentary behavior and increasing activity on weight change in obese children. *Health Psychol* 1995; 14: 109–15.
39. Epstein LH, Paluch RA, Gordy CC, Dorn J. Decreasing sedentary behaviors in treating pediatric obesity. *Arch Pediatr Adolesc Med* 2000; 154: 220–6.

DISCUSSION

Dr. Birch: Can you comment on the sex differences? What is going on here?

Dr. Robinson: We did not see sex differences in the TV reduction study, although it was a small study and there was limited power to detect a sex by treatment interaction. Although there were significant sex by treatment interactions in the Stanford Adolescent Heart Health study, there were significant effects in both sexes. The one study where we did see effects in girls only was a study of dance in 12-year-olds. My guess is that dance is probably not the behavior of choice for 12-year-old boys in terms of their motivation to participate.

Dr. Uauy: The question of effectiveness relates to what else is going on in the schools. One of the issues is snacks. How did you address the problem of snacking in school in your trials?

Dr. Robinson: To date, we haven't, although I agree it is a big problem. The snacks and à la carte foods that are now available did not become popular until after the high school study was done. Dr. Dietz may have some comments in his presentation on methods to change the school environment to try and reduce the effect of snacks obtained from vending machines and so on. There is room for creative approaches to try to change the food environment in schools, especially regarding what people are calling "competing foods"—that is, competing for what is normally served.

Dr. Endres: In some of your studies, especially in that using aerobics, it appeared that the control groups showed an increase in BMI. Why was that?

Dr. Robinson: I do not believe that any of the control groups increased their BMI in any way that was out of the ordinary. Children are naturally expected to increase in BMI as they grow. Therefore an effective prevention program is one that reduces excessive weight gain.

Dr. Gortmaker: Going back to your focus on shifting population distributions, I liked that perspective very much, and yet I feel that that the model should perhaps be modified a bit. Particularly in the context of, for example, China or some other countries where undernutrition is still a major issue, we would not want to move the entire distribution down and increase the underweight population. You might want to modify the model and think how to decrease obesity without moving the tail of the distribution to the left. Any comments on that?

Dr. Robinson: Those were hypothetical distributions, and there is nothing in the real world that actually looks like a true bell curve. I agree that you want to see larger changes at the higher levels. However, when countries change their distributions over time, the distributions really do move together, so while you may see a blunting of a tail at one end or another, in general the distribution does move as a whole.

Dr. Dietz: One of the points that has not been made here is that the distribution of obesity is skewed. We are really talking about maybe reducing this skew, which would lower the mean somewhat without affecting the median. Then the bottom half of the distribution would not change. Maybe that's the way to think about it.

Dr. Robinson: I may not have been as clear as I could have been in terms of describing the process. The idea is that most of the morbidity and mortality that occurs is really in those people to the left of (below) the cutoff, because problems like cardiovascular disease and cancer are so common. For example, in sheer numbers, most of the people who die from heart disease do not have high cholesterol levels. Thus moving the entire distribution by a small amount has a greater effect on morbidity and mortality than taking the small group of high-risk people and reducing their cholesterol levels.

Dr. Shi: How long is a suitable time for children to watch TV per day?

Dr. Robinson: Several expert groups have suggested that no more than 1 to 2 hours a day is recommended in the United States. I'm not sure we really know how much time children do watch TV because I don't necessarily believe the self-reports or the parental reports. Our approach was to ask what happens if you *reduce* television viewing, no matter where the starting point is. So I would say that if your child is watching what you think is an excessive amount of television, then first of all try to halve it.

Dr. Gortmaker: I can't resist following up on that. I'd just like to point out to everybody that there is no evidence whatsoever that watching more than an hour of TV a day is good for anybody, anywhere!

Obesity in Childhood and Adolescence, edited by
Chunming Chen and William H. Dietz. Nestlé
Nutrition Workshop Series, Pediatric Program,
Vol. 49. Nestec Ltd., Vevey/Lippincott
Williams & Wilkins, Philadelphia © 2002.

School Programs

Anna Jacob

Food and Nutrition Specialists Pte Ltd., Singapore, China

School-based programs that are carefully designed and implemented can play an important role in promoting lifelong physical activity and healthy eating among young people (1). The rationale for school health education programs is based largely on their potential ability to reduce preventable morbidity and mortality (2).

The advantage of school-based interventions is the extensive reach to a diverse group of children 5 to 17 years of age, cutting across socioeconomic, racial, and cultural lines; schools also provide opportunities for repeated exposure to intervention activities and access to the families of the participating children, spreading the benefits to other families and creating a positive environment at home.

A literature search suggests that school health education programs seem to have a long tradition in the United States (3,4), but only a few projects from Europe (5), Australia, and Asia are documented and published.

School-based health programs include short- and long-term trials as well as sustained programs. The school health education programs cited are diverse and not all directed at obese and overweight children. Many include the entire cohort of children, in order to promote physical activity, healthy eating, and healthy lifestyles, including prevention of smoking (5).

The purpose of this chapter is to provide an overview of school-based programs that primarily target obesity and overweight, that address obesity and overweight as risk factors for the development of cardiovascular diseases, and that use weight or body fat status as a variable in physical activity interventions among schoolchildren. Published reports of school-based health education programs and several programs in progress are included. School-based intervention programs are categorized by age group of intervention (Table 1).

PRIMARY OR ELEMENTARY SCHOOL PROGRAMS

The Child and Adolescent Trial for Cardiovascular Health (CATCH)

CATCH is the largest and most ambitious randomized controlled school health education intervention conducted in the United States. The goal of this 3-year randomized intervention trial, funded by the National Heart, Lung, and Blood Institute, was

TABLE 1. School health education programs categorized by age group and country of implementation

Primary/elementary school programs

School program	Implementation	Objective	Target population	Components	Time frame
The Child and Adolescent Trial for Cardiovascular Health (CATCH)	National Heart Lung and Blood Institute, USA	Impact of health education on cardiovascular risk factors and risk-related behaviors	5,000 ethnically diverse students from 96 schools in four states	• Manual for food service • Guidebook for teachers to increase moderate-to-vigorous physical activity • Activity box with 350 easy-to-teach activities • Three exercise videotapes • Classroom curriculum modules for third, fourth, and fifth graders • Family involvement component	3-year randomized intervention trial
Sports, Play, and Active Recreation for Kids (SPARK)	National Heart Lung and Blood Institute, USA	Create, implement, and evaluate a curriculum and staff development program	Over 350 schools in 12 states	• PE curriculum for K1 through 2 and grades 3 to 6 with a minimum of 30 minutes of PE, 3 days a week throughout the entire school year • Self-management program to be active outside of schools	2 years physical education and one semester for self-management
Know Your Body (KYB)	Los Angeles, USA	Improve knowledge and belief about health, increase physical activity	1,400 students in over 18 schools	• 30–50 hours of health education each year	3 years

Program	Location	Objective	Sample	Components	Duration
Go for Health (GH)	USA	Foster healthful diet and exercise	409 students in four schools	• Classroom health education • Changes in school lunch • Physical education	2 years
Nebraska School Study	Rural Nebraska, USA	Reduce obesity and improve fitness by promoting physical activity	Grades 3 to 5 in two schools	• Enhanced physical activity • Grade specific nutrition education	2 year study
Cardiovascular Health in Children Study (CHIC)	North Carolina, USA	Effects of classroom-based and risk-based interventions to reduce multiple VCD risk factors	2,109 schoolchildren in 18 randomly selected schools	• Lower fat and sodium school education • Knowledge, attitude, and physical activity components taught by teachers	8-week intervention
Eat Well and Keep Moving (EWKM)	USA	Impact of a school-based interdisciplinary health behavior education on diet and physical activity	Grades 4 and 5	• Training and wellness programs for the teachers • Intervention material to decrease fat and saturated fat, increase fruit and vegetable, reduce television viewing, and increase physical activity	2 years
Take 10™	ILSI's Center for Health Promotion, Atlanta, USA	Opportunities for physical activity during the school day	Over 200 schools in Georgia from kindergarten through 5th grade	• 10 different grade-specific activity cards • One coll-down lesson • Teacher's manual • Tracking poster	Ongoing since 1999

(continued)

TABLE 1. *Continued*

School program	Implementation	Objective	Target population	Components	Time frame
Primary/elementary and secondary/high school programs					
Trim and Fit (TAF) Program	Ministries of Health and Education, Singapore	Promote healthy lifestyle and enhance quality of life, starting with the nation's youth	All school children in primary and secondary schools and junior college Remedial program for over- and underweight children	• Physical education • Extracurricular activities • Improved the school environment • Healthier tuckshops • TAF club for overweight children • Obesity clinic for severely over- and underweight children	Ongoing since 1992
Power Kids Eat Smart™ Power kids on the go™	ILSI Southeast Asia Ministries of Health and Education, School of Physical Education, Singapore	Resource tool for TAF club teachers to educate and empower TAF club students	All TAF club students in elementary schools	• Nutrition education module • Physical education module • Self-management module	Launched 2001
Australia School Project	New South Wales, Australia	Increase the proportion of students who do more than 1 hour of exercise outside school	Over 3,200 students in one high school and two primary schools	• CVD screening • Curricula	2 years
Secondary/high school program					
The Stanford Adolescent Heart Health Program	USA	Create, implement, and test a school-based multiple-risk factor reduction program	1,447 students from four senior high schools	• Special 20-session CVD risk reduction intervention	2 months

Abbreviations: CVD, cardiovascular disease; PE, physical education.

to demonstrate the effectiveness of health education in producing modest changes in cardiovascular risk factors and risk-related behaviors in schoolchildren. CATCH involved more than 5,000 ethnically diverse students from 96 schools (56 intervention and 40 control) in four states in the United States (6).

The curricula that were developed for CATCH provide skills training in healthier eating, physical activity, and nonsmoking behaviors. The CATCH program includes a manual for food service directors and cooks on ways to lower total fat (30% of energy), saturated fat (10% of energy), and sodium (600 to 1000 mg per serving) in the school meals. It includes methods for planning menus, purchasing products, and promoting school lunch. The CATCH physical education (PE) module consists of a guidebook for elementary school teachers to help them increase moderate to vigorous physical activity of their students by 40% (2). The CATCH PE module also includes an activity box with 350 easy-to-teach activities and three videotapes that include warm-up, aerobics, strength-building activities, and cool-down activities. In addition, CATCH consists of classroom curriculum modules for third, fourth, and fifth graders. These sessions include messages on healthy eating, physical activity, and smoking prevention. The family involvement component consists of activity packets and family "fun nights" (7).

The result of extensive process evaluation confirmed that the CATCH curricula were delivered with adequate fidelity, with more than 90% of the curriculum completed and more than 88% of the lessons completed without modification (8). The mean percentage of energy from fat and saturated fat in the food served at school lunches fell by 6.8% and 2.8%, respectively, but sodium goals were not achieved (9). CATCH schools showed a significant increase in moderate-to-vigorous physical activity during PE class, from 37% to 52% (10). Total cholesterol, blood pressure, and body mass index (BMI) did not show significant change (11).

Sports, Play, and Active Recreation for Kids (SPARK)

SPARK is a physical education program for elementary schoolchildren. Also funded by a research grant from the National Heart, Lung, and Blood Institute, the aim of this project was to create and evaluate a curriculum and staff development program that can be implemented in real-world settings by both classroom teachers and physical education specialists. To date, more than 350 schools in 12 states in the United States have adopted SPARK (12).

The SPARK curriculum offers packages in two levels—for K2 and grades 3 to 6. SPARK recommends a minimum of 30 minutes of PE 3 days a week throughout the entire school year. One unique feature of SPARK is the self-management program that teaches children skills and techniques necessary to be active outside of schools, on the weekends, during vacations, and ultimately for the rest of their lives (12).

More than 24 papers have been published on a variety of topics about SPARK, ranging from methodology to impact. One study of 955 grade 4 and 5 students in seven schools in San Diego that took part in the SPARK curriculum showed that sessions led by physical education specialists and trained teachers provided more moderate-to-vigorous physical activity during PE than sessions led by regular teachers. No change was noted in out-of-school physical activity or self-management in any group (13,14). Researchers found that incentives provided as self-reward in this program had no effect on physical activity outside the school but succeeded in increasing moderate-to-vigorous physical activity in PE classes (13).

Know Your Body (KYB)

The KYB program, a multiple-risk-factor school health education curriculum, involved 1,400 students in more than 18 schools in Los Angeles. This program is targeted at elementary school students and aims to improve knowledge and belief about health and to increase physical activity (15).

The KYB program delivers 30 to 50 hours of health education each year for 3 years. Three major evaluations of the program carried out at the end of 3 years showed a significant difference in total cholesterol levels in two trials, and in systolic and diastolic blood pressure in all three trials, but no difference in BMI or skinfold thickness measurements (2).

Go for Health

The Go for Health program from the United States includes classroom health education and environmental changes in school lunch and physical education to foster a healthy diet and exercise among elementary schoolchildren.

In-depth study of 409 students in four schools who took part in the program showed increased knowledge and a better attitude, with an increase in moderate-to-vigorous physical activity in PE classes from less than 10% at baseline to about 40% of class time after intervention. No change was observed in out-of-school physical activity (16). In the two intervention schools, school lunches showed reductions from baseline in total fat (by 15.5% and 10.4%), saturated fat (by 31.7% to 18.8%), and sodium (by 40.2% and 53.6%) (17).

Nebraska School Study

Cohorts from grades 3 to 5 in two schools in rural Nebraska in the United States participated in this 2-year study of enhanced physical activity, grade-specific nutrition education, and a school lunch that was lower in fat and sodium. The aim of this school-based intervention was to reduce obesity and improve fitness by promoting physical activity (6).

By year 2, the investigators found that the intervention group was consuming significantly less energy (9%), fat (25%), and sodium (21%), and more fiber (17%) during lunch. However, 24-hour recalls showed differences for sodium alone (18). The researchers also found that compensation for lower-fat meals by the intervention schoolchildren was not evident, as the percentage of energy from fat in the diet as a whole was only 1.3% greater that the percentage in the lunch that was served (19).

Physical activity was 6% greater in the intervention group in the classroom and 16% lower outside of school when compared with controls. Body weight and body fat were also not different between normal and obese children in the two groups. However, high-density lipoprotein (HDL) cholesterol was significantly greater, and the total cholesterol-to-HDL ratio was significantly lower in the intervention group (18).

Cardiovascular Health in Children Study (CHIC)

The Cardiovascular Health in Children (CHIC) study sought to determine the population effects of both classroom-based and risk-based interventions designed to reduce multiple cardiovascular disease risk factors in children. The study involved 2,109 elementary school children in 18 randomly selected schools across North Carolina. The children were randomized by school to a classroom-based intervention for all third and fourth graders, a risk-based intervention group (which included children with one or more cardiovascular risk factors), or a control group. Regular teachers conducted an 8-week intervention that included knowledge, attitudes, and physical activity components (20).

Results showed that physical activity in the risk-based group and posttest knowledge in the classroom group were higher than in the control. Cholesterol, the primary outcome measure, fell in the classroom group by 11.7 mg/dl (0.30 mmol/l), in the risk-based group by 10.1 mg/dl (0.26 mmol/l), and in the control group by 2.3 mg/dl (0.06 mmol/l). Both intervention groups had greater health knowledge and a small reduction in body fat. Skinfold thickness decreased by 2.9% in the classroom group and by 3.2% in the risk-based group compared with the control (20).

Eat Well and Keep Moving (EWKM)

The Eat Well and Keep Moving (EWKM) project, also from the United States, aimed to evaluate the impact of a school-based interdisciplinary health behavior education on diet and physical activity among children in grades 4 and 5. Classroom teachers taught the EWKM program over 2 years in mathematics, science, language, arts, and social studies classes. Materials provided links to school food services and families. EWKM also provided training and wellness programs for the teachers and staff members. Intervention materials focused on decreasing consumption of foods high in total fat and saturated fat and increasing fruit and vegetable intake, as well as on reducing television viewing and increasing physical activity (21).

A quasi-experimental field trial with six intervention schools and eight matched control schools was conducted. The study showed that percentages of total energy from fat and saturated fat were reduced among students in intervention compared with control schools. There was also an increase in fruit and vegetable intake (0.36 serving per 1,000 kcal) as well as vitamin C and fiber intakes. Television viewing was marginally reduced by 0.55 h/day (21).

Take 10

Take 10 is a physical activity program specifically designed by the International Life Sciences Institute's (ILSI) Center for Health Promotion in Atlanta. It is designed to give children opportunities for physical activity during the school day. This program promotes 10-minute periods of moderate to vigorous physical activity in the classroom. Created by teachers, it includes graded packages that cover the elementary school, from kindergarten through fifth grade. The materials include 10 different grade-specific activity cards, one cool-down lesson, a teacher's manual, and a tracking poster. The activities suggested have been validated and proven effective for use in a classroom setting, and are linked to the core curriculum objectives (22). Approximately 2,600 students and 108 teachers from four Atlanta elementary schools participated in a 10-week pilot intervention and assessment in October 1999. Currently, implemented in over 200 schools in Georgia, various aspects of the Take 10 program are being evaluated.

Nutrifit

The Nutrifit program consists of nutrition education and physical training modules. The program was tested among 514 schoolchildren 8 to 9 years of age who were enrolled in two provincial government schools and two private schools in the Bangkok metropolitan area.

Health-related fitness tests using a Fitnessgram were administered in all four schools, followed by the Nutrifit intervention program. The intervention included 10 nutrition and physical education training classes held during regular PE class. During the 7-month program period, the nutritional status of children, as assessed by weight-for-height, did not show a significant change. However, there was definite improvement in health-related fitness tests in both intervention and control schools.

The investigators found that the fitness test scores alone inspired the school authorities to create opportunities for those who failed to take up extra training, even in the control groups. Plotting their own weight and height seemed to increase interest among the children to attain ideal weight-for-height. Use of "star labels" and "recognition" as incentives seemed to generate peer pressure to improve fitness in Thai children (23).

PRIMARY OR ELEMENTARY AND SECONDARY OR HIGH SCHOOL PROGRAMS

Trim and Fit (TAF) Program

The Trim and Fit (TAF) program in schools is part of the national integrated strategy to combat childhood obesity in Singapore. The TAF program was launched in 1992 as a motivational strategy to promote healthy lifestyle and enhance quality of life, starting with the nation's youth. The TAF program involves all schools—primary, secondary, and preuniversity. It encourages schools to develop strategies to reduce obesity and improve physical fitness of the entire student population.

Although national guidelines provide a framework for the school, each school is given the flexibility to develop strategies and plans for physical education and extracurricular activities and for improving the school environment. The program also creates a healthier tuckshop, with guidelines and workshop for vendors, green food labeling, water coolers, guidelines for food service, and monitoring of food sold.

In the TAF remediation program, children who are overweight, underweight, or unfit are managed at school level through a fitness group called the TAF Club, whereas severely overweight and underweight children are managed at a specialized clinic at the School Health Services by a team of health professionals. TAF Club includes a 30-week annual structured program of activities with proper record maintenance. The activities are designed to be fun and challenging and include brisk walks, aerobics, modified games, and even hiking. Children are also guided to make healthier food choices. Monthly monitoring of weight and height supports the TAF Club. Managed through a collaborative effort of several government departments such as the ministries for health and education in Singapore, the TAF program educates and trains implementers systematically.

National tracking of the program has shown that the overweight percentage has fallen from 14.0% in 1992 to 9.9% in 1998. Fitness of children, as assessed by the National Physical Fitness Awards test, showed improvement from 60% in 1992 to more than 70% in 1998. The program aims to improve the management of individuals whose weight is more than 160% of national standards, to introduce the elements of the TAF program to preschool and kindergarten levels, and to devise innovative ways to improve weight management that would appeal to children (24).

Power Kids Eat Smart and Power Kids on the Go

Responding to the government's call for innovative ways to educate and empower TAF Club students, ILSI Southeast Asia—along with the Ministries of Health and Education and the School of Physical Education in Singapore—developed a resource tool for TAF Club teachers in primary schools.

The aim was to conduct fun activity classes for children to promote overall health and fitness and create lifelong habits that will form the basis of healthy adult behaviors. The Power Kids resource tool consists of a nutrition education module called Power Kids Eat Smart and a physical education package called Power Kids on the Go. Power Kids Eat Smart consists of nutrition messages delivered through stories and reinforced through activity sheets and goal-setting exercises. Power Kids on the Go allows the teachers to develop varied, safe, and effective physical activity sessions that promote moderate to vigorous physical activity. Parental involvement and self-management feature strongly in the program.

Piloted in three schools in the year 2000, the program is now available to all 210 primary schools in Singapore. Process and impact evaluations are in progress (25).

Australia School Project

The Australia School Project covered more than 3,200 students in one high school and two primary schools in New South Wales. The sample included both girls and boys from the lower socioeconomic class. The experimental program aimed to increase the proportion of students who do more than 1 hour of exercise outside school. At the end of the project, it was reported that this proportion increased by 17.5% in the intervention group and by 6.5% in the control group (6,26).

Other Programs

Other school-based intervention programs in progress (all in the United States) include Pathways, Stanford Obesity Prevention for Preadolescents, Planet Health, Middle School Physical Activity and Nutrition, Lifestyle Education for Activity Project, and Adolescent Computer-Based CVD Curriculum and Advocacy (6).

SECONDARY OR HIGH SCHOOL PROGRAMS

The Stanford Adolescent Heart Health Program

The Stanford Adolescent Heart Health program was designed to create, implement, and test a school-based multiple-risk factor reduction program for high school students. All tenth graders from four senior high schools (1,447 students) from two school districts in the United States participated in the study. Within each district, one school was assigned at random to receive a special 20-session cardiovascular disease risk reduction intervention and one school served as the control. At a 2-month follow-up, knowledge gains were significantly greater for students in the treatment group on each of the risk factor domains tested—nutrition, physical activity, and cigarette smoking. A higher proportion of those in the treatment group started to exercise regularly and also reported that they were more likely to choose a heart-healthy snack item. Resting heart rate ($p < 0.0001$), BMI ($p = 0.05$), triceps skinfold thickness ($p = 0.003$), and subscapular skinfold thickness ($p = 0.01$) also showed improvement (27).

SYNTHESIS

The school-based programs in this paper include programs and intervention trials. Although most have been conducted in the United States, examples from Asia and Australia are included. The sample size of these programs ranged from as few as two schools to more than 400 schools. The duration ranged from short trials of 8 weeks to programs sustained for more than 8 years.

Only two programs included reduction in obesity or overweight as the major goal. Other studies addressed changes in weight status and/or body fatness as risk factors for cardiovascular diseases or as a result of physical activity interventions. Study design varied greatly in length and scope. Sampling ranged from random to nonrandomized assignment of schools to programs. Few programs included follow-up studies beyond the period of intervention.

The largest and the longest school program that addressed fitness of students and obesity was the Trim and Fit program in Singapore. CATCH and SPARK are the two school-based intervention trials with the most papers published in peer-reviewed journals. Each school-based health education program used a different approach to effect change in the food and activity behaviors of children. The design and components of the program were tailored to the environment in which the program was implemented. Newer programs are taking a more holistic approach to addressing health-related behavior change in the individual and address environmental change and involvement of parents to support newly learned behaviors.

The results of school-based interventions are mixed, with some showing no significant change as a result of intervention (Table 2). Success seems to be associated with direction and organizational support from the government related institutes, environmental change, provision of trained physical education teachers, a strong physical education program, and the inclusion of family-based components. Almost all studies that looked at knowledge and attitudes of the intervention group showed improvement. The results on overall increase in physical activity and improved nutrition were mixed: There were more consistent data on improvement in physical activity intensity during PE classes, no improvement in physical activity outside school, and a reduction in the fat and saturated fat content of school meals.

CHALLENGES

In the past, the creation, implementation, and evaluation of effective school programs has presented a challenge to public health officials, school authorities, and health educators. Study of successful school health programs has highlighted key strategies essential for success. The Center for Disease Control (CDC) reports (*Guidelines for School Health Programs to Promote Lifelong Healthy Eating* and *Guidelines for School and Community Programs to Promote Lifelong Physical Activity among Young People*) incorporate several of these effective and promising strategies for schools.

The CDC guidelines address the school policy on nutrition, a sequential and coordinated curriculum, appropriate instruction for students, integration of school food service and nutrition education, staff training, family and community involvement, and program evaluation (28). School-based interventions that have been highlighted include intramural sports, facilities that promote physical activity, psychosocial support for physical activity, food and beverages available in school outside the school meals program, and healthy eating (29).

As weight management in children does not focus on weight loss as much as it does on the prevention of weight gain, school programs need to be sustained for a sufficient length of time. Many health educators involved in school health education programs are now concerned about identifying strategies that ensure that school-based programs are sustainable beyond the intervention period. Renewing programs,

TABLE 2. *Selected outcomes of school health education programs*

School program	Impact of intervention
Primary/elementary school programs	
The Child and Adolescent Trial for Cardiovascular Health (CATCH)	• Mean percentage of energy from fat and saturated fat of school lunches dropped • Sodium goals were not achieved • Significant increase in MVPA during PE class • Total cholesterol, blood pressure, and BMI did not show significant changes
Sports, Play, and Active Recreation for Kids (SPARK)	• Sessions by trained teachers provided more MVPA during PE than those by regular teachers • No change was noted in out-of-school physical activity
Know Your Body (KYB)	• Increase in knowledge • Significant difference in total cholesterol levels • Systolic and diastolic blood pressure lowered • No difference in body mass index or skinfold measures
Go for Health (GH)	• Increased knowledge and a better attitude • Increased MVPA in PE classes • No change observed in out-of-school physical activity • School lunches lower in total fat, saturated fat, and sodium
Nebraska School Study	• Less energy, fat, and sodium and more fiber during lunch • Physical activity greater in the classroom and lower outside of school • Body weight and body fat not different • HDL cholesterol significantly greater • Total cholesterol to HDL ratio significantly lower
Cardiovascular Health in Children Study (CHIC)	• Physical activity and posttest knowledge higher • Reduced cholesterol • Small reduction in body fat • Skinfold decreased
Eat Well and Keep Moving (EWKM)	• Percentages of total energy from fat and saturated fat reduced • Increase in fruit and vegetable intake • Television viewing marginally reduced
Primary/elementary and secondary/high school programs	
Trim and Fit (TAF) Program	• Overweight percent has dropped from 14.0% in 1992 to 9.9% in 1998 • Fitness improvement from 60% in 1992 to over 70% in 1998
Australia School Project	• Students with more than 1 hour of exercise outside school increased
Secondary/high school programs	
The Stanford Adolescent Heart Health Program	• Knowledge gains significantly greater • Regular exercise increased • More likely to choose a heart healthy snack item • Resting heart rate, BMI, triceps skinfold, and subscapular skinfold thickness improved

Abbreviations: BMI, body mass index; HDL, high-density lipoprotein; MVPA, moderate to vigorous physical activity; PE, physical education.

sustaining interest of implementers and children, involving the community, and ensuring cost-efficacy are new challenges being discussed.

CONCLUSIONS

The recent epidemic of obesity among children presents formidable challenges for those seeking to develop, implement, and evaluate effective prevention and treatment programs. Major impediments to creating effective and sustainable intervention programs have been the lack of knowledge about the determinants of physical activity and dietary patterns in young people, and in particular, the understanding of the causes of obesity.

Three recent CDC guidelines for school health programs aimed at promoting lifelong physical activity among young people conclude that school programs are among the most effective strategies for reducing the public health burden of chronic disease associated with sedentary lifestyles and unhealthy eating patterns (28).

Although few published studies of long-term school programs address obesity or overweight in children, enough is known to merit continued implementation and ongoing refinement. More research is needed to study the impact of these programs on student physical activity, healthy eating, and weight management in children, as well as on the development and maintenance of healthy behaviors in adulthood.

Although school-based health promotion programs help children develop skills that encourage lifetime health and fitness, healthcare professionals, school authorities, and community partners play invaluable roles in reinforcing these behaviors.

REFERENCES

1. McGraw SA, Sellers D, Stone E, *et al.* Measuring implementation of school programs and policies to promote healthy eating and physical activity among youth. *Prev Med* 2000; 31: 86–97.
2. Resnicow K, Robinson TN, Frank E. Advances and future directions for school-based health promotion research: commentary on the CATCH intervention trial. *Prev Med* 1996; 25: 378–83.
3. Brownell KD, Kaye FS. A school based behavior modification, nutrition education and physical activity program for obese children, *Am J Clin Nutr* 1982; 35: 277–83.
4. Figueroa-Colon R, Franlin FA, Lee JY, van Alemen TK, Suskind RM. Feasibility of a clinic based hypocaloric dietary intervention implemented in a school setting for obese children. *Obes Res* 1996; 4: 419–29.
5. Zwiauer KFM. Intervention for prevention of overweight and obesity in children and adolescents, cited in ILSI Europe mini workshop on overweight and obesity in European children and adolescents: causes and consequences—prevention and treatment. Brussels, Belgium, ILSI Europe, 1998.
6. Stone EJ, McKenzie TL, Welk GJ, Booth ML. Effect of physical activity interventions in youth—review and synthesis. *Am J Prev Med* 1998; 15: 298–315.
7. CATCH (1995).National Heart Lung and Blood Institute Information Center, PO Box 30105, Bethesda, MD 20824-0105, USA.
8. Luepker RV, Perry CL, McKinlay SM, *et al.* Outcomes of a field trial to improve children's dietary patterns and physical activity. *JAMA* 1996; 275: 768–76.
9. Osganian SK, Ebzery MK, Montgomery DH, *et al.* Changes in the nutrient content of school lunches: results from CATCH eat smart food service intervention. *Prev Med* 1996; 25: 400–12.
10. McKenzie TL, Nader PR, Strikmiller PK, *et al.* School physical education: effect of the Child and Adolescent Trial for Cardiovascular Health. *Prev Med* 1996; 25: 423–31.
11. Webber LS, Osignan SK, Feldman HJ, *et al.* Cardiovascular risk factors in children after 2.5 years of intervention—the CATCH study. *Prev Med* 1996; 25: 432–41.

12. SPARK Physical Education (1993). San Diego State University, 6363 Alvarado Court, Suite 250, San Diego, California 92120, USA.
13. Sallis JF, McKenzie TL, Alcaraz JE, Kolody B, Faucette N, Hovell MF. Effects of a two-year health-related physical education program on physical activity and fitness in elementary school students: SPARK. *Am J Public Health* 1997; 87: 1328–34.
14. McKenzie TL, Sallis JF, Kolody B, Faucett FN. Long term effect of a physical education curriculum and staff development work: SPARK. *Res Q Exerc Sport* 1997; 68: 280–91.
15. Marcus AC, Wheeler RC, Cullen JW, Crane LA. Quasi-experimental evaluation of the Los Angeles Know Your Body Program: knowledge, beliefs, and self-reported behaviors. *Prev Med* 1987; 16: 803–15.
16. Simons-Morton B, Parcel GS, Baranowski T, Forthofer R, O'Hara NM. Promoting physical activity and a healthful diet among children: results of a school-based intervention study. *Am J Public Health* 1991; 81: 986–91.
17. Parcel GS, Simons-Morton B, O'Hara NM, Baranowski T, Wilson B. School promotion of healthful diet and physical activity: impact on learning outcomes and self reported behavior. *Health Educ Q* 1989; 16: 181–99.
18. Donnelly JE, Jacobsen DJ, Whatley JE, *et al.* Nutrition and physical activity program to attenuate obesity and promote physical and metabolic fitness in elementary school children. *Obes Res* 1996; 4: 229–43.
19. Whatley JE, Donnelly JE, Jacobsen DJ, Hill JO, Carlson MK. Energy and macronutrient consumption of elementary school children served modified lower fat and sodium lunches or standard higher fat and sodium lunches. *J Am Coll Nutr* 1996; 15: 602–7.
20. Harrell JS, McMurray RG, Gansky SA, Bangdiwala SI, Bradley CB. A public health vs risk-based intervention to improve cardiovascular health in elementary school children: the cardiovascular health in children study. *Am J Public Health* 1999; 89: 1529–35.
21. Gortmaker SL, Cheung LW, Peterson KE, *et al.* Impact of a school-based interdisciplinary intervention on diet and physical activity among urban primary school children: eat well and keep moving. *Arch Pediatr Adolesc Med* 1999; 153: 975–83.
22. Take 10! ILSI Center for Health Promotion, 2295 Parklake Drive, Suite 450, Atlanta, GA 30345, USA.
23. Kijboonchoo K, Thasansuwan W, Yamborisut, U. Nutrifit program to improve health-related fitness among young Thai schoolchildren. *Food Nutr Bull* 1999; 20: 231–7.
24. Frances C. Prevention and management of obesity in Singapore school children cited in Workshop on Obesity in China. April 24–26, 2000. ILSI and ILSI Focal Point on China.
25. Power Kids Eat Smart and Power Kids on the Go. ILSI Southeast Asia, 03-45 Goldhill Plaza Podium Block, 1 Newton Road, Singapore 308899.
26. Homel PJ, Daniels P, Reid TR, Lawson JS. Results of an experimental school-based health development program in Australia. *Int J Health Educ* 1981; 21: 263–70.
27. Killen JD, Robinson TN, Telch MJ, *et al.* The Stanford Adolescent Heart Health program. *Health Educ Q* 1989; 16: 263–83.
28. Mendlein JM, Baranowski T, Pratt M. Physical activity and nutrition in children and youth: opportunities for performing assessments and interventions. *Prev Med* 2000; 31: 150–3.
29. Wechsler H, Devereaux RS, Davis M, Collins J. Using the school environment to promote physical activity and healthy eating. *Prev Med* 2000; 31: 121–37.

DISCUSSION

Dr. Uauy: What is the cost of this program per child per year?

Mrs. Jacob: Nobody has ever done that evaluation. For the Trim and Fit program, there is intensive input from the Ministry of Education and the school health services. The government in Singapore is willing to carry the cost for now. They have never said it costs too much. Children are considered very important.

Dr. Endres: In relation to those parents who did not change their diet at home, was this because they could they not afford to, or did they resist change for cultural reasons?

Mrs. Jacob: Some parents will always be resistant to change. In other cases, though the teachers were doing many things with the children in school, they did not reach out to the parents. Through the Power Kids resource we made an effort to keep the parents up to speed with what was going on in the schools. I would not say there was a cultural problem or that they couldn't afford it in Singapore; it's mainly lack of interest.

Dr. Endres: I have heard from Dr. Roulet that parents were against his school programs in Lausanne, Switzerland. Perhaps he could comment?

Dr. Roulet: We have tried to establish a weight control program in schools in Lausanne, but many parents refused to allow their children to take part. They say it's not the role of a school to check on children's weight or what they are eating at home. It can be quite a problem to involve the family, and this might be the same in Singapore.

Mrs. Jacob: We have had experience of parents who argue with you about whether their child is overweight or not, but the majority of parents appreciate that the school is interested and the teachers are willing to give up their busy time to care about the children in this way.

Dr. Baerlocher: You said that only a few programs had been described from Europe. It is true that not many have been reported in international journals, but there are in fact many programs in Europe. They have been published in one or other of the European languages in the form of booklets or reports that are available for teachers and institutions but have not appeared in medical journals. In Germany for example, the state of Baden-Würtenberg has been running nutrition education programs for children from 3 to 12 years for the last 25 years, supervised by nutritionists and dietitians. In Switzerland we have recently carried out a survey of nutritional programs throughout the country which has shown that nutrition education is a part of the regular curriculum in all schools for 10 to 16-year-old children; they even have cooking lessons. There are also specific programs that have evolved in the context of a European network for health promotion in schools. In this network, schools can send in their own programs for evaluation and use in other European countries. One of these programs is called "Pausenkiosk," which is a snack food service run by the children themselves. They buy foods at local farms and prepare the snacks that they sell to the other children. While doing this they learn about nutrition from their teachers. In another state there is a program called "energy management," which lasts for 4 years and has the goal of improving physical activity and nutrition. In Switzerland, there is also a nutrition museum established by Nestlé in Vevey, called "Alimentarium." This museum includes nutritional education programs for children that are very interactive. Children really enjoy going there and learning about nutrition.

Mrs. Jacob: Thank you. One of the things about school programs is that not all of them do get published, so if we limit our search for successful programs to those that have been published in scientific journals we will probably miss some effective and culturally specific programs.

Dr. Ma: Was the nutrition education program integrated with classroom teaching and is there any special school policy for the program? As you know, in China all schools are focused on academic achievement, so if there are no specific school policies it may be hard for health educators work in the schools.

Mrs. Jacob: In Singapore, we have a standard health education curriculum. It is not easy to change that unless you are part of the education system and can exert an influence on educators. It is simpler to set up extracurricular activities, which give you greater flexibility. On the other hand, there are many opportunities outside the curriculum area, and we can make use of these in Singapore.

Dr. Robinson: One of the problems that has led to school programs being less effective than they could be is that we put a lot of our energy into developing interventions for children or families and forget that we need to develop interventions for schools. We need to pay the same attention to identifying the factors that affect teacher behavior in school, administrators' behavior, and Department of Education behavior as we do to looking at the individual behavior of children. The things that motivate teachers or parents are just as important as the things that motivate children. For example, schools may not be impressed by being told that reducing TV watching may prevent obesity, because from their point of view that is not particularly important. However, if you could tell them that reducing TV would improve school performance and test scores, they would take notice. You need to think about what the needs of the schools are, and then address those needs as part of the program.

Dr. Dulloo: Dr. Birch mentioned the importance of portion size in nutrition education. In your Singapore program, how was that taken into account?

Mrs. Jacob: Our school portions are much smaller than the portions served in outlets outside the school environment. For example, a bowl of noodles in school would be around a cupful only, but if you were to order noodles outside of school, you would get a double or two and a half times that amount. In our curriculum, we have a healthy diet pyramid, with prescribed serving sizes. We use these consistently so that the children do not get mixed messages. We incorporated Ministry of Health serving size guidelines in this program.

Obesity in Childhood and Adolescence, edited by Chunming Chen and William H. Dietz. Nestlé Nutrition Workshop Series, Pediatric Program, Vol. 49. Nestec Ltd., Vevey/Lippincott Williams & Wilkins, Philadelphia © 2002.

Policy and Environmental Changes Related to the Prevention and Treatment of Childhood and Adolescent Obesity

William H. Dietz

Division of Nutrition and Physical Activity, Centers for Disease Control and Prevention, Atlanta, Georgia, USA

Policy is defined as an "organizational guideline intended to modify behavior." Historically, the most effective strategies for preventing nutritional diseases have relied on policy or environmental changes. For example, environmental changes— such as fortification of milk with vitamin D—provided an effective strategy for preventing rickets. In those cases, fortification of the food supply promptly eradicated existing disease and provided effective prevention of new cases. Although obesity is a more complex problem, because excess energy consumption relative to expenditure has not been linked to a single product, it appears worthwhile to explore environmental strategies that promote reduced energy intake or increase energy expenditure.

The current worldwide epidemic of obesity and its associated effects suggest that the time has come to begin to identify and implement policy and environmental changes that effectively address the epidemic. Several caveats are essential at the outset of this discussion. First, changes in policy and the environment should be science based, to the extent that is possible. However, because the epidemic of obesity has progressed so rapidly and because its consequences are severe, it may be necessary to implement some changes based on their logical association with obesity before compelling evidence becomes available. Second, because the causes of obesity and its cultural context may vary from country to country, policy and environmental changes that are effective in one country may not be so in others. Third, because political systems differ from country to country, the changes proposed for one country may not be appropriate in others. The suggestions presented here reflect my own views, not those of the US government, but necessarily address conditions in the United States.

FAMILY PRACTICES RELATED TO OBESITY

As discussed elsewhere in this volume, childhood and adolescent obesity occurs in a family context. Although the familial clustering of obesity may have a genetic basis,

TABLE 1. *Family strategies for preventing obesity in children*

Breast-feeding
Reduction of television time
Feeding interactions
   Parents decide what children are offered
   Children decide whether to eat it or not
   No encouragement to eat
   No forbidden foods
   Small portions
   Family meals

it may also reflect family patterns of food availability, preparation, or consumption. Strategies within families for preventing obesity are shown in Table 1. These include promotion of breast-feeding, the control of television time, and the division of responsibility between parents and children over meals. Each of these will be considered in turn.

Breast-feeding has not been consistently associated with a reduction in the risk of obesity. However, until recently, most of the studies that examined this relation included unreliable measurements of the duration of breast-feeding. Two recent studies (one published [1,2]) with large samples, reliable measures of breast-feeding, and sound follow-up found that breast-feeding reduces the incidence of childhood obesity in a dose-dependent fashion. At least two potential mechanisms could mediate the relation between breast-feeding and obesity. First, in breast-fed infants, the duration of feeding and the quantity of breast milk consumed are almost exclusively under the infant's control, in contrast to bottle-feeding, where the parent may continue to prompt the infant to feed until an expected quantity of formula has been consumed. Second, infants who are breast-fed adapt more readily to the introduction of new foods (3), probably because the taste of breast milk varies in response to the maternal diet. As a result, infants who are breast-fed may consume a more varied diet or a diet higher in fruits and vegetables. No data are available to confirm either of these hypotheses. Nonetheless, because breast milk is the best food for infants and may prevent obesity, breast-feeding should be promoted as the most appropriate choice of feeding for most infants.

As shown in other chapters in this volume, the duration of television viewing is associated with the prevalence of obesity in the United States (4) and other countries (5). Furthermore, reductions in television viewing time appear to be an effective means of preventing obesity (6) or reducing obesity in those who are already overweight (7,8). These data emphasize the fact that parental control of television time may be an effective strategy for preventing or treating obesity.

The final family-based strategy depends on the division of responsibility between parents and children with regard to meals. Parents should be responsible for what children are offered, and children are responsible for whether to eat the foods that are offered (9). This approach addresses many of the practices that discourage the intake of certain foods or impair the child's capacity to regulate energy intake. For example, the more children are encouraged to eat a food, the less likely they may be to do so (10). Therefore parental efforts to persuade children to increase their intake of fruits and vegetables may decrease the likelihood that they will do so. Second, several studies have now shown that parents who control their child's energy intake have children who are less capable of doing so themselves (11). Although the directionality of this relation remains unclear, some studies now suggest that the likelihood of obesity among such children is greater (12). Furthermore, family meals appear to decrease the quantity of fat, fast food, and soda, and to increase the quantities of fruits and vegetables, that children eat (13).

POLICY CHANGES IN MEDICAL SETTINGS

Because parents of young children represent the most appropriate target for these efforts, the most appropriate individual to engage parents around these strategies is probably the primary care provider. Another potential change agent is the dietitian who counsels families in the Supplemental Foods for Women, Infants, and Children (WIC) program, the program in the United States that provides supplemental foods to low-income children and nutritional education for their parents. Primary care and WIC clinics offer access to children and parents. Thus, children at risk of developing obesity can be identified and parents can be counseled around preventive strategies. Children at risk are those whose BMI is the 85th centile or more, or who have at least one obese parent (14). As indicated earlier, reasonable strategies for prevention in primary care settings are parental control of television time and the division of responsibility for feeding between parents and children.

The most important shift necessary to increase the promotion of these strategies by primary care providers is the acceptance of the BMI cutoff point for identifying children at risk of obesity and the demonstration that counseling about television time and the division of mealtime responsibility between parents and children are effective strategies for preventing obesity. However, before the effectiveness of anticipatory guidance can be tested, the interaction of families and physicians may require revision. Providers must be educated about how to counsel families in these areas. Current counseling usually consists of the provider expressing concern about a problem and telling parents how they should respond. This approach does not acknowledge the important role that feeding interactions or television may play in family functioning, and provides little incentive for families to change. More effective mechanisms to engage families about the need to change these behaviors must be established. For example, conflict resolution around eating may be a more effective way of promoting the division of responsibility than concern about the development of obesity. Likewise, concern about televised violence may be perceived as a greater concern than exposure to food advertising on television. Thus the implementation of these strategies will require alterations in the training of medical students, junior doctors, and practitioners. Likewise, changes in WIC practices will require specific directives to address these issues.

Because 10% to 15% of children are already overweight, effective treatment protocols are also essential. An expert committee in the United States has already recommended an approach to the evaluation and treatment of overweight children (15). Nonetheless, because few managed-care organizations consider the treatment of childhood obesity to be a member benefit and few insurance companies reimburse for the care of overweight children or adolescents, compensation for providers is a major barrier. The time required for treatment will probably require changes in the policies of insurance or managed-care companies, either to provide such counseling as a member benefit or to reimburse for it. Reimbursement will depend not only on demand, but also on the demonstration that treatment is effective. However, the efficacy of the guidelines recommended by the expert committee has not been examined in a randomized controlled clinical trial. How one should define *effective treatment* for children and adolescents also remains unclear. Because obesity-associated hypertension, diabetes, or dyslipidemia in children and adolescents is less prevalent than in adults, remission or improvement of these comorbidities cannot be used routinely as measures of effectiveness.

Although reimbursement and effective programs represent important barriers to treatment, a significant question remains about who should best provide these services. Although pediatricians play a major role in the delivery of anticipatory guidance, it is unclear that they represent the most cost-effective providers of treatment. The role and effectiveness of nutritionists or nurse practitioners should also be explored.

POLICY AND ENVIRONMENTAL CHANGES IN WORK SITES

One of the most important factors that appears to reduce the duration of breast-feeding in the United States is the return of the employed mother to work. Sustained breast-feeding after a new mother returns to work requires either child care facilities in the work site, with policies that permit the mother to feed her child during the work day, or facilities and policies that enable the mother to pump and store her breast milk during the day. Maintenance of breast-feeding is not a high priority for many businesses in the United States. Additional data showing that maternal absenteeism is lessened because of the reduced frequency of illness in the breast-fed child or that mothers who can continue to nurse after they return to work are more satisfied may provide important incentives for businesses to support breast-feeding.

POLICY AND ENVIRONMENTAL CHANGES IN SCHOOLS

Schools offer an important setting in which to modify children's food and physical activity patterns. Children spend substantial amounts of time in school, and in the United States they may consume two meals a day in school, often provided by the school without cost or at a low price. Furthermore, schools usually have the facilities to support PE programs and provide opportunities for physical activity as part of the curriculum, as well as before and after school. Nonetheless, neither the food nor the physical activity environments within schools are optimal for the prevention of obesity. I will consider each of these areas in turn.

Food Environment

As indicated earlier, schools are an important source of food intake for children. High-energy-density foods have become a staple in many schools, through *à la carte* foods available in cafeterias and through the choices available in vending machines. As shown in Table 2, the major items sold in cafeterias and vending machines are foods of high energy density. Lower-energy alternatives are rarely available. For example, in California, a student survey disclosed that 24% of students reported that their school cafeteria regularly served fast foods from commercial vendors (16). Furthermore, children who reported eating fast food on a typical school day consumed twice as many high-fat snacks as students in schools that did not serve fast food. Although at present no data link these practices to an increased prevalence of obesity, such observations suggest that the provision of fast foods in school feeding programs may be associated with an increased energy intake and with a less healthy eating pattern.

The financial viability of many school feeding programs is heavily dependent on the sales of *à la carte* and vending machine foods. Therefore environmental strategies to provide lower-energy choices must be cost-neutral. The availability of alternatives to the high-energy-density products sold in cafeteria lines and vending machines provides one important strategy. Subsidies provided for fruit and vegetables, as well as more attractive alternatives offered in cafeteria lines, have been associated with increased consumption of those foods (17). A similar strategy applied to vending machines increased the consumption of lower-energy alternatives (18). A variant of this approach has been instituted in a novel program known as the Farmer's Market Salad Bar (19). In this project, the school food service purchased fruits and vegetables directly from producers twice a week and offered them in an attractive salad bar as an alternative to the school lunch. Data from the first several years of the project indicate dramatic increases in fruit and vegetable consumption, even among children in poorer communities. Although no data yet link consumption of fruit and vegetables to lower rates of obesity, these observations indicate that food consumption patterns can be modified either by manipulation of prices or by the provision and

TABLE 2. *Foods and beverages most commonly consumed in school cafeterias (à la carte) and vending machines*

A la carte cafeteria foods
  Baked desserts
  Juices and juice drinks
  Ice cream
  Potato chips
Vending machines
  Sodas
  Potato chips and salty snacks
  Baked dessert
  Candy

promotion of attractive lower-energy-density alternatives. The Farmer's Market Salad Bar also provides an important example of how agricultural production can be directly linked to healthy eating patterns of children.

Strategies that rely on financial subsidies cannot be considered cost-neutral as long as financial subsidies are required to modify patterns of consumption. A potentially viable alternative may be to increase the price of higher-energy-density foods, thereby making the prices of the fruits and vegetables more competitive. Although this approach has not been rigorously tested, data from the Santa Monica School System suggest that the strategy may maintain a high level of fruit and vegetable consumption without affecting the total revenue from a school feeding program (Taylor R, School Food Service and Nutrition Director, Santa Monica-Malibu Unified School District, personal communication, 2001).

Physical Activity

Physical education (PE) programs in schools provide an important opportunity for children to be physically active. Nonetheless, in the United States there has been a sharp reduction in the number of schools that offer daily PE programs. For example, in 1991, 42% of schools offered daily PE programs, but by 1999 only 29% of schools did so (20). Even when state policies recommend PE programs, school systems are not obliged to follow the state's recommendations. For example, in California, 17% of children reported that they received no PE classes in school, and on average the number of PE classes and time in PE was only about half of the state's recommendation of 200 minutes every 10 days (16). A second strategy within PE programs is to make them more active. In many schools, PE programs are not taught by trained instructors. Furthermore, estimates suggest that children are not moving for much of the time they are in PE class. The use of strategies that keep all children engaged in physical activity, rather than the typical activities that engage small numbers of children while the remainder of the class are spectators awaiting their turn, will increase physical activity levels further in schools that have retained PE classes.

As with the strategies outlined previously to address food practices in schools, few studies suggest that strategies to improve the frequency or character of PE programs effectively prevent obesity. In fact, in comprehensive school-based cardiovascular risk reduction programs that included both PE and food-based strategies, no effects on obesity rates in children were observed (21,22), despite self-reported changes in behavior. One of the potential problems with these programs was that obesity prevention was not targeted as a primary goal.

In contrast, when obesity was the principal target of school-based interventions and when reduced sedentary behavior has been included as a strategy, the prevalence of obesity decreased (8) or less rapid rates of weight gain were observed (6). Several important differences distinguished these two school-based interventions from those addressed earlier. First, obesity was an explicit target in both interventions, whereas in earlier studies obesity was only one of a number of cardiovascular disease risk factors. Second, reductions in television time and other media use were a prominent feature of both interventions. These represent the first interventions directed at reductions in sedentary behavior rather than increased physical activity.

POLICY AND ENVIRONMENTAL CHANGES WITHIN COMMUNITIES

Communities offer additional opportunities for the design and implementation of strategies to reduce obesity.

Food Intake

Although no data yet link specific dietary practices with obesity, various strategies may be employed to make lower-energy foods available to children. It would seem logical that high-energy-density foods are more likely to be consumed when they are the least expensive and most readily available foods, and that the converse will be true for foods of low energy density. For example, fruit and vegetable consumption is unlikely to be substantial in neighborhoods that lack large supermarkets where attractive and varied fruits and vegetables can be purchased at reasonable practices. Likewise, unless access to inexpensive fruit and vegetables exists in poor neighborhoods, campaigns to promote their consumption are unlikely to be successful. Nonetheless, almost nothing is known about the relation of the availability of high-energy-density foods to either their consumption or the risk of obesity. Despite these limitations, there are ample reasons for promoting fruit and vegetable consumption and for exploring strategies to reduce the barriers that limit fruit and vegetable consumption as potential community strategies for health promotion.

Physical Activity

There is more justification for promoting physical activity as a strategy to address obesity. For example, sedentary behavior promotes the development of obesity (23), and increased physical activity in adults improves many of the comorbidities associated with obesity, such as diabetes, hypertension, or hyperlipidemia. Thus community strategies to increase physical activity may be effective in the prevention and treatment of obesity. Several sources of data suggest that community design may be associated with alterations in physical activity. Recent studies of travel behaviors in the United States show that less than one-third of children who live within a mile of school walk to school (Ham S, personal communication). Furthermore, although 25% of all trips in the United States are less than 1 mile, 75% of those trips are taken by car (24). These observations probably reflect recent changes in community design in the United States. For example, car use is inversely related to the age of communities, and directly to population density. Many newer suburban communities in the United States lack sidewalks and centralized shopping facilities or schools, although other facilities to support physical activity may be available. We currently lack data that provide insight into the relative contribution of these elements to daily physical activity levels among the residents of such communities.

Communities with resources like parks or recreation facilities that support physical activity are also more likely to have physically active residents. The development of a series of walking trails in the Bootheel area of Missouri has been associated with an increase in self-reported walking (25). Strategies to make walking trails or increase the use of recreation facilities include better urban planning and the use of schools for community physical activities after school hours. Facilities are also needed to provide alternatives to television viewing in children, as viewing is unlikely to be reduced unless alternatives are available. Nonetheless, the effects on physical activity of making schools available for physical activity after school hours, developing walking trails, and building new parks or recreational facilities have not been carefully examined.

A final strategy involves changes in building design to promote physical activity. Stairs offer a daily opportunity for activity, and studies in adults show that frequent stair use can have beneficial health effects. Furthermore, several studies have now shown that signs promoting stair use increase the use of stairs as opposed to that of escalators or elevators. These observations suggest that locating stairs in a central position and promoting their use may represent an effective strategy for increasing physical activity.

The incentives to introduce such shifts remain unclear. However, several potential strategies might be pursued. For example, housing developments that support physical activity such as recreational facilities are viewed as highly desirable by new-home buyers (26), which suggests that linkages of public health practitioners with developers and builders may be mutually beneficial. The role that alternative forms of transport could play in the reduction of car use and the consequent reduction of air pollution suggests that nontraditional allies in the transportation industry may share an interest in walking and bicycling. Increased interest in living in communities with cluster housing, central shops, and central schools has implications for urban design. Community projects that encourage adults to help children identify and use safe routes to walk to school are promising strategies for increasing physical activity as part of daily living (27) and may enhance community livability. A notable example is California, which provided $22 million for building sidewalks to enable children to walk to school.

Communication Strategies

The rapid increase in the prevalence of obesity is unlikely to be arrested by any single strategy. One of the first steps necessary to prevent obesity is to understand how families perceive excess weight and how to engage them in the need to avoid or lose excess weight. Several recent focus groups conducted in children of different ages suggest that excess weight is not defined in terms of where the child appears on a growth chart but by whether the excess weight affects the child's self-esteem. Under these circumstances, the parents may not share a provider's concern about the child's weight. Although we know little about how children and adolescents perceive the risks of obesity, a recent study conducted by Discovery Health and the American Heart Association (28) showed that less than 30% of adults recognized that obesity, inactivity, and high blood pressure were associated with increased risk of cardiovascular disease. Because few obese children and adolescents develop an acute complication of their obesity and because so many of the health effects occur in adulthood, concerns about the health effects of obesity may not motivate children and parents to change their behavior in relation to food intake or physical activity. Unless providers and parents agree that a problem exists, efforts to change diet or physical activity are unlikely to succeed. Similarly, communication campaigns will require an improved understanding of the public's perception of obesity, its risks, and the strategies necessary to prevent it. Because of the risks of stigmatization of overweight children, it seems unlikely that obesity will be the focus of any media campaigns.

CONCLUSIONS

The epidemic of childhood obesity is unlikely to respond to any single approach. Starting to make healthy choices easy will require additional research into efficacy and a great deal of creativity. Identification of causal behaviors will be essential. However, in contrast to adult obesity, where preventive strategies remain uncertain, several strategies in children and adolescents appear promising. These include increased rates of breast-feeding and a reduction in television viewing time. However, to achieve these strategies, policy and environmental changes will be required in medical settings, schools, worksites, and communities.

REFERENCES

1. Von Kreiz R, Koletzko B, Sauerwald T, *et al.* Breast feeding and obesity: a cross sectional study. *BMJ* 1999; 319; 147–50.
2. Gillman MW, Rifas-Shiman SL, Camargo CA Jr, *et al.* Risk of overweight among adolescents who were breastfed as infants. *JAMA* 2001; 285: 2461–7.
3. Sullivan SA, Birch LL. Infant dietary experience and acceptance of solid foods. *Pediatrics* 1994; 93: 271–7.
4. Dietz WH, Gortmaker SL. Do we fatten our children at the TV set? Obesity and television viewing in children and adolescents. *Pediatrics* 1985; 75: 807–12.
5. Hernandez B, Gortmaker SL, Colditz GA, Peterson KE, Laird NM, Parra-Cabrera S. Association of obesity with physical activity, television programs and other forms of video viewing among children in Mexico City. *Int J Obes* 1999; 23: 845–54.
6. Robinson TN. Reducing children's television viewing to prevent obesity: a randomized trial. *JAMA* 1999; 282: 1561–7.
7. Epstein LH, Valoski AM, Vara LS, *et al.* Effects of decreasing sedentary behavior and increasing activity on weight change in obese children. *Health Psychol* 1995; 14: 109–15.
8. Gortmaker SL, Peterson K, Wiecha J, *et al.* Reducing obesity via a school-based interdisciplinary intervention among youth: Planet Health. *Arch Pediatr Adolesc Med* 1999; 153: 409–18.
9. Dietz WH, Stern L. *A guide to your child's nutrition; peace at the dinner table.* New York: Villard, 1999.
10. Birch LL, Marlin DW, Rotter J. Eating as the "means" activity in a contingency: effects on young children's food preference. *Child Dev* 1985; 55: 431–9.
11. Johnson SL, Birch LL. Parents' and children's adiposity and eating style. *Pediatrics* 1994; 94: 653–61.
12. Birch LL, Fisher JO. Mothers' child-feeding practices influence daughters' eating and weight. *Am J Clin Nutr* 2000; 71: 1054–61.
13. Gillman MW, Rifas-Shiman SL, Frazier AL, *et al.* Family dinner and diet quality among older children and adolescents. *Arch Fam Med* 2000; 9: 235–40.

14. Whitaker RC, Wright JA, Pepe MS, Seidel KD, Dietz WH. Predicting obesity in young adulthood from childhood and parental obesity. *N Engl J Med* 1997; 337: 869–73.
15. Barlow SE, Dietz WH. Assessment and treatment of obesity in children and adolescents: recommendations of an expert committee. URL, 1998: http://www.pediatrics.org/cgi/content/full/102/3/e29.
16. Public Health Institute. Special Report to the California Endowment; findings from the 1999 California Children's Healthy Eating and Exercise Practices Survey: *Childhood overweight, dietary and physical activity disparities, and policy implications.* Berkeley, CA: Public Health Institute, 1999.
17. French SA, Story M, Jeffery RW, *et al.* Pricing strategy to promote fruit and vegetable purchase in high school cafeterias. *J Am Dietet Assoc* 1997; 97: 1008–10.
18. French SA, Jeffery RW, Story M, Hannan P, Snyder MP. A pricing strategy to promote low-fat snack choices through vending machines. *Am J Public Health.* 1997; 87: 849–51.
19. Mascarenhas M, Gottlieb R. The Farmer's Market Salad Bar: assessing the first three years of the Santa Monica-Malibu Unified School District Program. Los Angeles: Community Food Security Project, Occidental College, Los Angeles, 2000.
20. US Department of Health and Human Services. *Physical activity and fitness. Healthy people 2010,* 2nd ed. Washington, DC: US Government Printing Office, 2000; v2, section 22.
21. Resnicow K, Robinson TN. School-based cardiovascular disease prevention studies: review and synthesis. *Ann Epidemiol* 1997; S7: 14–31.
22. Nader PR, Stone EJ, Lytle LA, *et al.* Three-year maintenance of improved diet and physical activity; the CATCH cohort. *Arch Pediatr Adolesc Med* 1999; 153: 695–704.
23. Ching PLYH, Willett WC, Rimm EB, Colditz GA, Gortmaker SL, Stampfer MJ. Activity level and risk of overweight in male health professionals. *Am J Public Health* 1996; 86: 25–30.
24. US Department of Transportation, Federal Highway Administration, Research and Technical Support Center. *1995 nationwide personal transportation survey.* Lanham, MD: Federal Highway Administration, 1997.
25. Brownson RC, Housemann RA, Brown DR, *et al.* Promoting physical activity in rural communities; walking trail access, use, and effects. *Am J Prev Med* 2000; 18: 235–41.
26. Fletcher J. Is this Disneyland? No, the new suburbs. *Wall Street J* 1999; June 4: w12.
27. Centers for Disease Control and Prevention. *Kids walk-to-school.* Atlanta: US Department of Health and Human Services, Centers for Disease Control and Prevention, 2000.
28. Anon. Aware of risk factors. *USA Today* 2000; Feb 22: section 6D.

DISCUSSION

Dr. Uauy: I'm surprised that you did not include the food aspect. I know that physical activity is probably just as important, but what can we do to orient consumers toward healthy foods and healthy dietary habits in a world where the opposite is being promoted?

Dr. Dietz: That's a good question. The only food-related strategy that I think we can implement at the population level for chronic disease prevention is the promotion of fruit and vegetable consumption, although there are no published data showing that fruit and vegetables consumption is related to reduced obesity. Although there have been various changes in the food supply that have accompanied the epidemic of obesity—such as fast foods, increased soda and sugared beverage consumption, skipping meals, or greater variety of foods available to us—there isn't yet any evidence that these are causal. For implementation of policy change at the governmental level, we need that evidence. It may be coming. We have seen the one study that shows that soda and sugar beverage consumption is linked to obesity (1), and we have evidence that family meals provide better food choices not yet linked to obesity. Part of the problem is that the traditional means of analysis has focused on nutrients and not on food patterns, but that is starting to change.

Dr. Bellizzi: In relation to breast-feeding, our experience in Scotland shows that the initiation and continuation of breast-feeding needs a multisector approach. Many women start to breast-feed but then stop long before they even begin to go back to work. Thus, although I would agree that workplace policies are essential, we need to look at other areas. For instance, in the health sector, the primary care setting is important, but we do not have the resources to enable health professionals to support women for the long period they may need that support—which may involve just sitting there and giving confidence. Nonprofessional peer group supporters may even be better at helping nursing mothers to continue breast-feeding. Indeed, research shows that women who are having problems with breast-feeding would rather *not* talk to health professionals, but prefer to talk to friends or family members. Those are important groups that we need to access in order to help with the promotion of breast-feeding.

Children can also be targeted. We recently had a poster competition on breast-feeding in our region, and it became clear that there were children who actually did not know that babies *can* be breast-fed. That is perhaps not surprising when children are given dolls that come with bottles, and that's all they are exposed to.

We should also try to influence the media. There was a study in the *BMJ* looking at the media and how they portray infant feeding in the United Kingdom (2). This showed that in the soap opera programs on television, when there was a baby involved it was usually being bottle-fed. On the occasions when a baby was being breast-fed, the scenario was usually one in which there were problems with the feeding. I really believe that a multifaceted approach is needed in order to improve breast-feeding.

Dr. Dietz: I agree. I did not mean to imply that one single strategy was going to be effective. The broad outline that you have given is helpful. Thank you.

Dr. Kumar: The Malaysian practice is to provide education and counseling about breast-feeding from early on in pregnancy, as early as the first trimester. Intensive promotion extends the period of exclusive breast-feeding for up to 6 months to 1 year.

Dr. Dietz: I'm not sure I would want to promote exclusive breast-feeding for a year, but early counseling makes good sense (3,4).

Dr. Rolland-Cachera: You mentioned that environmental changes are essential, so we should build sidewalks, parks, and so on. But we have those, so what else can we do to promote change?

Dr. Dietz: I think what we lack is promotion for physical activity in the way we promote other types of behavior. We know from our own experience in Atlanta, for example, that just rebuilding a park, or putting in a walking path or bicycle trail, or redecorating stairways is not enough to get people to use these facilities. They really need to be promoted. I would like to know more about the reasons why children are watching a lot of television in Paris, where there are alternatives, compared with other areas where there are not. My examples were taken largely from the United States obviously, where many neighborhoods lack sidewalks or bicycle trails or central parks, and in those neighborhoods there *is* no alternative but to get in your car and drive somewhere—and that's not the best way to facilitate physical activity. What we need from around the world are studies of urban and rural environments that begin to examine more closely why children are watching so much television and what kinds of alternatives are available. I don't pretend to have the answer, but I do think that's a strategy we can employ.

Dr. Dulloo: As students, we learned from the energy balance equation that if you increase energy expenditure intensively, by being a lumberjack for example, your food intake will also increase. Bringing this to the community level, you have focused almost entirely on the energy expenditure side by trying to encourage physical activity, creating parks, and so on. But one could argue that as people go outside and take more exercise, food consumption will increase in parallel. The tendency will be to maintain static weight and the problem will not really be solved.

Dr. Dietz: That's a good point. I think we know more about the relation of the physical environment to physical activity than we do about the food environment and food consumption.

One of the strategies we are now funding is to begin to look at the infrastructure of communities and how this relates to food consumption and physical activity. Dr. Gortmaker has made the point that it makes little sense to go out for a walk if the only place you are walking to is a McDonalds! I think that's a sound point, but we actually don't know the relation between the availability of fast food restaurants and fast food consumption. I suspect the manufacturers do, but we don't. We have some evidence that the food environment affects food-related behaviors—fruit and vegetable consumption, for example, which is reduced among inner-city populations that lack access to large supermarkets where fruits and vegetables can be purchased inexpensively. So I think this is a logical direction to follow in terms of a research agenda. I contend that we have more information about the relation of the physical environment to physical activity than we do about the food environment.

Dr. Maffeis: Has the relation between the breast-feeding duration and the prevalence of obesity in children been controlled for obesity in the mothers?

Dr. Dietz: In the two studies I quoted the answer is yes.

Dr. Maffeis: What about the variation in the BMI of the mothers between parturition and the point at which the obesity was assessed in the child?

Dr. Dietz: We don't have those data. The offspring of the Nurses' Health Study were linked to maternal obesity at age 18 and subsequently. The Hain study only had obesity of the mother at the time the survey was conducted. The children in that study were younger than the ones in the Nurses' Health Study, so they weren't exactly comparable in terms of age.

Dr. Endres: In relation to maternal weight and breast-feeding: mothers who breast-feed for longer—that is, more than 6 months—lose a little more weight than mothers who breast-feed for 4 months or less. They also store more iron, because they are amenorrheic and so do not lose so much blood.

Dr. Dietz: The other problem related to breast-feeding is that overweight mothers initiate breast-feeding less often and breast-feed for a shorter time. So it's really a circular problem: if the mothers are overweight, they tend not to breast-feed, and I think will have children who are more likely to be overweight, and so the cycle continues. That cycle can be broken.

Dr. Ma: The Chinese Academy of Preventive Medicine is undergoing reform. Later this year, it is to be replaced by the Chinese Center for Disease Control and Prevention. I would like to know what role the CDC plays in the United States in developing health-related policies.

Dr. Dietz: The CDC is the United States agency for prevention, but in order to be effective it needs resources that are either allocated by the administration—the president and his staff—or by Congress. One of the things that has changed dramatically in the last 3 years is the awareness of obesity as a public health problem, and the willingness of Congress to begin to fund it. Three years ago, our budget was $2 million a year specifically for obesity; last year it was $16 million. The increase in our budget indicates that Congress is responsive to these needs. At the end of this year, we will be funding 12 states for nutrition and physical activity programs to prevent obesity and other chronic diseases. Our strategy is not simply to focus on obesity, because many of the physical activity and nutrition strategies act across a variety of diseases—they are just as effective for diabetes and cardiovascular disease control as they are for obesity. So we are moving toward what is really for the first time an effective nutrition and physical activity program based in state health departments. The question is, "How do we make those as effective as possible?" What we are trying to do is to build linkages between public health departments and universities, so that not only in the design but also in the evaluation phase there is more science brought to bear and we can begin to identify promising models that can then be disseminated.

Dr. Nguyen-Howles: We have heard about the key role of parents. How else can we promote education on nutrition and physical activity?

Dr. Dietz: One area that is very promising and was mentioned earlier in this meeting is the development of daycare centers. Such centers provide care for children and in many cases are just as important as the parents in terms of promoting physical activities and appropriate foods for the children. One of the things we have thought about but don't have a model for is using daycare providers not only as a locus for intervention but as people who can teach *parents* about their children and their children's needs. The other advantage of thinking about daycare is that daycare policies relating to nutrition and physical activity already exist in the United States, and if policies exist they can be examined and modified to affect the health of the children who are participating in those programs. At the moment all of that is theoretical, but I think it is a promising direction in which to move. As far as schools are concerned, my understanding is that there has been difficulty in getting parents to come to meetings to educate them. A final thought is that, as with smoking, children themselves may be effective agents for change. We haven't heard about that, and I'm not sure if we have any models in the nutrition/physical activity area, but some of the models in the smoking cessation field have promise. If children learn about physical activity or fruit and vegetable consumption as part of their curriculum, they may bring home those attitudes and change their parents' practices.

Dr. Buenaluz: A measure that could be adopted would be that would-be parents, such as high school students, could be enrolled in a health promotion curriculum, so that they would be taught about the principles of child care, with emphasis on health and proper diet. In the Philippines, we have many teenage pregnancies and the young mothers usually have no knowledge at all about the advantages of breast-feeding and proper nutrition, or even how to cook. They only know about buying foods already cooked, and nothing at all about their nutritional value.

Dr. Dietz: I think that's a good point. We are raising a generation that does not know how to cook in the United States. That plus the shift in lifestyle has increased the reliance on fast foods.

REFERENCES

1. Ludwig DS, Peterson KE, Gortmaker SL. Relation between consumption of sugar-sweetened drinks and childhood obesity: a prospective, observational analysis. *Lancet* 2001; 357: 505–8.
2. Henderson L, Kitzinger J, Green J. Representing infant feeding: content analysis of British media portrayals of bottle-feeding and breastfeeding. *BMJ* 2000; 321: 1196–8.
3. Gillman MW, Rifas-Shiman SL, Camargo CA Jr, *et al.* Risk of overweight among adolescents who were breastfed as infants. *JAMA* 2001; 285: 2461–67.
4. Hediger ML, Overpeck MD, Kuczmarski RJ, *et al.* Association between infant breastfeeding and overweight in young children. *JAMA* 2001; 285: 2453–60.

Subject Index

Page numbers in italics denote figures; those followed by "t" denote tables.

Prevention (*contd.*)
  reasons for, 245
  sedentary behaviors, 251, 279
  strategies for, 138–139
  summary overview of, 252–254
  television viewing reduction, 251–252
Program(s)
  community-based, 248
  description of, 223
  evaluation of, 218
  primary care–based, 247
  school (*See* School programs)
Programming hypothesis
  cold exposure, 88
  description of, 83
  environmental temperatures, 88
  future studies of, 93
  growth, 84–85
  intrauterine environment effects, 87
  lean tissue, 85–87
  leptin concentrations, 89–92
  maternal factors associated with, 87–88
  mechanisms, 89
Protein intake
  adiposity rebound and, 108
  energy requirements, 133–134
  self-regulation, 134
Protein-sparing modified fast diet,
  226–227
Puberty
  body composition changes during, 122
  body fat distribution in, 124

Q

Quantile regression, 8

R

Race, body composition differences based
  on, 123
Risk factors for obesity
  activity patterns, 54–55 (*See also*
    Physical activity)
  Chilean studies of, 52–56
  description of, 56–57
  food availability, 56
  race/ethnicity influences, 71
  sedentarism, 57

  social expenditures, 54, 56
  socioeconomic changes, 53, 56
Roux-en Y gastric bypass, 236–238,
  237

S

School programs
  advantage of, 257
  Australia School Project, 260t, 266, 268t
  Cardiovascular Health in Children
    Study, 259t, 263, 268t
  CDC guidelines, 267
  challenges for, 267, 269
  Child and Adolescent Trial for
    Cardiovascular Health, 257, 258t,
    261, 267, 268t
  classroom curriculum, 249–250
  description of, 248, 257
  Eat Well and Keep Moving, 259t, 263,
    268t
  elementary, 257, 258t–259t, 261–264
  food service interventions, 250,
    277–278
  foods commonly consumed, 277t
  Go for Health, 259t, 262, 268t
  high school, 264–267
  Know Your Body, 258t, 262, 268t
  Nebraska School Study, 259t, 262–263,
    268t
  Nutrifit, 264
  outcomes of, 268t
  physical education interventions,
    250–251, 278–279
  policy changes in, 277–278
  Power Kids Eat Smart, 260t, 265
  Power Kids on the go, 260t, 265
  primary school, 257, 258t–259t,
    261–264
  Sports, Play, and Active Recreation for
    Kids, 258t, 261–262, 268t
  Stanford Adolescent Heart Health
    Program, 249, 260t, 266, 268t
  studies of, 248–249
  Take 10, 259t, 264
  Trim and Fit, 260t, 264–265, 268t
Secular trends
  adiposity rebound and, 107
  body mass index, 65